Sample Size Determination and Power

Sample Size Determination and Power

THOMAS P. RYAN

Institute for Statistics Education, Arlington, Virginia and
Northwestern University, Evanston, Illinois

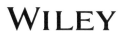

Library of Congress Cataloging-in-Publication Data:

Ryan, Thomas P., 1945–
   Sample size determination and power / Thomas P. Ryan.
      p. ; cm.
   Includes bibliographical references and index.
   ISBN 978-1-118-43760-5 (cloth)
   I. Title.
   [DNLM: 1. Sample Size.   2. Clinical Trials as Topic.   3. Mathematical Computing.   4. Regression
Analysis.   5. Sampling Studies. WA 950]
   615.5072′4–dc23

                                                                                      2013000329

Printed in the United States of America

10 9 8 7 6 5 4 3 2 1

Contents

3 Means and Variances   57

Preface

Determining a good sample size to use in a scientific study is of utmost importance, especially in clinical studies with some participants receiving a placebo or nothing at all and others taking a drug whose efficacy has not been established. It is imperative that a large enough sample be used so that an effect that is large enough to be of practical significance has a high probability of being detected from the study. That is, the study should have sufficient *power*. It is also important that sample sizes not be larger than necessary so that the cost of a study not be any larger than necessary and to minimize risk to human subjects in drug studies.

Compared to other subjects in the field of statistics, there is a relative paucity of books on sample size determination and power, especially general purpose books. The classic book on the subject has for decades been Jacob Cohen's *Statistical Power Analysis for the Behavioral Sciences*, the second edition of which was published in 1988. That book is oriented, as the title indicates, toward the behavioral sciences, with the statistical methodology being quite useful in the behavioral sciences. The second edition has 567 numbered pages, 208 of which are tables, reflecting the "noncomputer" age in which the two editions of the book were written. In contrast, the relatively recent book by Patrick Dattalo, *Determining Sample Size: Balancing Power, Precision, and Practicality* (2008), which is part of the series in Pocket Guides to Social Work Research Methods, is 167 pages with more than 20% consisting of tables and screen displays reflecting the now heavy reliance on software for sample size determination. An even smaller book is *Sample Size Methodology* (1990) by Desu and Raghavarao at 135 pages, while *How Many Subjects: Statistical Power Analysis in Research* (1987) by Kraemer and Thiemann is just 120 pages and was stated in a review as being an extension of a 1985 journal article by Kraemer. *Sample-Size Determination* (1964) by Mace is larger at 226 pages and *Sample Size Choice: Charts for Experimenters*, 2nd ed. (1991) by Odeh and Fox is 216 pages. Thus, some rather small books have been published on the subject, with almost all of these books having been published over 20 years ago.

At the other extreme in terms of size, focus, and mathematical sophistication, there are books on sample determination for clinical studies, such as *Sample Size Calculations in Clinical Research*, 2nd ed. (2008) by Chow, Shao, and Wang, that are mathematically sophisticated, with the title of this book perhaps suggesting that. A similar recent book is *Sample Sizes for Clinical Trials* (2010) by Julious, whereas *Sample Size Calculations: Practical Methods for Engineers and Scientists* (2010) by Mathews is oriented toward engineering and industrial applications.

There are additional statistical methods that are useful in fields other than behavioral sciences, social sciences, and clinical trials, however, and during the past two decades new needs for sample size determination have arisen in fields that are part of the advancement of science, such as microarray experiments.

Although many formulas are given in Cohen's book, they are not derived in either the chapters or chapter appendices, so the inquisitive reader is left wondering how the formulas came about.

Software is also not covered in Cohen's book, nor is software discussed in the books by Mathews, Julious or Chow, Shao, and Wang. Software and Java applets for sample size determination are now fairly prevalent and, of course, are more useful than tables since theoretically there are an infinite number of values that could be entered for one or more parameter values. There was a need for a book that has a broader scope than Cohen's book and that gives some of the underlying math for interested readers, as well as having a strong software focus, along the lines of Dattalo's book, but is not too mathematical for a general readership. No such book met these requirements at the time of writing, which is why this book was written.

This book can be used as a reference book as well as a textbook in special topics courses. Software discussion and illustration is integrated with the subject matter, and there is also a summary section on software at the end of most chapters. Mixing software discussion with subject matter may seem unorthodox, but I believe this is the best way to cover the material since almost every experimenter faced with software determination will probably feel the need to use software and should know what is available in terms of various software and applets. So the book is to a significant extent a software guide, with considerable discussion about the capabilities of each software package. There is also a very large number of references, considerably more than in any other book on the subject.

THOMAS P. RYAN

Smyrna, Georgia
October 2012

CHAPTER 1

Brief Review of Hypothesis Testing Concepts/Issues and Confidence Intervals

Statistical techniques are used for purposes such as estimating population parameters using either point estimates or interval estimates, developing models, and testing hypotheses. For each of these uses, a sample must be obtained from the population of interest. The immediate question is then "How large should the sample be?" That is the focus of this book. There are several types of sampling methods that are used, such as simple random sampling, stratified random sampling, and cluster sampling. Readers interested in learning about these methods are referred to books on sampling. Such books range from books with an applied emphasis such as Thompson (2012) to an advanced treatment with some theoretical emphasis as in Lohr (2010). Readers interested in an extensive coverage of sample survey methodology may be interested in Groves, Fowler, Couper, Lepkowski, Singer, and Tourangeau (2009).

1.1 BASIC CONCEPTS OF HYPOTHESIS TESTING

If sampling is very inexpensive in a particular application, we might be tempted to obtain a very large sample, but settle for a small sample in applications where sampling is expensive.

The cliché "the bigger the better" can cause problems that users of statistical methods might not anticipate, however. To illustrate, assume that there are two alternative methods that could be employed at some stage of a manufacturing

Sample Size Determination and Power, First Edition. Thomas P. Ryan.
© 2013 John Wiley & Sons, Inc. Published 2013 by John Wiley & Sons, Inc.

process, and the plant manager would like to determine if one is better than the other one in terms of process yield. So an experiment is performed with one of the methods applied to thousands of units of production, and then the other method applied to the same number of units.

What is likely to happen if a hypothesis test (also called a significance test) is performed, testing the equality of the population means (i.e., the theoretical average process yield using each method), against the alternative hypothesis that those means are not equal? Almost certainly the test will lead to rejection of the (null) hypothesis of equal population means, but we should know that the means, recorded to, say, one decimal place are not likely to be equal before we even collect the data! What is the chance that any two U.S cities, randomly selected from two specified states, will have exactly the same population? What is the probability that a company's two plants will have exactly the same proportion of nonconforming units? And so on. The bottom line is that null hypotheses (i.e., hypotheses that are tested) are almost always false. This has been emphasized in the literature by various authors, including Nester (1996) and Loftus (2010).

Other authors have made similar statements, although being somewhat conservative and less blunt. For example, Hahn and Meeker (1991, p. 39) in pointing out that hypothesis tests are less useful than confidence intervals stated: "Thus, confidence intervals are usually more meaningful than statistical hypothesis tests. In fact, one can argue that in some practical situations, there is really no reason for the statistical hypothesis to hold exactly."

If null hypotheses are false, then why do we test them? [This is essentially the title of the paper by Murphy (1990).] Indeed, hypothesis testing has received much criticism in the literature; see, for example, Nester (1996) and Tukey (1991). In particular, Loftus (1993) stated "First, hypothesis testing is overrated, overused, and practically useless as a means of illuminating what the data in some experiment are trying to tell us." Provocative discussions of hypothesis testing can also be found in Loftus (1991) and Shrout (1997). Howard, Maxwell, and Fleming (2000) discuss and endorse a movement away from heavy reliance on hypothesis testing in the field of psychology. At the other extreme, Lazzeroni and Ray (2012) refer to millions of tests being performed with genomics data.

Despite these criticisms, a decision must be reached in some manner about the population parameter(s) of interest, and a hypothesis test does directly provide a result ("significant" or "not significant") upon which a decision can be based. One of the criticisms of hypothesis testing is that it is a "yes–no" mechanism. That is, the result is either significant or not, with the magnitude of an effect (such as the effect of implementing a new manufacturing process) hidden, which would not be the case if a confidence interval on the effect were constructed.

Such criticisms are not entirely valid, however, as the magnitude of an effect, such as the difference of two averages, is in the numerator of a test statistic. When we compute the value of a test statistic, we can view this as a linear transformation of an effect. For example, if we are testing the null hypothesis,

H_0: $\mu_1 = \mu_2$, which is equivalent to $\mu_1 - \mu_2 = 0$, the difference in the two parameters is estimated by the difference in the sample averages, $\bar{x}_1 - \bar{x}_2$, which is in the numerator of the test statistic,

$$ t = \frac{(\bar{x}_1 - \bar{x}_2) - 0}{S_{\bar{x}_1 - \bar{x}_2}} \tag{1.1} $$

with $S_{\bar{x}_1 - \bar{x}_2}$ denoting the standard error (i.e., estimator of the standard deviation) of $\bar{x}_1 - \bar{x}_2$, and 0 is the value of $\mu_1 - \mu_2$ under the null ypothesis. Thus, the "effect," which is estimated by $\bar{x}_1 - \bar{x}_2$, is used in computing the value of the test statistic, with every type of t-statistic having the general form: $t =$ estimator/standard error of estimator.

Many practitioners would prefer to have a confidence interval on the true effect so that they can judge how likely the true (unknown) effect, $\mu_1 - \mu_2$, is to be of practical significance. For example, Rhoads (1995) stated that many epidemiologists consider confidence intervals to be more useful than hypothesis tests. Confidence intervals are reviewed in Section 1.2.

In using the test statistic in Eq. (1.1) to test the null hypothesis of equal population means, we must have either a reference value in mind such that if the test statistic exceeds it in absolute value, we will conclude that the means differ, or, as is commonly done, a decision will be based on the "p-value," which is part of the computer output and is the probability of obtaining a value of the test statistic that is more extreme, relative to the alternative hypothesis, as the value that was observed, conditioned on the null hypothesis being true. As discussed earlier in this section, however, null hypotheses are almost always false, which implies that p-values are hardly ever valid. Therefore, the p-values contained in computer software output should not be followed slavishly, and some people believe that they shouldn't be used at all (see, e.g., Fidler and Loftus, 2009).

If we use the first approach, the reference value would be the value of the test statistic determined by the selected significance level, denoted by α, which is the probability of rejecting a (conceptually) true null hypothesis. This is also called the probability of a Type I error. If the test is two-sided, there will be two values that are equal in absolute value, such as ± 1.96, with the null hypothesis rejected if the test statistic exceeds 1.96 or is less than -1.96. If we adopt the second approach and, for example, $p = .038$, we may (or may not) conclude that the null hypothesis is false, whereas there would be no doubt if $p = .0038$, since that is a very small number and in particular is less than .01. (Recall the discussion about null hypotheses almost always being false, however.)

There are four possible outcomes of a hypothesis test, as the null hypothesis could be (1) correctly rejected, (2) incorrectly rejected, (3) correctly not rejected, or (4) incorrectly not rejected. The latter is called a Type II error and the probability of a Type II error occurring is denoted by β. Thus, $1 - \beta$ is the probability of correctly rejecting a false null hypothesis and this is termed "the power of the test." An experimenter must consider the costs associated with each type of error and the cost of sampling in arriving at an appropriate sample size to be used in hypothesis tests, as well as to determine an appropriate sample size for other purposes.

Some practitioners believe that the experiments should be conducted with the probability of a Type I error set equal to the probability of a Type II error. Although the former can literally be "set" by simply selecting the value, the latter depends on a number of factors, including the difference between the hypothesized parameter value and the true parameter value α, the standard deviation of the estimator of the parameter, and the sample size. We cannot literally set the probability of a Type II error because, in particular, the standard deviation of the estimator of the parameter will be unknown. So even though we may think we are setting the power for detecting a certain value of the parameter with the software we use, we are not literally doing so since the value for the standard deviation that the user must enter in the software is almost certainly not the true value.

Since $\alpha \leq .10$, typically, and usually .05 or .01, this would mean having power $\geq .90$ since power $= 1 - \beta$, as stated previously. Although this rule-of-thumb may be useful in some applications, it would result in a very large required sample size in many applications since increased power means increased sample size and power of .95 or .99 will often require a much larger sample size than power $= .90$, depending on the value of the standard error. Thus, in addition to being an uncommon choice for power, .95 or .99 could require a sample size that would be impractical. The increased sample size that results from using .95 or .99 is illustrated in Section 3.1.

Regarding the choice of, α one of my old professors said that we use .05 because we have five fingers on each hand, thus making the point that the selection of .05 is rather arbitrary. Mudge, Baker, Edge, and Houlahan (2012) suggested that α be chosen to either (a) minimizing the sum of the probability of a Type I error plus the probability of a Type II error at a critical effect size, or (b) "minimizing the overall cost associated with Type I and Type II errors given their respective probabilities."

There are various misinterpretations of hypothesis test results and p-values, such as concluding that the smaller the p-value, the larger the effect or, for example, the difference in the population means is greater if the equality of two means is being tested. A p-value has also been misinterpreted as the probability that the null hypothesis is true. These types of misinterpretations have been discussed in the literature, such as in Gunst (2002) and Hubbard and Bayarri (2003). There have also been articles about p-value misconceptions in which the author gives an incorrect or at least incomplete definition of a p-value. Goodman (2008) is one such example, while giving 12 p-value misconceptions. Hubbard and Bayarri (2003) stated: "The p-value is then mistakenly interpreted as a frequency-based Type I error rate." They went on to state that "confusion over the meaning and interpretation of p's and α's is almost total . . . this same confusion exists among some statisticians." The confusion is indeed apparent in some introductory statistics textbooks, some of which have defined a p-value as "the smallest Type I error rate that an experimenter is willing to accept." Berk (2003), in discussing Hubbard and Bayarri (2003), quoted Boniface (1995, p. 21): "The *level of significance* is the probability that a difference in means has been erroneously declared to be significant. Another name for significance level is p-value." See also the discussion in Seaman and Allen (2011). Additionally, Casella and Berger (1987, p. 133) stated that "there are a great many statistically naive users who are interpreting p-values as probabilities of Type I error."

The bottom line is that p-values are completely different conceptually from the probability of a Type I error (i.e., significance level) and the two concepts should never be intermingled. There has obviously been a great deal of confusion about these concepts in the literature and undoubtedly also in practice.

There has also been confusion over what can be concluded regarding the null hypothesis. If the sample data do not result in rejection of it, that does not mean it is true (especially considering the earlier discussion of null hypotheses in this chapter), so we should not say that it is accepted. Indeed, the null hypothesis can never be proved to be true, and for that matter, it can never be proved that it isn't true (with absolute, 100% certainty), so we should say that it is "not rejected" rather than saying that it is "accepted." This is more than just a matter of semantics, as there is an important, fundamental difference. (The alternative hypothesis also cannot be "proved," nor can *anything* be proved whenever a sample is taken from a population.) The reader who wishes to do additional reading on this may wish to consult Cohen (1988, pp. 16–17).

A decision must be reached as to whether a two-sided test or a one-sided test will be performed. For the former, the alternative hypothesis is that the parameter or the difference of two parameters is not equal to the value specified in the null hypothesis. A one-sided test is a directional test, with the parameter or the difference of two parameters specified as either greater than or less than the value specified in the null hypothesis. Bland and Altman (1994) stated that a one-sided test is sometimes appropriate but further stated the following:

> In general a one sided test is appropriate when a large difference in one direction would lead to the same action as no difference at all. Expectation of a difference in a particular direction is not adequate justification. In medicine, things do not always work out as expected, and researchers may be surprised by their results.... Two sided tests should be used unless there is a very good reason for doing otherwise.

1.2 REVIEW OF CONFIDENCE INTERVALS AND THEIR RELATIONSHIP TO HYPOTHESIS TESTS

Many practitioners prefer confidence intervals to hypothesis tests, especially Smith and Bates (1992). Confidence intervals do provide an interval that will contain the parameter value (or difference of parameter values) of interest with the stated probability, such as .95. Many types of confidence intervals are symmetric about the estimate of the parameter for which the interval is being constructed. Such intervals are of the form

$$\hat{\theta} \pm t(\text{or } Z)\hat{\sigma}_{\hat{\theta}}(\text{or } \sigma_{\hat{\theta}})$$

where θ is the parameter for which the confidence interval is being constructed, $\hat{\theta}$ is the estimator of that parameter, $\hat{\sigma}_{\hat{\theta}}$ is the estimator of the standard deviation of the estimator ($\sigma_{\hat{\theta}}$), and either t or Z is used in constructing the interval, depending on which should be used.

A confidence interval is constructed by taking a single sample, but, speaking hypothetically to add insight, if we were to take a very large number of samples and construct a 95% confidence interval using the data in each sample, approximately 95% of the intervals would contain the (unknown value) of the parameter since the probability that any one interval will contain the parameter is .95. (Such statements can of course be verified using simulation.) Such a probability statement must be made before a sample is obtained because after the interval has been computed the probability is either zero or one that the interval contains the parameter, and we don't know which it is because we don't know the value of the parameter.

A confidence interval does have the advantage of preserving the unit of measurement, whereas the value of a test statistic is a unitless number. There is a direct relationship between a hypothesis test and the corresponding confidence interval, as emphasized throughout Ryan (2007). In particular, we could use a confidence interval to test a hypothesis, as there is a direct relationship between a two-sided hypothesis test with significance level α and a $100(1 - \alpha)\%$ confidence interval using the same data. Similarly, there is a direct relationship between a one-sided hypothesis test and the corresponding one-sided confidence bound.

Specifically, if H_0: $\mu_1 = \mu_2$, equivalently H_0: $\mu_1 - \mu_2 = 0$, is not rejected using a two-sided test with significance level α, then the corresponding $100(1 - \alpha)\%$ confidence interval will contain zero. Similarly, if the hypothesis test had led to rejection of H_0, then the confidence interval would not have included zero. The same type of statements can be made regarding what will happen with the hypothesis test based on the confidence interval. This relationship holds true for almost all hypothesis tests. An argument could be made that it is better to test a hypothesis by constructing the confidence interval because the unit of measurement is not lost with the latter, but is lost with the former.

Although an alternative hypothesis value for the parameter of interest is not specified in confidence interval construction because power is not involved, since the form of a confidence interval is just a rearrangement of the components of the corresponding hypothesis test, values of those components must be specified before the sample size for a confidence interval can be determined, just as is the case with hypothesis tests. So confidence intervals share this obstacle with hypothesis tests.

Software for sample size determination is primarily oriented toward hypothesis testing, however. For example, although Power and Precision provides a 95% confidence interval in addition to the necessary sample size for the specified power value, in addition to the capability for obtaining a tolerance interval for a future 95% confidence interval for the mean, there is no way to solve for the sample size such that a confidence interval will have a desired expected width, a topic that is usually presented in introductory statistics texts. This capability is also absent in some multipurpose statistical software that can be used for sample size determination, such as Stata. Sample size for confidence intervals can be determined using MINITAB, however.

Among software specifically for sample size determination and power, the capability for solving for sample size for specified confidence interval widths is available in PASS, as well as the capability to obtain a tolerance interval for a future confidence interval. nQuery also provides the capability for determining sample size for confidence intervals, with the user specifying the desired half-width of the interval.

Software capability for sample size determination and power is discussed in detail in subsequent chapters.

If a null hypothesis is false, the experimenter either correctly rejects it or makes what has been termed a Type II error in failing to reject it. (A Type I error occurs, conceptually at least, when an experimenter rejects a true null hypothesis.) If the true parameter value, or difference of two parameter values, is very close to the hypothesized value, there is a high probability of making a Type II error, but that is not of any consequence since it should be understood that the true value is almost certainly not equal to the hypothesized value. Thus, there is some true, unknown parameter value that is presumably close to the hypothesized value. What is important, however, is to detect a difference between the hypothesized and assumed parameter value that is of practical importance, recognizing the difference between statistical significance and practical significance.

Of course, experimenters are going to know what is of practical significance in their studies, and they might frown on tests that show a statistically significant result that they know to be not of practical significance. The first sentence of the article Thomas and Juanes (1996) states: "Statistical significance and biological significance are not the same thing."

The probability of correctly detecting the difference between the true and hypothesized parameter values is called the *power of the test*, which is $1 - \beta$, with β representing the probability of a Type II error. The latter is computed by determining the probability that the value of the random variable that is the

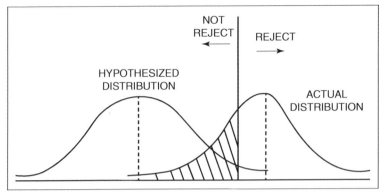

Figure 1.1   Illustration of Type II error probability.

estimator of the parameter being tested falls in the nonrejection region for the curve of the hypothesized distribution of the random variable, which contains the hypothesized parameter value. This is illustrated in Figure 1.1, for which a one-sided test is assumed.

The probability of a Type II error is represented by the shaded area. The smaller this area, the greater the power of the test. It should be apparent, however, that the shaded area will not be small when there is only a small difference between the true parameter value and the hypothesized value. The area can be decreased by increasing the sample, which will cause the spread of each curve to be less, but a very large sample size can make a test too sensitive to small differences between the true and hypothesized parameter values.

There is a trade-off between Type I and Type II errors because increasing one will decrease the other. An experimenter can decide which is the more important of the two in a particular application. Students in a statistics course might be exposed to this in a courtroom setting, where the null hypothesis of course is that the person on trial is innocent (until proved guilty). For example, see Feinberg (1971) and Friedman (1972). So a Type I error would be convicting an innocent person and a Type II error would be not convicting a guilty person. While either error could have dire consequences, in the United States, avoidance of a Type I error would be considered most important. In drug testing, the Food and Drug Administration naturally wants to see a small Type I error, whereas a drug developer of course wants to see a small Type II error, which means high power. Thomas and Juanes (1996) stated: "What constitutes 'high power' is best judged by the researcher . . . ." Another important statement is: "There are no agreed conventions as to what constitutes a biologically significant effect; this will depend upon the context of the experiment and the judgment of the researcher." That paper, which seems to have been intended to be a guide for researchers, contains some excellent practical advice.

1.3 SPORTS APPLICATIONS

Professional sports teams do a form of testing all of the time when they make decisions regarding individual players (making the team, being benched, etc.) Frequently, there are statements made in the media regarding the comparison of two players competing for a position based on a small sample size, with the latter discussed frequently in print. For example, the April 20, 2009 edition of the *The New York Times* had an article with the headline "Over the Wall and Under the Microscope in the Bronx," referring to the number of home runs (20) hit in the new Yankee Stadium during the first four games of the 2009 season, compared to only 10 home runs being hit in the first six games at Citi Field, the new home of the New York Mets. Regarding the latter, the chief operating officer of the Mets stated: "It's a small sample size . . . ."

Similarly, a player's batting average might be over .400 after the first week of a season, but he almost certainly won't hit over .400 for the entire season. The problem, of course, is the small sample size.

1.4 OBSERVED POWER, RETROSPECTIVE POWER, CONDITIONAL POWER, AND PREDICTIVE POWER

We should restrict our attention to thinking of power as being a concept that is applicable *before* the data have been collected. Unfortunately, the term "observed power" (see, e.g., Hoenig and Heisey, 2001) is used to represent the power *after* the data have been collected, acting as if parameter values are equal to the observed sample statistics. That is poor practice because such equality will rarely exist. Hoenig and Heisey (2001) stated that "observed power can never fulfill the goals of its advocates" and explained that this is because observed power is a 1:1 function of the p-value. Similarly, Thomas (1997) stated: "Therefore calculating power using the observed effect size and variance is simply a way of re-stating the statistical significance of the test." Since "power" is a probability and a p-value is a sample statistic, the latter cannot in any way be equated with the former. The practice of using retrospective power has also been debunked by Lenth (2001, 2012), who additionally used the term "retrospective power" in referring to observed power.

Various other prominent scholars have said the same thing, including Senn (2002), who stated that power is irrelevant in interpreting completed studies. The esteemed Sir David Cox also stated that power is irrelevant in the analysis of data (Cox, 1958). Zumbo and Hubley (1998) went further and stated (p. 387): "Finally, it is important to note that retrospective power cannot, generally, be computed in a research setting." Zumbo and Hubley (1998) explained that "we know that retrospective power can be written as a function of two unconditional probabilities. However, the unconditional probabilities are not attainable in a research setting." They further stated: "We suggest that it is nonsensical to make power calculations *after* a study has been conducted and a decision has been made." Yuan and Maxwell (2005) found that observed power is almost always a biased estimator of the true power. Unfortunately, bad advice regarding this can be found in the literature. For example, in an editorial explaining what researchers should know about sample size, power, and effect size, Hudson (2009) stated: "If data is not available in the literature, then a pilot study is justified. If, for whatever reason, sufficient subjects are not recruited, then power can be conducted on a post hoc basis." Somewhat similarly, Thomas (1997) also presented retrospective power as an option and indicated that it can be useful for certain study goals.

Conditional power, as proposed by Lan and Wittes (1988), is prospective rather than retrospective in that it is essentially a conditional probability of rejecting the null hypothesis in favor of the alternative hypothesis at the end of a study period, conditional on the data that have been accumulated up to the point in time at which the conditional power is computed. It is applicable when data are slowly accruing from a nonsequentially designed trial. See also the discussion in Zhu, Ni, and Yao (2011) and Denne (2001), with the latter determining the number of additional observations required at the end of the main study to gain the prescribed power, conditional on the data that had been observed to that point. This is in the same general spirit as Proschan and Hunsberger (1995).

Predictive power, which takes all uncertainties into account, parts of which are ignored by standard sample size calculations and conditional power, might seem preferable, but Dallow and Fina (2011) pointed out that the use of predictive power can lead to much larger sample sizes than occur with the use of either conditional power or standard sample size calculations.

1.5   TESTING FOR EQUALITY, EQUIVALENCE, NONINFERIORITY, OR SUPERIORITY

In traditional hypothesis testing, as presented in introductory level textbooks and taught in introductory courses, the null hypothesis in comparing, say, two means or two proportions is that they are equal, which implies that the difference between them is zero. If there is no prior belief that one mean is larger than the other mean, the alternative hypothesis is that the means are unequal, with a directional alternative hypothesis used if there is prior information to suggest that one mean is larger than the other one.

The difference between the means in the null hypothesis need not be specified as zero, and in practice the difference almost certainly won't be zero, as was mentioned earlier in the chapter. Equivalence testing simply formalizes this approach, although it is really just a part—although an unorthodox part—of hypothesis testing. That is, with equivalence testing, the means from two populations are considered to be "equivalent" if they differ only slightly, and of course this would have to be quantified, with the acceptable difference determined by the specific application.

Reeve and Giesbrecht (1998) stated: "Many questions that are answered with hypothesis testing could be better answered using an equivalence approach." The latter is used with dissolution tests and in other applications. Whereas equivalence tests are often presented as being different from hypothesis tests, they are really a form of a hypothesis test, as discussed later in this section. Bioequivalence testing, which is discussed in Chapter 10 in Chow, Shao, and Wang (2008), is an important part of hypothesis testing. That source also contains theoretical details and sample size computations for equivalence, noninferiority, and superiority in other chapters. There is also material on these topics in subsequent chapters of this book, including software capability and output.

Mathematically, if the absolute value of the difference of the two means is less than δ, then the means are considered to be equivalent. This is the alternative hypothesis, with the null hypothesis being that the absolute value of the difference between the two means is at least equal to δ. A few examples of equivalence testing, with the appropriate sample size formula, are given in later chapters.

As stated by Schumi and Wittes (2011), "non-inferiority trials test whether a new product is not unacceptably worse than a product already in use." Of course, the obvious question is: "Why would anyone be interested in a new treatment that is worse by any amount than the standard treatment?" The answer is that a new treatment that is only slightly worse than the standard treatment relative to the intended benefit of each may be less costly to produce and less costly to the consumer than the standard treatment, and might also have fewer side effects. See Pocock (2003) and Schumi and Wittes (2011) for additional information on noninferiority testing.

Since "noninferiority" thus essentially means "not much worse than" and the latter implies a one-sided test, noninferiority can be tested with either a one-sided hypothesis test or a one-sided confidence interval.

In superiority testing, the objective is to show that the new drug is superior, so the null hypothesis is $\mu_T - \mu_S \leq \delta$ and the alternative hypothesis is $\mu_T - \mu_S > \delta$. Of course, the objective is to reject the null hypothesis and accept the alternative hypothesis.

1.5.1 Software

Software for equivalence, noninferiority, or superiority testing is not widely available; nQuery Advisor has some capability, most of which is for t-tests. PASS, on the other hand, has over 20 routines for determining sample size for equivalence testing and about the same number for noninferiority tests.

REFERENCES

Berk, K. N. (2003). Discussion (of a paper by Hubbard and Bayarri). *The American Statistician*, **57**(3), 178–179.

Bland, J. M. and D. G. Altman (1994). Statistics Notes: One and two-sided tests of significance. *British Medical Journal*, **309**, 248.

Boniface, D. R. (1995). *Experiment Design and Statistical Method for Behavioural and Social Research*. Boca Raton, FL: CRC Press.

Casella, G. and R. L. Berger (1987). Reconciling Bayesian and frequentist evidence in the one-sided testing problem (with comments). *Journal of the American Statistical Association*, **82**, 106–139.

Chow, S.-C., J. Shao, and H. Wang (2008). *Sample Size Calculations in Clinical Research*, 2nd ed. Boca Raton, FL: Chapman & Hall/CRC.

Cohen, J. (1988). *Statistical Power Analysis for the Behavioral Sciences*. Philadelphia: Lawrence Erlbaum Associates.

Cox, D. R. (1958). *Planning of Experiments*. New York: Wiley.

Dallow, N. and P. Fina (2011). The perils with the misuse of predictive power. *Pharmaceutical Statistics*, **10**(4), 311–317.

Denne, J. S. (2001). Sample size recalculation using conditional power. *Statistics in Medicine*, **20**(17-18), 2645–2660.

Feinberg, W. E. (1971). Teaching the Type I and Type II errors: The judicial process. *The American Statistician*, **25**, 30–32.

Fidler, F. and G. R. Loftus (2009). Why figures with error bars should replace *p*-values: Some conceptual arguments and empirical demonstrations. *Zeitschrift für Psychologie [Journal of Psychology]*, **217**(1), 27–37.

Friedman, H. (1972). Trial by jury: Criteria for convictions, jury size, and Type I and Type II errors. *The American Statistician*, **26**, 21–23.

Goodman, S. (2008). A dirty dozen: Twelve *p*-value misconceptions. *Seminars in Hematology*, **45**(3), 135–140.

Groves, R. M., F. J. Fowler, M. P. Couper, J. M. Lepkowski, E. Singer, and R. Tourangeau (2009). *Survey Methodology*, 2nd ed. Hoboken, NJ: Wiley.

Gunst, R. F. (2002). Finding confidence in statistical significance. *Quality Progress*, **35** (10), 107–108.

Hahn, G. J. and W. O. Meeker (1991). *Statistical Intervals: A Guide for Practitioners*. New York: Wiley.

Hoenig, J. M. and D. M. Heisey (2001). The abuse of power: The pervasive fallacy of power calculations for data analysis. *The American Statistician*, **55**(1), 19–24.

Howard, G. S., S. E. Maxwell, and K. J. Fleming (2000). The proof of the pudding: An illustration of the relative strengths of null hypothesis, meta-analysis, and Bayesian analysis. *Psychological Methods*, **5**(3), 315–332.

Hubbard, R. and M. J. Bayarri (2003). Confusion over measures of evidence (*p*'s) versus errors (*α*'s) in classical testing. *The American Statistician* **57**(3), 171–178.

Hudson, Z. (2009). Sample size, power, and effect size—What all researchers need to know (editorial). *Physical Therapy in Sport*, **10**, 43–44.

Lan, K. K. G. and J. Wittes (1988). The B-value: A tool for monitoring data. *Biometrics*, **44**, 579–585.

Lazzeroni, L. C. and A. Ray (2012). The cost of large numbers of hypothesis tests on power, effect size, and sample size. *Molecular Psychiatry*, **17**, 108–114.

Lenth, R. V. (2001). Some practical guidelines for effective sample size determination. *The American Statistician*, **55**(3), 187–193.

Lenth, R. (2012). Sample size determination using applets. Talk given at the American Statistical Association Conference on Statistical Practice. Orlando, FL. Feb. 18.

Loftus, G. R. (1991). On the tyranny of hypothesis testing in the social sciences. *Contemporary Psychology*, **36**(2), 102–105.

Loftus, G. R. (1993). A picture is worth a thousand *p*-values: On the irrelevance of hypothesis testing in the computer age. *Behavior Research Methods, Instrumentation and Computers*, **25**, 250–256.

Loftus, G. R. (2010). The null hypothesis. In *Encyclopedia of Research Design*, pp. 939–943. Thousand Oaks, CA: Sage Publications.

Lohr, S. L. (2010). *Sampling: Design and Analysis*, 2nd ed. Boston, MA:Brooks/Cole, Cengage Learning.

Mudge, J. F., L. F. Baker, C. B. Edge, and J. E. Houlahan (2012). Setting an optimal α that minimizes errors in null hypothesis significance tests. *PLoS One*, **7**(2), 1–7.

Murphy, K. R. (1990). If the null hypothesis is impossible, why test it? *American Psychologist*, **45**, 403–404.

Nester, M. R. (1996). An applied statistician's creed. *Applied Statistics*, **45**, 401–410.

Pocock, S. (2003). The pros and cons of noninferiority trials. *Fundamental and Clinical Pharmacology*, **17**, 483–490.

Proschan, M. A. and S. A. Hunsberger (1995). Designed extension of studies based on conditional power. *Biometrics*, **51**, 1315–1324.

Reeve, R. and F. Giesbrecht (1998). Dissolution method equivalence. In *Statistical Case Studies: A Collaboration Between Academe and Industry* (R. Peck, L. D. Haugh, and A. Goodman, eds.). Alexandria, VA: American Statistical Association and Philadelphia, PA: Society for Industrial and Applied Mathematics.

Rhoads, G. G. (1995). Reporting of power and sample size in randomized controlled trials. *Journal of the American Medical Association*, **273**(1), 22–23.

Ryan, T. P. (2007). *Modern Engineering Statistics*. Hoboken, NJ: Wiley.

Schumi, J. and J. T. Wittes (2011). Through the looking glass: Understanding noninferiority. *Trials*, **12**, 106.

Seaman, J. E. and E. Allen (2011). Not significant, but important? *Quality Progress*, 58–59 (August).

Sedgwick, P. (2011). Sample size and power. *British Medical Journal*, **343**, 5579.

Senn, S. J. (2002). Power is indeed irrelevant in interpreting completed studies. *British Medical Journal*, **325**, 1304–1304.

Shrout, P. E. (1997). Should significance tests be banned? Introduction to a special section exploring the pros and cons. *Psychological Science*, **8**, 1–2.

Smith, A. H. and M. N. Bates (1992). Confidence limit analyses should replace power calculations in the interpretation of epidemiologic studies. *Epidemiology*, **3**, 449–452.

Thomas, L. (1997). Retrospective power analysis. *Conservation Biology*, **11**(1), 276–280.

Thomas, L. and F. Juanes (1996). The importance of statistical power analysis: An example from *Animal Behaviour*. *Animal Behaviour*, **52**, 856–859.

Thomson, S. (2012). *Sampling*, 3rd ed. Hoboken, NJ: Wiley.

Tukey, J. W. (1991). The philosophy of multiple comparisons. *Statistical Science*, **6**, 100–116.

Yuan, K. and S. E. Maxwell (2005). On the post hoc power in testing mean differences. *Journal of Educational and Behavioral Statistics*, **30**(2), 141–167.

Zhu, L., L. Ni, and B. Yao (2011). Group sequential methods and software applications. *The American Statistician*, **65**(2), 127–135.

Zumbo, B. D. and A. M. Hubley (1998). A note on misconceptions concerning prospective and retrospective power. *The Statistician*, **47**(2), 385–388.

EXERCISES

1.1. Explain what a *p*-value is. Why do you think there are so many misconceptions about what a *p*-value really is?

1.2. Why would you not want to have a hypothesis test that has high power (such as .90) for detecting a very small difference in two population means?

1.3. Why would a confidence interval be preferred over the corresponding hypothesis test when they can both be used to test a hypothesis and the results will agree?

1.4. Although a statistical null hypothesis is generally not true, assume that a particular null hypothesis *is* true. If $\alpha = .05$, what is the probability of a Type II error, or does it make any sense to talk about the probability of a Type II error for this scenario? What would be the approximate probability if the null hypothesis were for a single parameter whose mean differed from the hypothesized mean by approximately 10^{-5}, with the standard deviation of the estimator of the parameter being of the order 10^{-2}?

1.5. Perform the following exercise to verify what was stated in Section 1.2. Write appropriate computer code to generate 1000 samples of size 100 from the standard normal distribution (i.e., normal distribution with mean zero and standard deviation one) and construct a 95% confidence interval for each sample, using the form: $\bar{x} \pm 1.96\, s/\sqrt{100}$, with $\bar{x}$ denoting the sample mean and s the sample standard deviation. How many intervals would you expect to contain the population mean of zero? How many did contain zero? Comment.

1.6. An experimenter rejects a null hypothesis and explains that he was not surprised that happened since the probability of it happening was .05, the chosen significance level of the test. Comment on that statement.

1.7. Sedgwick (2011) provided a tutorial question in a journal column that involved power for a clinical setting. Four statements were given and the reader was asked to determine which statements, if any, were true. The one statement that was declared to be true was "Power is the probability of observing the smallest effect of clinical interest, if it exists in the population." One might view this as a "short answer," although it was adequate relative to the context. If you were trying to explain to someone what power is, in general, what must be added to this in order to have a full explanation?

CHAPTER 2

Methods of Determining Sample Sizes

Sample size and power determinations are an important and necessary component of research grant proposals, including proposals involving clinical trials
submitted to the National Institutes of Health (NIH). Biostatisticians often assist
in the statistical part of grant proposals and are often a member of the research
team. The guidelines for researchers provided by the Quantitative Methods Core
of the Department of Quantitative Health Sciences in the University of Mas-
sachusetts Medical School may be of interest (http://www.umassmed.edu/
uploadedFiles/QHS/QMCGuidelinesforGrantApplications2.pdf).

Before embarking on a study of sample size determination and power, it is
worth noting that there are two relatively recent papers that rattle conventions
and that should be read by anyone faced with the task of determining sample
size, whether it be infrequently as in writing grant proposals, or for more frequent
applications as might be involved with a company's operations. Those two papers
are Bacchetti, Deeks, and McCune (2011) and Bacchetti (2010). Quoting from the
latter: "Inaccuracy of sample size calculations is not only theoretically inevitable
(Kraemer, Mintz, Noda, Tinklenberg, and Yesavage, 2006; Matthews, 1995) but
also empirically verified." Bacchetti (2010) went on to relate that Vickers (2003)
found in a study of assumed values for standard deviations for randomized clinical
trials published in four leading general medical journals that about one-fourth
had more than a fivefold inaccuracy in sample size and more than half had
more than a twofold inaccuracy. Bacchetti (2010) also stated that it is difficult
to estimate a standard deviation accurately unless there is such a large amount
of preliminary data available that the planned study is unnecessary! The author
debunks the idea of a minimum acceptable power of .80 and instead advocates
Value of Information methods, for which sample size is determined to maximize
the expected value of the information produced minus the total cost of the study.

Sample Size Determination and Power, First Edition. Thomas P. Ryan.
© 2013 John Wiley & Sons, Inc. Published 2013 by John Wiley & Sons, Inc.

The author pointed out that it is easier to estimate cost than to estimate a standard deviation. This is a very important point since estimation of "other" parameters is necessary when determining sample size. A similar approach is advocated by Bacchetti, McCulloch, and Segal (2008), who stated that "we see no justification for ignoring costs." The response to Bacchetti (2010) by Schulz, Moher, and Altman (2010) may also be of interest, in addition to Bacchetti's reply. See also the determination of sample size when there is a cost constraint, as discussed by Guo, Chen, and Luh (2011)

The same general line of thinking is found in Bacchetti et al. (2011), who stated: "Studies of new ideas often must start small (sometimes even with an n of 1) because of cost and feasibility concerns, and recent statistical work shows that small sample sizes for such research can produce more projected scientific value per dollar spent than larger sample sizes." Glick (2011a) reviewed sample size and power formulas for cost-effectiveness analyses that have been given in the literature and Glick (2011b) explained the relationship between sample size and power and "maximum willingness to pay."

The methods espoused in these recently published papers, almost all of which have had Bacchetti as a co-author, may eventually lead to the use of new methods of determining sample size. That may take some time, however, so the emphasis in this book is on the conventional approach of determining sample size using power considerations, in addition to determining sample size for confidence intervals. There is also an emphasis, for simplicity and for space considerations, on determining a single sample size for a given problem, while recognizing the importance of the following quote from Sahu and Smith (2006): "A single reported sample size is not very informative on its own and its sensitivity with respect to many different assumptions should be investigated. In a practical situation this sensitivity needs to be explored and matched with the practical information that is available to decide the sample size."

Determining sample size does require overcoming certain obstacles. In particular, whether our objective is to determine a sample size so as to have a desired degree of power for a hypothesis test, to have a confidence interval with a specified width, or to estimate a parameter with a maximum error of estimation for a specified probability, it is necessary to specify values of the parameters that are involved in the distribution of the estimate of the parameter for which the hypothesis test, confidence interval, or point estimate is being constructed. Since the other parameters will also generally be unknown, some type of estimate must be provided for them. For example, in the outline given in the link provided in the first paragraph of this chapter, note B2(b): Continuous outcomes: need standard deviation. Of course, a sample estimate won't work (unless from a previous study) since the sample whose size is being determined hasn't been taken yet!

This naturally leads to consideration of Bayesian approaches, as pointed out by Adcock (1997), who discussed both frequentist and Bayesian approaches, as well as to sequential approaches, in general, as discussed by Betensky and Tierney (1997). A frequentist approach is the standard textbook approach to sample size determination and data analysis, with Bayesian approaches being more involved. Their one obvious commonality, however, is that both are used to provide a prior estimate of parameters other than the parameter that is being either tested in a hypothesis test or for which a confidence interval is to be constructed.

Inoue, Berry and Parmigiani (2005) pointed out that an increasing number of submissions for approval of drugs and medical devices, for example, are using Bayesian approaches. These authors also indicated, though, that "one of the problems in Bayesian submissions is that there is no standard method for calculating sample size from a Bayesian perspective." This coupled with possible difficulty in justifying a selected prior distribution for the parameters that must be specified may limit the number of studies in which Bayesian methods will be used. Joseph, du Berger, and Bélisle (1997) reviewed the use of a Bayesian approach to sample size determination and provided a good motivation for such an approach, with their focus being confidence interval width rather than hypothesis tests. Lindley (1997) also gave a Bayesian approach using a utility function, with Pezeshk, Nematollahi, Maroufy, and Gittins (2009) being related work. Earlier work on a Bayesian approach to sample size determination included Goldstein (1981), Adcock (1988), Weiss (1997), and Joseph and Bélisle (1997). See also Dendukuri, Rahme, Bélisle, and Joseph (2004) for Bayesian sample size determination with nonidentified models and Gustafson (2006), who considered sample size determination when model bias is modeled rather than ignored. Wang and Gelfand (2002) proposed a generic Bayesian approach that would be applicable to a wide range of models. A Bayesian sample size determination for equivalence testing and noninferiority testing was given by Wang and Stamey (2010). See also De Santis (2004, 2006), Pham-Gia and Bekker (2005), Stüger (2006), and Yin, Choudhary, Varghese, and Goodman (2008).

Although the use of Bayesian methods in sample size determination can thus be easily motivated, they are covered briefly in this chapter and in certain subsequent chapters because the methods are generally not available in the leading software for sample size determination. Readers who desire a more detailed and technical discussion of Bayesian sample size determination methods are referred to Chapter 13 of Chow, Shao, and Wang (2008).

Hare (2008) touched upon the problems that can be encountered with nonexperts who will say things like not to bother with a statistically rigorous approach to sample size determination, or that the sample size used should be "the industry standard," or that the sample size should be "where the numbers stabilize." None of these responses are valid, as Hare (2008) noted.

Similarly, ad hoc approaches can be found in fields in which methods are employed that lack mathematical rigor. For example, Ariola (2006, p. 140) stated: "These formula [sic] may either be Slovin's formula, Parten's formula, Ibe's formula, or the majority rule formula." None of these formulas are given in sampling books. On page 79, the author stated: "If there is ignorance of population, use Slovin's formula"

$$n = \frac{N}{\left(1 + Ne^2\right)}$$

with n = sample size, N = population size, and e = "desired margin of error." There are multiple problems with such a formula, which we might call a nonparametric sample size formula because there is no indication of a distributional assumption. While it is certainly true that there is no distributional assumption when nonparametric statistical methods are used, the size of a sample must certainly be a function of the population variability of whatever is being measured, and here there is no variability represented by the formula. If the numbers in a population differ very little, a small sample size could lead to a good estimate of the population mean, whereas a larger sample would be needed if the variability was not small. This point is made in every book on sampling.

Another obvious problem with Slovin's formula is that there is no indication of what the "margin of error" is for—a mean, a proportion, a parameter estimate? Although simple approaches will generally be preferred by practitioners, simple approaches that are flawed and not statistically justifiable should be eschewed.

One thing that should be kept in mind is that subjects may drop out of an experimental study, and/or some subjects may not comply with the stipulated conditions of the study. So the initial sample size and the "final" sample size may be quite different, and this should be taken into consideration in selecting the sample size for the beginning of a study. Furthermore, in various applications, such as medical applications, there will be sequential sample size selection because more than one phase will be involved, such as in clinical trials, and sequential sample size determination can also be used within a given phase. That is, sample size reestimation can occur as a study progresses. Shih (2001) provided an invited commentary on sample size reestimation, and the following quote (p. 515), in reference to clinical trials, should be noted: "Hence, one would very much like to utilize the information from the current trial at an interim stage to update the initial estimates and make adjustment of the sample size, if necessary, to ensure that the study's objective is accomplishable with adequate power."

2.1 INTERNAL PILOT STUDY VERSUS EXTERNAL PILOT STUDY

This leads to consideration of an internal pilot study versus an external pilot study. The former is part of the main study, whereas the latter is conducted for the purpose of obtaining necessary parameter estimates. For example, if a test of a population mean is being conducted, the sample size cannot be determined without having an estimate of the population standard deviation. A small (external) pilot study might be conducted before the main study for the express purpose of obtaining data that would be used to provide an estimate of any so-called nuisance parameter, such as the standard deviation. (A nuisance parameter is any parameter that is not the parameter of interest.) Wittes and Brittain (2008) cautioned against the use of external pilot studies for parameter studies, at least for clinical trials, however, as they stated, "external pilot studies are often very unrepresentative of the population to which they refer." Instead, they recommended that internal pilot studies be used for parameter estimation. That is, at a certain point in the study/trial, the data that had been accumulated to that point would be used for parameter estimation, which would then enable the sample size to be recalculated, assuming that an initial estimate of sample size was used before the internal pilot study began.

The idea of using an internal pilot study for parameter estimation has also been discussed by many other authors, including Coffey and Muller (2001), Posch and Bauer (2000), Denne and Jennison (1999), and Browne (1995), as mentioned by Machin and Campbell (2005). Day (2000) reviewed previous work on internal pilot studies and addressed the question of the point at which to stop collecting data in an internal pilot study.

The general idea of an internal pilot study is to use an initial group of subjects, such as patients, with the sample size for the full study reestimated based on data from this initial group. The difference between this type of pilot study and a standard (external) pilot study is that with the latter the subjects are not part of the sample that is used in the regular study, whereas with an internal pilot study they are part of the sample and are thus "internal" to the study. This does have a consequence, however, as the Type I error rate is slightly inflated (Lancaster, Dodd, and Williamson, 2004) since the pilot study and the main study are not independent, as is tacitly assumed when the pilot study is used to estimate sample size for the main study. Wittes, Schabenberger, Zucker, Brittain, and Proschan (1999) found that the Type I error rate inflation is often negligible, however. Wittes and Brittain (1990) and Birkett and Day (1994) gave simulation results that quantified the extent to which the Type I error rate is inflated under certain conditions. Coffey and Muller (2001) gave analytical results that agreed with the simulation results of Wittes and Brittain (1990) and gave exact results that apply to any general linear univariate model with fixed predictors, such as regression models with fixed predictors, mentioned in Chapter 5, and ANOVA models of Chapter 6. Kieser and Friede (2000) explained that the t-test that results from use of a pilot study does not have a central t-distribution and derived the actual distribution, in addition to providing the expression for the actual Type I error and methods for controlling the Type I error level. Denne and Jennison (1999) stated that, when using an internal pilot study, the power of a t-test is not robust to misspecification of the variance and proposed a t-test for a two-treatment comparison that was based on Stein's (1945) two-stage test.

Similarly, Lancaster et al. (2004) stated that in some situations patients involved in an external pilot study are later included in the main study, as a way of minimizing the number of people who must be recruited. This would also inflate the Type I error rate.

If the initial variance estimate that resulted in the initial sample size was at least equal to the sample variance from the internal pilot study, then there would be no adjustment to the initial sample size. If, however, the sample variance exceeded the initial variance estimate, there would be an appropriate adjustment in the sample size. The study would then continue using either the original sample size or a revised sample size obtained using the pilot study parameter estimates.

This obviously raises the question of the point at which the study should be stopped to obtain the parameter estimates. Wittes and Brittain (1990) do not address this issue. If the study is stopped too soon, there will be a large variance associated with the estimate of the population variance, so the latter might be poorly estimated, which in turn would produce a sample size that is either too large or too small. A conservative approach would be to construct a confidence interval for the population variance and use the upper limit of the interval in determining the sample size. While focusing on external pilot studies, Lancaster et al. (2004) cited Browne (1995) as recommending at least an 80% upper one-sided confidence limit, while also citing Browne (1995) as stating that a general rule of thumb is to use at least 30 patients. (That rule of thumb might be based on what is discussed in an introductory statistics book regarding large versus small samples.) Of course, these suggestions could also be applied to an internal pilot study, with the use of confidence limits for σ^2 also suggested by Dudewicz (1972), with this resulting in approximate confidence limits on power.

Whether or not this would be a reasonable approach would depend on the costs, both tangible and intangible, of using a larger-than-necessary sample size since the larger the variance estimate, the larger the sample size.

Some insight as to desirable sizes of internal pilot studies can be gleaned from the Pilot Study routine in Lenth's applet, which is mentioned briefly in Section 2.11 and is used in succeeding chapters. The applet routine essentially allows a user to see how the size of a pilot study will determine how well the sample size for the main study is determined. Specifically, the user enters the degrees of freedom for the "error term," with the latter being just σ for a test of one mean, specifies the percent by which the sample size is underestimated, and then sees as output an approximation of the probability that the percent underestimation is exceeded, with the probability being exact under certain conditions.

For example, if the degrees of freedom for error is 19 and the percent underestimation is 10, the applet gives a 41.69% chance that the percent underestimation will exceed 10, whereas this drops to 24.68% when the degrees of freedom is 100, and drops to only 9.44% when the degrees of freedom is 335. Of course, the latter might be prohibitively large for an external pilot study, but perhaps not for an internal pilot study, depending on the nature of the study. If the sample size percent underestimation was 15, a pilot study sample size of only 140 would be necessary for the percent risk to be (barely) less than 10, but such a percent underestimation could cause a study to be significantly underpowered.

Those numbers are obtained as follows. Consider the test of a population mean under the assumption of a normal distribution and an internal pilot study of n observations.

A well-known result from statistical theory is that $[(n-1)s^2]/\sigma^2 \sim \chi^2_{n-1}$, with "$\sim$" read "is distributed as" and χ^2_{n-1} denoting a chi-square random variable that has the chi-square distribution with $(n-1)$ degrees of freedom. The expected value (i.e., mean) of that random variable is $(n-1)$, which of course is what $[(n-1)s^2]/\sigma^2$ is equal to if $s^2 = \sigma^2$. Similarly, $s^2 \sim [\sigma^2/(n-1)]\chi^2_{n-1}$, so that $E(s^2) = \sigma^2$, taking the expected value of each side. If, for example, we knew that $s^2 = 0.9\sigma^2$, so that the use of s^2 to estimate σ^2 would, in expectation, underestimate the latter by 10%, then we need the value of χ^2_{n-1} such that

$$E\left[\left(\frac{\sigma^2}{n-1}\right)\chi^2_{n-1}\right] = 0.9\sigma^2$$

which means that we need $E\left(0.9\chi^2_{n-1}\right) = 0.9(n-1)$. Using the example with degrees of freedom $= 100$ from the ' preceding paragraph and still assuming that the percent underestimation is 10%, we need to obtain $P\left(\chi^2_{100} < 90\right)$. The use of statistical software shows that this probability is 0.2468, in agreement with the probability obtained using Lenth's applet. [*Note*: Here we are looking at the percent underestimation of σ^2, not σ, but it is the former that is most relevant because sample size formulas are a function of σ^2, as will be seen, for example, in Eq. (2.4) in Section 2.3.]

Table 2.1 shows the probability of underestimating the required sample size for selected values of n for the hypothesis test of a population mean, assuming a normal distribution. Such a table might be used to select the size of an internal pilot study.

These numbers are exact for the underestimation of the degrees of freedom for estimating σ and are thus approximations relative to the required sample size. The numbers show that it is highly desirable to have a reasonably large internal pilot study, but certainly not so large that the required sample size for the full study is less than the size of the internal pilot study.

Of course, this leads to the question of the extent to which an undersized full study results in the full study being underpowered. Power depends on other factors in addition to the sample size, specifically the significance level, the difference between the value of the mean under the null hypothesis and the value that is to be detected with the prescribed power if the null hypothesis is false, and σ. Therefore, a simple result cannot be given and further discussion of the effect on power is deferred to the examples that are given in later sections of this chapter. Some insight is given by Anderson (2006), however.

Table 2.1 Probability of Underestimating Required Sample Size[a]

Size of Internal Pilot Study	Percent by Which d.f. (σ) Is Underestimated	Probability of Exceeding Percentage
10	10(0.9)	.4759
	25(2.25)	.3369
	50(4.5)	.1245
	75(6.75)	.0131
25	10(2.4)	.3969
	25(6.0)	.1970
	50(12.0)	.0201
50	10(4.9)	.3279
	25(12.25)	.0985
	50(24.5)	.0013
100	10(9.9)	.2480
	25(24.75)	.0298
	50(49.5)	<.0001
200	10(19.9)	.1589
	25(49.75)	.0034
500	10(49.9)	.0532

[a]Note that since d.f. $= n - 1$, all of the percentages except the last two for size $= 25$ result in a degrees of freedom that is not an integer, which would correspond to the sample size for the full study being a noninteger value. No adjustment was made for that since Lenth's applet gives d.f. (σ).

2.2 EXAMPLES: FREQUENTIST AND BAYESIAN

A frequentist approach is contrasted with a Bayesian approach in Example 2.1, but Bayesian sample size determination techniques are not emphasized in this book, nor are they incorporated into the leading sample size determination software. Such software is available, however, as functions written for R and for S-Plus. See http://www.medicine.mcgill.ca/epidemiology/joseph/Bayesian-Software-Bayesian-Sample-Size.html.

Bayesian sample size determination is discussed further in this chapter in Section 2.1.1 and is also discussed, albeit somewhat briefly, in some of the subsequent chapters. Readers with an interest in Bayesian approaches to sample size determination are referred, in particular, to the references at the end of these chapters and to Chapter 13 of Chow, Shao, and Wang (2008). Also recommended is Inoue et al. (2005), who provided a general framework that allowed Bayesian approaches to sample size determination to be contrasted and compared with frequentist approaches.

We will start with a very simple, hypothetical example to illustrate the frequentist approach.

■ **EXAMPLE 2.1**

Let's assume that a manufacturing process yield is standardized in such a way that 100 has been the long-term value and this value has been acceptable. If intended improvements are made, however, there is a good chance that the yield will reach 101, and it is desired to determine the number of units of production to sample so that such an improvement can be detected, if it has occurred, with a probability of .80 (i.e., the power is to be .80, a value that is customarily used but will be critiqued in later sections).

That is, a hypothesis test will be performed such that the null hypothesis is $\mu = 100$ and the alternative hypothesis is $\mu > 100$.

What should be the sample size? We will assume an infinite population size for this example, as populations are frequently so large that they are practically countably infinite, and thus might as well be considered as infinite. Later we will look at how to proceed when populations are finite and the population size is known. We will also assume that the population can be adequately represented by a normal distribution and that σ, the standard deviation of the individual observations, is the same for both the distribution with the hypothesized mean and the distribution with the true mean. This is a reasonable assumption in the absence of any prior information to suggest otherwise, especially if the true mean does not differ greatly from the hypothesized mean.

The starting point is to look at the probability statement that leads to the sample size expression. If we use a significance level of .05, the statement is

$$P(\overline{X} > 100 + 1.645\sigma/\sqrt{n}|\mu = 101) = .80 \tag{2.1}$$

with $\sigma/\sqrt{n}$ being $\sigma_{\bar{x}}$ and $\overline{X}$ denoting the average of the individual observations, X, in a sample of size n. The value of $100 + 1.645\sigma/\sqrt{n}$ is the value for $\overline{X}$ such that values of $\overline{X}$ greater than this will result in the null hypothesis, $\mu = 100$, being rejected and the conclusion will be that $\mu > 100$. The constant 1.645 is determined by the .05 significance level and the fact that the test is one-sided, and is based on the assumption that either the individual observations have approximately a normal distribution (as stated for this example), or that the sample size, n, to be determined, will be large enough that the distribution of $\overline{X}$ will be approximately normal. The probability of the null hypothesis being rejected is .80 when $\mu = 101$ because the sample size will be determined so as to (approximately) produce that power if in fact $\mu = 101$. Note that we will conclude that $\mu > 100$ with probability .05 when $\mu = 100$ because we have selected .05 as the significance level. Note also that $1.645\sigma/\sqrt{n}$ goes to zero as $n \to \infty$, so if n was somewhat arbitrarily selected and made very large, eschewing sample size determination formula, the probability that $\overline{X}$ exceeds $100 + 1.645\sigma/\sqrt{n}$ could, depending on the value of σ, be virtually 1.0 not only for $\mu = 101$ but also for values of $\mu < 101$ that would not be of practical interest. Thus, the test would be too sensitive. This is one reason why a sample size should not be arbitrarily or haphazardly chosen, such as a sample size that uses all of the money that has been committed to a study.

A value for σ must be used unless the experimenter is willing to express in standard deviation units the shift that is to be detected with whatever probability is selected. The use of standard deviation units in sample size determination is not advocated here, however, and has also been criticized by Lenth (2001). The reason for this is perhaps obvious: standard deviation units enable the experimenter to avoid facing the question of what threshold parameter value defines practical significance in a given setting, plus the estimation of the standard deviation is avoided. Since the improvement of processes entails reducing variability, trying to avoid thinking about variability is not a good idea.

If a pilot study had been conducted, the sample standard deviation, s, could be used in estimating σ if the pilot study was of at least moderate size, although it should be kept in mind that s is a statistically biased estimator of σ. If the data were normally distributed (as assumed here), $E(s) = c_4\sigma$, with "$E(s)$" denoting the expected value of s and the value of c_4 is dependent on the sample size, being less than 1.0 for all sample sizes. For example, $c_4 = 0.9727$ for $n = 10$ and $c_4 = 0.9896$ for $n = 25$. Thus, for small samples it would be better to use s/c_4 to estimate σ, although it might be even better to use the upper limit of a confidence interval for σ, depending on the application. Tables of c_4 values are given in statistical quality control and improvement books, such as Ryan (2011). When $n \geq 10$, a reasonable approximation for c_4 is $c_4 = 1 - 1/4n - 7/32n^2$. There is not much point in using c_4 when n is much larger than 25, provided that there is evidence of at least approximate normality.

It is well known that $\mathrm{Var}(s) = \sigma^2(1 - c_4^2)$, so a large value of σ^2 coupled with a small pilot study could result in sampling variability in s of such a magnitude that it cannot be ignored. Nevertheless, Sims, Elston, Harris, and Wanless (2007) stated: "In fields such as the physical and chemical sciences and engineering, detailed knowledge of the variance can often be obtained from a pilot study reasonably quickly and efficiently, and it is considered acceptable to regard the estimate as the true population variance. In some areas of biological research, such as clinical trials where variance information can be cumulated across trials with identical protocols,the assumption of known variance may also be valid." Since $\mathrm{Var}(s) \rightarrow 0$ as $c_4 \rightarrow 1$, which occurs as $n \rightarrow \infty$, it is really a question of how much data is available for estimating σ before the major study is performed. At the other extreme, Sims et al. (2007) also stated: "In contrast to other fields of science, ecological pilot studies can be financially expensive and, where years act as a basic unit of replication, only accrue information very slowly." Thus, practitioners need to think about the field in which they are working in terms of the cost of pilot studies and the amount of data available for estimating σ. If in doubt, it would be best to *not* act as if σ is known and to incorporate sampling variability into the determination of power and sample size. Of course, this is even more important when multiple parameters must be estimated in the course of determining sample size. Incorporating sampling variability is discussed and illustrated in Chapter 3 and to a lesser extent in succeeding chapters.

If the observations are approximately normally distributed, then the range of possible observations divided by six will provide a reasonable estimate of σ. This assumes that the largest possible observation is at approximately $\mu + 3\sigma$ (the 99.865 percentile of a normal distribution) and the smallest value is at approximately $\mu - 3\sigma$ (the 0.135 percentile of a normal distribution). The difference between them is thus $(\mu + 3\sigma) - (\mu - 3\sigma) = 6\sigma$, so σ is estimated by Range/6. [Some writers have recommended that four be used as the divisor and others have indicated that either might be used (e.g., Lohr, 1999, p. 41), but six is the better choice, in my opinion, provided that there is sufficient information available regarding the largest possible value likely to be encountered as well as the smallest possible value. We will illustrate later how this can affect sample size determination.] Note that there is no sampling variability with the range method of estimating σ because the largest and smallest values likely to be encountered are assumed to be known.

Similarly, it is also possible to estimate σ if two percentiles of a normal distribution are known. For example, if the 90th percentile is believed to be 18 and the 20th percentile is considered to be 10, the 90th percentile is at $\mu + 1.28\sigma$ and the 20th percentile is at $\mu - 0.84\sigma$, with the difference between them thus being 2.12σ. So for this example we would estimate σ as $\hat{\sigma} = (18 - 10)/2.12 = 3.77$. [The software PASS can be used to estimate σ in this manner, as well as to estimate σ as (population range)/4.] Similarly, nQuery also has this capability. For example, if the option "Estimate standard deviation from sample percentiles" is selected in nQuery and "1" is entered for "Percentile" and 20 entered for the "lower observed value" and 80 entered for the "upper observed value," the software acts as if 1 is the population first percentile and 80 is the population 99th percentile, and further assumes that the population has a normal distribution. That is, it gives $\hat{\sigma} = 12.896$, which is obtained from $(80 - 20)/[2(2.32635)]$, with 2.32635 being the 99th percentile of the standard normal distribution and -2.32635 being the first percentile. Hand computation gives $\hat{\sigma} = 12.8957$, in agreement with the result given by nQuery.

Here process yield is being measured and let's assume that daily measurements are made, with past records indicating that almost all daily yield measurements have been between 91 and 109. Then we can estimate σ as $\hat{\sigma} = (109 - 91)/6 = 3.0$.

With σ estimated in this manner and approximate normality assumed, as stated, the test statistic is

$$Z = \frac{\bar{X} - 100}{3/\sqrt{n}}$$

Since we want $P(\bar{X} > 100 + 1.645\sigma/\sqrt{n})$, substituting $(100 + 1.645(3)/\sqrt{n})$ for $\bar{X}$ in the expression for Z of course produces 1.645, the threshold value for the test statistic, Z, such that any Z-value larger than 1.645 would result in rejection of the null hypothesis. Approximate normality for the distribution of $\bar{X}$ would have to be assumed in order to use Z, but in this example approximate normality of the individual observations was assumed in the estimation of σ. Approximate normality of the individual observations implies approximate normality of $\bar{X}$, and indeed the distribution of $\bar{X}$ will always be closer to a normal distribution than will the distribution of X (i.e., the individual observations).

Since 100 is the value for μ that forms the null hypothesis but 101 is assumed to be the true value of μ, we need to perform appropriate algebra starting from Eq. (2.1) to obtain an equation that will be used to solve for n. Subtracting 101 from both sides of the inequality and then dividing by $\sigma/\sqrt{n}$ produces

$$P\left(\frac{\bar{X} - 101}{3/\sqrt{n}} > 1.645 + \frac{100 - 101}{3/\sqrt{n}} \,\middle|\, \mu = 101\right) = .80$$

Thus,

$$1 - \Phi\left(1.645 + \frac{100 - 101}{3/\sqrt{n}}\right) = .80,$$

so that

$$\Phi\left(1.645 + \frac{100 - 101}{3/\sqrt{n}}\right) = .20$$

with $\Phi(\cdot)$ denoting the cumulative normal probability density function (*pdf*). Then

$$1.645 + \frac{100 - 101}{3/\sqrt{n}} = \Phi^{-1}(.20) = \Phi^{-1}(\beta) = -Z_\beta$$

with β denoting, in general, the probability of failing to reject the null hypothesis when it is false, with Z_β denoting the value of the standard normal variate with an area, β, to be specified, in the right tail of the distribution. (Later Z_α and $Z_{\alpha/2}$ will be used and the same general definition applies to these expressions.)

Thus, $\beta = 1 -$ power. Since $-Z_\beta = -Z_{.20} = -0.84$, the desired value of n is thus obtained by solving the equation

$$1.645 + \frac{100 - 101}{3/\sqrt{n}} = -0.84 \qquad (2.2)$$

Doing so produces $n = [2.485*3/(101 - 100)]^2 = 55.58$. The value $n = 56$ would then be used so that the power is at least .80.

Of course, this result is conditional on $\sigma = 3$, so that .80 is the assumed power. What if the true value of the standard deviation was $\sigma = 2$? Then the actual power should be much greater than .80 since the smaller the standard deviation, the more powerful the test if everything else is kept constant. The power is

$$1 - \Phi\left(1.645 + \frac{100 - 101}{2/\sqrt{n}}\right) = .982$$

This large increase in the power should be expected since we are using a value for σ that is 33% smaller than the previous value.

What would the sample size have been if the range had been divided by 4 instead of by 6? Then $\hat{\sigma} = 4.5$ and following this same sequence of steps in PASS would lead to $n = 126$—more than twice the sample size when 6 was used as the divisor. How can there be such a huge difference? Since $n = 56$ was obtained from the calculation $n = [(2.485)(3)/(101 - 100)]^2$ and since $4.5 = 3(1.5)$ and the 1.5 would be squared in the formula, this means that the sample size obtained using $\hat{\sigma} = 4.5$ will be $(1.5)^2 = 2.25$ times the sample size obtained using $\hat{\sigma} = 3.0$. Here one could verify that $2.25(56)$ does equal 126. This shows how very sensitive the sample size is to the estimate of σ! Therefore, it is imperative that a "good" and perhaps conservative estimate of σ be used. This is pursued in Chapter 3, especially Section 3.3, in discussing how data from a pilot study might be used in determining sample size.

If we write Eq. (2.2) in the general form

$$Z_\alpha + \frac{\mu_0 - \mu}{\sigma/\sqrt{n}} = -Z_\beta \tag{2.3}$$

with μ denoting the actual mean and μ_0 denoting the hypothesized mean, we can see by performing some simple algebra that the general form of the solution for n for a one-sided test is

$$n = \left[\frac{(Z_\alpha + Z_\beta)\sigma}{(\mu - \mu_0)}\right]^2 \tag{2.4}$$

Notice from Eq. (2.4) that n is inversely related to the difference between the actual value of μ and the hypothesized value. This is quite intuitive because if the true value is much greater than the hypothesized value, that should not be hard to detect, so a large sample size would not be needed. Notice also that when the other components are fixed, the required sample size varies directly with the specified power, as 1.28 would be used in Eq. (2.4) instead of 0.84 if the specified power had been .90. Then $Z_\alpha + Z_\beta$ would have been 2.925 instead of 2.485. Of course, this is also intuitive because we would expect to need a larger sample size to have greater power in detecting a given difference between the hypothesized value and the true value.

Regarding the relationship between sample size and power, if we start from Eq. (2.3) and solve for power as a function of sample size, we obtain

$$\Phi\left[Z_\alpha - \frac{\sqrt{n}(|\mu - \mu_0|)}{\sigma}\right] = \beta$$

so

$$\text{Power} = 1 - \Phi\left[Z_\alpha - \frac{\sqrt{n}\,(|\mu - \mu_0|)}{\sigma}\right] \tag{2.5}$$

If the sample size is too small, then the fraction in the brackets is too small and the bracketed expression is too large, so that the power is then too low. To illustrate, let $\delta = |\mu - \mu_0| = 2$, $Z_\alpha = 1.645$, $\sigma = 8$, and $n = 90$. We will assume that the sample size was underestimated by (only) 10%, so that a sample size of 100 should have been used. The power, using either hand calculation or software such as PASS, can be shown to be .7663. If $n = 100$ had been used, then the power would have been .8038. If the user insists on having power of at least .80 in every application, then the underestimation of sample size for this example would be a problem.

It should be apparent from this example with slight sample size underestimation and from the results of Table 2.1 that the use of an internal pilot study of an appropriate size is very important. We will return to this topic with more examples in later chapters. ∎

2.2.1 Bayesian Approaches

Bayesian sample size determination methods were reviewed in a general way at the beginning of this chapter. How would a Bayesian statistician or a person who wishes to use a Bayesian approach have proceeded relative to Example 2.1? Prior distributions are used in Bayesian statistics and here it is necessary to assign a prior probability to μ_0 and to a value for μ for which power is to be specified. In the current example, μ_0 and μ are 100 and 101, respectively. A simple assignment of prior probabilities would be to use 1/2 for each of the two values. As discussed by Inoue et al. (2005), a decision regarding the null hypothesis under the Bayesian approach would be based on the posterior probabilities for each of the two values. (Posterior probabilities are computed by combining the prior probabilities with sample data. In sample size determination, data from a pilot study might constitute the Sample data.") A decision rule might be to not reject the hypothesized value if its posterior probability is at least $1/(1 + k)$ for a suitably chosen value of k. Let $\pi = P(\mu = \mu_0)$ and $\delta = \mu - \mu_0$. Bayesian sample size determination is then made using (π, K, δ, σ).

Inoue et al. (2005) gave an example with $\sigma = 1$, $\delta = .10$, $\alpha = .05$, and $\beta = .10$. The use of Eq. (2.4) produces $n = 856.385$, so $n = 857$ would be used. They showed how the same sample size is obtained with the Bayesian approach if the "minimum rate of correct classification" (i.e., the probability of making the right decision) is .9283. Of course, an experimenter would be more apt to select a number such as .80, .90, or .95 rather than .9283, so sample sizes obtained with frequentist and Bayesian approaches will generally differ.

What if σ could not be estimated in the preceding manner? The effectiveness of that method depends on (a) approximate normality of the individual observations and (b) information on the range of possible values. [What was tacitly assumed in obtaining the estimate of σ in Example 2.1 is that approximately 27 of every 10,000 observations is outside the interval (91, 109).] We would generally expect that information would be available to construct such an interval. If not, the process engineer and other workers involved in a manufacturing process or whatever type process was involved would presumably be able to provide a reasonable estimate of the process standard deviation. Therefore, a Bayesian approach, specifying some prior distribution for σ, should usually be unnecessary.

De Santis (2007) considered the use of data from similar studies in discussing a Bayesian approach to sample size determination but that could become a bit tricky because the populations and study conditions would need to be identical, or at least very similar.

Sahu and Smith (2006) considered a Bayesian approach to sample size determination, motivated by a practical application in clinical trials and in a financial audit. See also the Bayesian approach for sample size determination proposed by Berg (2006) for auditing property value appraisals to determine whether state accuracy guidelines are met.

Walker (2003) considered a Bayesian nonparametric approach that utilized decision theory and specifically solved for the sample size using the "maximization of expected utility." The author argues for a nonparametric approach because "a sample size is advocated without the benefit of observed data." The advocated approach is rather involved and complicated, however, and accordingly is likely to be primarily only of academic interest. (Sample size determination for nonparametric methods is covered in Chapter 10.)

Bayesian sample size determination methods for clinical trials were reviewed by Pezeshk (2003). This paper and many other papers on Bayesian sample size determination methods for clinical trials are discussed briefly in Section 7.8.

2.2.2 Probability Assessment Approach

As discussed by, for example, Chow et al. (2008, p. 18), for rare events, it may not be appropriate to determine sample size based on power, because the necessary sample size may be impractically large and small changes may not be of practical interest. Therefore, it may be more practical to determine sample size based on a probability statement that, say, a treatment group sample mean will be less than/greater than a control group sample mean. (Of course, no probability statement can be made about population means, at least with a frequentist approach, since population means are not random variables.) See Section 1.3.4 of Chow et al. (2008) for further details.

2.2.3 Reproducibility Probability Approach

This approach is due to Shao and Chow (2002) and relates to the fact that the U.S. Food and Drug Administration (FDA) usually requires at least two well-controlled clinical trials for providing evidence of the effectiveness and safety of a new drug. The general idea is to compute the sample size for the second trial using the concept of reproducibility probability. The sample size for the second trial is a function of the value of the test statistic for testing the equality of the treatment group mean (μ_2) and the control group mean (μ_1) that produces the desired reproducibility probability, as well as ϵ and C, with the difference in the population means assumed to change from $\mu_1 - \mu_2$ in the first trial to $\mu_1 - \mu_2 + \epsilon$ in the second trial, and the assumed common population variance assumed to change from σ^2 in the first trial to $C^2\sigma^2$ in the second trial, with $C > 0$. See Shao and Chow (2002) and/or Section 1.3.5 of Chow et al. (2008) for details.

2.2.4 Competing Probability Approach

Rahardja and Zhao (2009) proposed a new approach to sample size determination, which they termed the *competing probability* (CP) *approach,* with particular applications in clinical trials. Accordingly, the method is discussed and illustrated in Section 7.7. Briefly, the authors stated that "CP can be interpreted as the probability of the experimental treatment being more efficacious than the control treatment." Thus, the focus is on this probability rather than a specified minimum effect size that an experimenter wishes to detect with a hypothesis test. See Lautoche and Porcher (2007) for somewhat related work.

2.2.5 Evidential Approach

Another method of determining sample size is to use an "evidential framework," as described by Strug, Rohde, and Corey (2007). This utilizes the likelihood function, with evidence about a parameter classified as strong, weak, or misleading. See also Sutton, Cooper, Jones, Lambert, Thompson, and Abrams (2007).

2.3 FINITE POPULATIONS

In determining sample size it is generally sufficient to act as if the population is infinite and ignore the *finite population correction* (fpc) *factor,* which is $(N - n)/(N - 1)$, with N denoting the population size. More specifically,

$$\sigma_{\bar{x}}^2 = \frac{\sigma_x^2}{n}\left(\frac{N - n}{N - 1}\right) \tag{2.6}$$

Population sizes are unknown in most applications, so the fpc is generally ignored. In some applications, however, such as in accounting when the total number of records for a certain time period is known but it is too time consuming and costly to examine very record, the population size is known. If the sample size is to be a sufficiently large percentage of the population size (the usual rule of thumb is 5%), the fpc should be used in determining the sample size, whether a hypothesis test or a confidence interval is to be used.

When PASS is used for a hypothesis test of a single mean, the fpc is automatically used whenever the user specifies the size of the population rather than indicating that the population is infinite.

The use of the fpc in determining sample size for confidence intervals is discussed and illustrated in Section 2.4.1.

2.4   SAMPLE SIZES FOR CONFIDENCE INTERVALS

Although the relationship between confidence intervals and hypothesis tests was discussed briefly in Section 1.2, sample size could not be determined using a confidence interval so as to provide a specified power of the corresponding hypothesis test simply because power is not involved in confidence interval construction. As noted in Section 1.2, a confidence interval could be used to test a hypothesis and in some ways this is better than using a standard hypothesis test. (Sample size could be computed using a hypothesis test approach and then a confidence interval or one-sided confidence bound constructed rather than performing the hypothesis test, but that would be a mixture of a hypothesis testing approach and a confidence interval approach.) While stating a trend away from hypotheses tests and toward confidence intervals in epidemiologic analyses, Greenland (1987) notes that confidence intervals can be misleading indicators of the discriminatory power of a study if they are not properly centered and Jiroutek, Muller, Kupper, and Stewart (2003) presented what they claimed to be improved methods of determining sample size for confidence intervals. Specifically, with the term "Validity" defined as a confidence interval that contains the true parameter value, they addressed the question "Given validity, how many subjects are needed to have a high probability of producing a confidence interval that correctly does not contain the null value when the null hypothesis is false and has a width no greater than δ?"

Sample size can be determined so as to give a confidence interval of a specified width, or equivalently, a maximum error of estimation, which is just the halfwidth of the confidence interval. Bristol (1989) discussed the determination of sample size for confidence intervals of a specified width and compared that to the usual determination of sample size for hypothesis tests with a stated power.

To illustrate, consider a confidence interval for μ. The expression for the width of a confidence interval for μ using Z is obtained by taking the difference between the upper limit (*U.L.*) and the lower limit (*L.L.*). Specifically, the width, *W*, is given by

$$W = L.L. - U.L. = \bar{X} + Z_{\alpha/2}\sigma/\sqrt{n} - (\bar{X} - Z_{\alpha/2}\sigma/\sqrt{n})$$
$$= 2Z_{\alpha/2}\sigma/\sqrt{n}$$

Thus, $W = 2Z_{\alpha/2}\sigma/\sqrt{n}$. Solving this equation for *n* gives $n = (2Z_{\alpha/2}\sigma/W)^2$. Thus, *n* is inversely related to *W*, with a small value of *W*, relative to σ, producing a large value of *n*. Of course, an estimate of σ is needed, perhaps to be obtained using the method in Example 2.1, or from prior data such as historical records.

Since $\hat{\mu} = \bar{X}$ and the latter is in the middle of the confidence interval, this means that the maximum error of estimation is $E = W/2$, with probability $1 - \alpha$. Thus, sample size could be computed for a specified maximum error of estimation, with the expression for *n* being

$$n = (Z_{\alpha/2}\sigma/E)^2 \tag{2.7}$$

with *n* rounded to the next integer value since the result will almost certainly not be an integer. The choice between the use of *E* or *W* of course depends on the focus of the experimenter. We can see from Eq. (2.7) that if an experimenter has a value of *E* in mind but decides to switch to a value half as large, then the necessary sample will, on average, be four times the required value with the original value of *E*. Thus, extra precision could be quite expensive and there is no guarantee of what will happen on individual samples since $\bar{X}$ is a random variable. Thus, there is randomness involved even if σ were assumed to be known. This motivated Webb, Smith, and Firag (2010) to look at the probability of achieving improved accuracy with an increased sample size, extending the results of Gauch (2006). The results of Webb et al. (2010) showed that very large increases in the sample size are required in order for the probability that the error of estimation with the increased sample size, which they term the "gain probability," will be close to 1. (The gain probability is the probability that the estimator based on the larger of two sample sizes is closer to the true parameter than the estimator based on the smaller sample size.) Webb et al. (2010) stated that "it is known that setting sample size requirements to guarantee improved accuracy with a given probability can lead to an alarmingly high demand on sample size" and they quantified that statement, although they did so using graphs rather than tables. Their Figure 8 combined with some statistical work shows that the gain probability is well-approximated by $0.627 + 0.0751[\log(k/n)]$, assuming normality and essentially independent of *n*, with *k* denoting the number of additional samples and $2 \le k/n \le 10$. Thus, when $k/n = 10$ so that the sample size is being increased by 10 times the original sample size, the gain probability would be approximated by .80, whereas their Figure 8 suggests that the probability is approximately .81. It should be of concern that such an enormous increase in the sample size results in a gain probability that is considerably less than 1.

When viewed from a cost perspective, which Webb et al. (2010) did not consider, in addition to statistical considerations, this would likely be a very undesirable way of determining sample size.

The user does not have a choice when PASS is used for determining the sample size, however, as the user specifies the "distance from mean to limit(s)," which of course is E. To illustrate, let $\sigma = 2, E = 1$, an infinite population is assumed, and a 95% two-sided confidence interval for the mean is desired. The software gives $n = 16$ as the required sample size. We can see that hand computation would give $n = [1.96(2)]^2 = (3.92)^2 = 15.37$, so $n = 16$ would be used, as the software indicated.

Kupper and Hafner (1989) reported that this formula performed poorly in their numerical work. This requires some clarification. The sample size expression in Eq. (2.7) is an exact result *if* the individual observations have a normal distribution and if the population standard deviation, σ, is *known*. Of course, neither condition is likely to be met in practice. Kupper and Hafner (1989) stated that the use of $n = \left(Z_{\alpha/2}\sigma/E\right)^2$ "always leads to a serious underestimation of the required sample size. This surprising result can be illustrated by appealing to an overlooked, but nevertheless important, result due to Guenther (1965)." The result is really not surprising because if σ is later assumed unknown after solving for n for known σ, the sample size so determined will be too small since the variability resulting from using s to estimate σ will not have been accounted for! The reader is asked to show in Exercise 2.1 that this sample size formula does work as intended, when the *conditions for its use are met*. The discussion of Kupper and Hafner (1989) is not irrelevant, however, as there is at least one software package that solves for n using an inputted value of σ in the two-sample case, then allows the user to specify whether the test statistic to be used is for a pooled t-test (i.e, unknown common σ) or not. This is discussed further in Section 3.2. There is a definite inconsistency when software is used and any type of t-test is selected, for one sample or more than one sample, because σ must be indicated as known to solve for the sample size, but if we knew σ we wouldn't be using t in the first place! An important contribution of Kupper and Hafner (1989) is that they emphasized the need to use sample size formulas for simple confidence intervals that incorporate the appropriate expression for factoring in a tolerance or coverage probability for the estimation of σ by S. This is important because sample size determination software such as PASS assume that the value for the standard deviation that the user enters will be that value in all future samples when the menu item with the coverage probability is not selected. Obviously all future samples will not have the same standard deviation.

Note that this assumed two-sided confidence interval does not correspond directly to Example 2.1 because that was a one-sided hypothesis test, which corresponds to a one-sided confidence bound, not to a two-sided confidence interval. It is not possible to solve for n for a one-sided confidence bound of a desired width because such bounds of course do not have a finite width since no value is used for a bound on the other side.

We could, however, do something similar and solve for n such that there is a maximum error of estimation in the direction of interest. For a two-sided confidence interval, the maximum error of estimation (with the stated probability) is half the width of the confidence interval. For a one-sided confidence bound, the maximum error of estimation is given by the expression for the estimator and the expression for the confidence bound.

For example, assume normality for the sake of illustration, known σ, and that μ is to be estimated by $\bar{X}$ such that $\bar{X}$ should not exceed μ by more than two units with probability .95. Stated differently, we want the lower confidence bound on μ to be within two units of $\bar{X}$ with probability .95. Since the 95% lower confidence bound on μ is given by the expression $\bar{X} - 1.645\sigma/\sqrt{n}$, $\bar{X} - (\bar{X} - 1.645\sigma/\sqrt{n}) = 1.645\sigma/\sqrt{n}$. Since this difference is to be at most 2, $1.645\sigma/\sqrt{n} \leq 2$. Solving this inequality gives $n \geq 0.676\sigma^2$. Thus, if $\sigma = 10$, for example, $n = 68$ would be used.

Of course, normality does not exist in practice, so the user who wants to solve for the sample size to give a confidence interval of a specified width or a maximum error of estimation with a certain probability must also contend with nonnormality and consider how large the sample size would have to be to overcome the fact that normal theory methods are being used on nonnormal data. Boos and Hughes-Oliver (2000) addressed this issue and gave some recommendations that were based on the population skewness. They concluded, however, by stating that "These are rough generalizations and we encourage readers to find their own rules."

2.4.1 Using the Finite Population Correction Factor

As indicated in Section 2.2, it is sometimes necessary to use the finite population correction factor (fpc), which is $(N - n)/(N - 1)$, although some sources use $(N - n)/(N)$. Whichever quantity is used, it is multiplied times $\sigma_{\bar{x}}^2$ when $\bar{X}$ is the random variable that is used, as in estimating a population mean or total.

Of course, in solving for the sample size we won't know whether or not the fpc will be needed unless we know what fraction of the population will have to be sampled in order to obtain a desired confidence interval width or to reject the null hypothesis when the parameter being tested has a certain value.

To illustrate, let's assume that σ has been estimated by the range method, with the estimate being 2.0, so Z will be used in constructing a 95% confidence interval that is to have width $W = 1$, and $N = 1000$. From the development in Section 2.3 combined with Eq. (2.5), we have $2(Z_{\alpha/2})\sigma_{\bar{x}} = W$, so that

$$2(Z_{\alpha/2})\sqrt{\frac{\sigma_x^2}{n}\left(\frac{N - n}{N - 1}\right)} = W \tag{2.8}$$

Solving for n produces

$$n = \frac{4N Z_{\alpha/2}^2 \sigma^2}{(N-1)W^2 + 4Z_{\alpha/2}^2 \sigma^2} \tag{2.9}$$

Using $\hat{\sigma} = 2.0$, $W = 1$, $N = 1000$, and $Z_{\alpha/2} = 1.96$, we obtain $n = 57.96$, so $n = 58$ would be used. If the fpc had not been used, the solution would have been $n = 4Z_{\alpha/2}^2 \sigma^2 / W^2 = 61.47$, so $n = 62$ would have been used. Thus, there is a slight difference in this case. Here n/N was only .058, so it isn't much larger than .05. There would have been a greater difference in the two sample sizes if n/N had been larger.

If we wanted the sample size expression in terms of the maximum possible error of estimation, E, we would use the relationship between W and E noted in Section 2.4 ($E = W/2$), and substitute $2E$ for W in Eq. (2.9). Doing so produces

$$n = \frac{N Z_{\alpha/2}^2 \sigma^2}{(N-1)E^2 + Z_{\alpha/2}^2 \sigma^2} \tag{2.10}$$

Assume that a company wishes to estimate its average accounts receivable at some point in time. The company's computerized accounting system is not set up to easily generate this number, and since there are too many accounts to look at in order to do this manually, a sample will be taken. It might be necessary to stratify the population in applications such as this when there is a wide range of amounts, as a smaller sample size will be possible by sampling within well-determined strata rather than sampling at random from the population.

There are skeptics who believe that sample size determination in auditing is not a worthwhile endeavor. In particular, Wilburn (1984, p. 47) stated: "Any meticulous, absolutely exact or time consuming procedure with precisely determined sample size is neither justifiable nor desirable in most audits. Predetermined sample sizes are generally based on assumptions which may not be applicable in the audit circumstances." Of course, the last sentence applies to virtually *any* sampling situation, not just to auditing. There is evidence from documents available on the Internet, however, that statistical methods of determining sample size have fallen into disfavor with the auditing profession. Even though there are problems inherent in the statistical approach to sample size determination, worse results could easily result when a nonstatistical approach is used.

Nevertheless, there appears to be the growing realization that sample size determination is fraught with problems. One sign of this is the recent discussion in Noordzij, Dekker, Zoccali, and Jager (2011). In particular, they stated:

> These examples show the most important drawback of sample size calculations: investigators can easily influence the result of their sample size calculations by changing the components in such a way that they need fewer patients, as that is usually what is most convenient to the researchers. For this reason, sample size calculations are sometimes of limited value. Furthermore, more and more experts are expressing criticism of the current

methods used. They suggest introducing new ways to determine sample sizes, for example, estimating the sample size based on the likely width of the confidence interval for a set of outcomes.

Bland (2009) has argued in favor of determining sample size based on the width of a confidence interval, not the power of a hypothesis test. Such an approach would have considerable merit, but this probably won't happen to any great extent in practice until software for sample size determination moves in that direction.

2.4.1.1 Estimating Population Totals

In addition to means and other parameters, sampling books also cover the estimation of population totals. In order to estimate a population total, a population must be finite and known. We have used E to denote the maximum error of estimation in estimating μ by $\bar{X}$. Since a population total would be estimated by $N\bar{X}$, with N denoting the population size, it would be logical to use NE to represent the maximum error in estimating the corresponding population total.

Using NE, the sample size would be the same as the sample size for estimating μ with error E. This should be intuitively apparent, but we can also easily show it, as follows, with need for the fpc assumed. Since

$$\mathrm{Var}(N\bar{X}) = N^2 \mathrm{Var}(\bar{X}) = N^2 = N^2 \frac{\sigma_x^2}{n}\left(\frac{N-n}{N-1}\right)$$

then

$$\sigma_{N\bar{X}} = N\sqrt{\frac{\sigma_x^2}{n}\left(\frac{N-n}{N-1}\right)}$$

The sample size determination as a function of E would then be obtained by solving the equation

$$Z_{\alpha/2}N\sqrt{\frac{\sigma_x^2}{n}\left(\frac{N-n}{N-1}\right)} = NE \tag{2.11}$$

Since $E = W/2$, it can easily be seen that Eq. (2.11) is equivalent to Eq. (2.8).

Of course, a sample size formula could also be derived independent of the error expression for the population mean. Let E^* denote the selected maximum error of estimation for the population total. The sample size expression would then be obtained by substituting E^* for NE in Eq. (2.11) and then solving for n. Doing so produces

$$n = \frac{N Z_{\alpha/2}^2 \sigma^2}{(N-1)(E^*)^2 + Z_{\alpha/2}^2 \sigma^2}$$

It can be noted that it is never wrong to use the fpc in deriving the sample size expression for a finite population, as was done in deriving this expression. It is wise to use it whenever the population size is known because the effect that it has can't be determined until the value of n is obtained. If n/N is quite small, the use of the fpc in deriving the formula will have little effect; otherwise, the effect will be noticeable.

2.5   CONFIDENCE INTERVALS ON SAMPLE SIZE AND POWER

Since sample size is computed using an estimate of at least one other parameter, such as a variance being estimated, this means that the resultant sample size is a random variable, as is the assumed power. Therefore, a more realistic approach would be to construct confidence intervals for sample size and power, rather than assume that these are known. Although this is not built into sample size determination software and thus may be seldom used, the interested reader is referred to Taylor and Muller (1995).

2.6   SPECIFICATION OF POWER

There is no reason why .80 should be used, in general, for sample size calculations. Indeed, in statistics we generally prefer more "certainty" than that, such as a 95% or 99% confidence interval. Cohen (1988, p. 55) addressed the selection of a value for power and stated that "in the judgment of the author, for most behavioral science research (although admitting of many exceptions), power values as large as .90–.99 would demand sample sizes so large as to exceed an investigator's resources." Power depends on a number of factors, however, including the size of effect to be detected with high probability, and the standard deviation of the random variable that serves as the estimator of the parameter being tested. Thus, power values of at least .90 won't necessarily result in an impractically large sample size.

In pointing out problems with the assumptions and mechanics of sample size computations, Parker and Berman (2003) made a very valid point when they stated the following: "First, there is no a priori reason why one specific value of a difference... is worthy of detection with a certain power, while a slightly different value is worthy of less (or more) power of being detected." They feel that emphasis should shift from determining the sample size that is needed to detect a particular difference with a specified power to determining the information that is gained from using a particular sample size. Of course, we would ideally like to be able to detect the true value of the parameter with a high probability, rather than have a high probability of detecting a parameter value that might be somewhat arbitrarily chosen.

Their points are well taken. If we test that a population mean is 50 but a true value of μ between 49.5 and 50.5 is "close enough," why should there be a higher probability of rejecting the null hypothesis when $\mu = 50.4$ compared to $\mu = 50.3$ when both differences from 50 are deemed inconsequential, and thus the difference between 50.4 and 50.3 is also inconsequential? Debates such as this argue indirectly against the use of hypothesis testing, in general, and thus indirectly argue against the determination of sample size in a hypothesis testing context.

2.7   COST OF SAMPLING

Regardless of what methods are used to determine sample size, the cost of sampling must be considered. Remember that although increasing the sample size beyond what was originally envisioned will give increased power, it will also generally result in increased costs. So the marginal cost must be considered relative to the gain in precision/power. See `http://www.pmean.com/08/TooMuch Power.html` for a description of a study in which costs were considered, and note the following statement of Simon (2008): "The optimal sample size is one where the incremental value of improved precision is offset by the direct and indirect costs of obtaining an additional patient. No one does it this way, but they should." Of course, this assumes that the optimal sample size results in a cost that is within the budget for a study. If not, there is not much point in identifying a point of diminishing returns. See Chapter 7 of Brush (1988) for information on using costs and loss functions in the determination of sample size.

In addition to the explicit cost of sampling, it is recognized that sampling can simply be burdensome, especially when large samples are obtained. This point was made, for example, in the *2006–2007 Quality Assurance Program Sampling Guide* for Federal Student Aid, as educational institutions were required to sample 350 student records only every other year, rather than every year.

2.8   ETHICAL CONSIDERATIONS

Referring to clinical studies, various authors (e.g., Halpern, Karlawish, and Berlin, 2002) have claimed that many such studies do not have a power of at least .80 for detecting a minimum important effect, as discussed by Bacchetti, Wolf, Segal, and McCulloch (2005). [Readers may be interested in the response to that article by Halpern, Karlawish, and Berlin (2005).] See also Maxwell (2004) for a discussion of low power in psychological studies.

The argument has been that it is unfair to ask study participants to accept the risks and discomfort of being participants if the study does not have sufficient power to detect an effect of the minimum size that is considered to be important. Indeed, in referring to clinical trials, Altman (1980) stated: "If the sample size is too small there is an increased risk of a false-negative reading." See also the discussion of this in Lenth (2001).

That argument has received some criticism, however, as others have stated that such studies may still produce useful point estimates and confidence intervals, or contribute to meta-analyses. The latter was the point made by Chalmers, Levin, Sacks, Reitman, Berrier, and Nagalingham (1987). (Meta-analyses of clinical trials does present certain challengers, however, as discussed in Section 7.6.) Interestingly, Schulz and Grimes (2005) stated that Tom Chalmers considered Freiman, Chalmers, Smith, and Kuebler (1978) to be the most damaging paper he co-authored. Why? The paper was heavily cited (over 600 citations) and took the position that trials with low power were unethical. Many people were influenced by that paper and adopted the same position.

Bacchetti et al. (2005) have a different counterargument, explaining that "the balance between a study's value and the burdens accepted by its participants does not improve as the sample size increases. Thus, the argument for ethical condemnation of small studies fails even on its own terms." The authors conclude: "Indeed, a more legitimate ethical issue regarding sample size is whether it is too large."

Study participants are divided into two (or more) groups, so if the "treatment group" is receiving something that is beneficial, then by definition the other group does not receive it. So the larger the sample size, the greater the number of people who are not receiving a treatment that they may need, or at least an alternative to that treatment. So ethical considerations do have to be made, at least in a nonquantitative manner, for certain types of studies when sample size determination is being made.

Sample size computations depend on whether the test is one-sided or two-sided. This can be seen from Eq. (2.4). If Example 2.1 had been a two-sided test instead of a one-sided test, Z_α in Eq. (2.4) would be replaced by $Z_{\alpha/2}$. Since $\alpha/2$ is obviously less than α, $Z_{\alpha/2}$ is larger than Z_α since the former is further out into the right tail of the standard normal distribution than is the latter. Assume, as in Example 2.1, that power is to be .80. For $\alpha = 0.05$, $Z_{\alpha/2} = 1.96$ compared to $Z_\alpha = 1.645$. Since $(0.84 + 1.96)^2 = 7.84$, $(0.84 + 1.645)^2 = 6.175$ and $7.84/6.175 = 1.27$, the computed sample size for a two-sided test would thus be 27% greater than the sample size for a one-sided test. Stated differently, the necessary sample size for a one-sided test would be 79% of the sample size needed for a two-sized test.

Despite the popularity of one-sided testing in clinical research, Moyé and Tita (2002) argued in favor of two-sided tests and gave a graph that plotted the percentage against α, with 79% being one of the points on the graph. One point they made to support their contention is that a treatment may be harmful rather than helpful, and that harm often does occur. Of course, it would be important to detect that, and to detect it as soon as possible. An important quote from their paper is: "Here, the finding of harm in a one-tailed test designed to find benefit makes it ethically unacceptable but scientifically necessary to reproduce the result. This conundrum causes confusion in the medical community and could have been completely avoided by carrying out a two-tailed test from the beginning." They also stated that "a one-tailed test designed exclusively to find benefit does not permit the assessment of the role of sampling error in producing harm, a dangerous omission for a profession whose fundamental tenet is to first do no harm."

Knottnerus and Bouter (2001) offered a counterargument, stating that more people would receive the inferior treatment (in, say, a clinical study), but a study might be terminated early if there is strong evidence of benefit, as pointed out by Moyé and Tita (2002).

These are some important points and other important points regarding the choice of one-sided versus two-sided tests were also made by Bland and Altman (1994). While indicating that a one-sided test is sometimes appropriate, they strongly favor two-sided tests in clinical research "unless there is a very good reason for doing otherwise." Their statement—"If a new treatment kills a lot of patients we should not simply abandon it; we should ask why this happened"—is clearly a sizable understatement! Their paper prompted Letters to the Editor by R. Wolterbeek and M. W. Enkin in the October issue of that journal, with each expressing a dissenting opinion. This was followed by a response from Bland and Altman, who made the important point that in clinical research there is a definite need to determine why the results were in the opposite direction from what would have been specified in the alternative hypothesis if a one-sided test had been used.

Of course, algorithmic approaches to sample size determination in software and applets do not incorporate ethical considerations, so the reader may want to study the paper by Bacchetti et al. (2005) for ways in which ethical considerations should influence sample size. Similarly, sampling costs are also generally not incorporated in software, so it is up to practitioners to assume the initiative. As Simon (2008) stated: "No one does it this way, but they should." Of course, it would be helpful if software would allow the input of costs, but I am not aware of any statistical software that has ever had this capability, although surely there must be some software, perhaps little known, that allows the user to input costs for determining sample size.

2.9   STANDARDIZATION AND SPECIFICATION OF EFFECT SIZES

Effects are generally given as the difference between the hypothesized value of a parameter and a value that an experimenter wishes to detect with a high probability, standardized in some manner. For example, the difference between the hypothesized value of μ and a detectable value may be standardized by dividing that difference by σ. Let that standardized statistic be represented by d. For the comparison of two means, Cohen (1988) defined "small," "medium," and "large" values of d as .10, .30, and .50, respectively. We will see in later chapters that such designation will generally be inappropriate, and the use of these labels has been criticized by Lenth (2001) and others. In particular, note that Lenth (2006–2009) refers to these as "T-shirt effect sizes" and lists this as one of "two very wrong things that people try to do with my software." While admitting that the determination of effect size in ecological studies is difficult due to the paucity of relevant data, Fox, Ben-Haim, Hayes, McCarthy, Wintle, and Dunstan (2007) agree with Lenth (2006–2009) that "T-shirt effect sizes . . . is not the way to resolve this problem." They proposed the use of "info-gap theory," which is intended "to address the 'robustness' of decision making under uncertainty."

Using standardized effects enables a practitioner to avoid thinking about the magnitude of σ, which is not a good idea. Regarding the "shirt sizes approach," Thomas (1997) stated: "These conventions are widely used in psychology and other disciplines, where a medium standardized effect size may correspond with the median effect size found in psychological research (Sedlmeier and Gigerenzer 1989)."

Regarding effect sizes, van Belle (2008, Chap. 2) stated: "Some social science journals insist that all hypotheses be formulated in terms of effect size. This is an unwarranted demand that places research in an unnecessary straight jacket."

Cohen (1988) gave a different set of numbers for other types of hypothesis tests; as indicated in his Section 10.2.2. In general, however, it is unwise to try to associate various degrees of change with specific numbers. How the magnitude of a change would be assessed should certainly depend on what is being measured as well as the field of application.

2.10 EQUIVALENCE TESTS

In this section we introduce sample size determination for equivalence tests and also consider sample size determination for noninferiority and superiority tests, following the introduction and comparison of these different types of tests in Section 1.5.

Equivalence testing was proposed when the objective is to show the "equivalence," appropriately defined, between two population means or proportions. Garrett (1997) stated that "equivalence tests are perhaps the second most useful general class of hypothesis tests after the standard hypothesis testing framework."

The essential difference between traditional hypothesis testing (THT) when two populations are involved and equivalence testing is that in THT the focus is on the null hypothesis, which is often equality ("equivalence"), and seeing if it can be rejected in favor of one method, treatment, and so on being better than the other one, whereas in equivalence testing the objective is to show equivalence, appropriately defined. (Recall that, except in testing distributional assumptions, the null hypothesis is what we doubt to be true.)

In equivalence testing, the form of the equivalence could be stated in either the null hypothesis or the alternative hypothesis, but regardless of how it is set up, we can never "prove" equivalence (nor prove any hypothesis, in general, with sample data), contrary to such wording that is used in the literature, which is really a misnomer. What *can* be done, however, is to determine whether or not there is "essential equivalence" relative to a range of scientific or clinical indifference.

That is, if we take a sample from each of two populations, we don't know if the parameters of interest are either equal or differ by a very tiny amount without the sample being the entire population, so that there would then be no sampling variability.

As discussed by Dixon (1998), much of the statistical development of equivalence testing has been motivated by the regulatory requirement that a newly developed generic drug must be shown to be equivalent to the corresponding name-brand drug. This leads to the consideration of bioequivalence and sample size determination for it (see, e.g., Phillips, 1990). With AUC denoting the plasma concentration time curve and C_{max} denoting the peak concentration, the FDA has considered a test product to be bioequivalent to a standard (reference) product if a 90% confidence interval for the geometric mean ratio of AUC and C_{max} between the test and reference products falls within the interval 80% to 125%. Alternatively, a hypothesis test could be performed using an upper bioequivalence limit of 1.25 and a lower bioequivalence limit of .80.

Equivalence testing has applications beyond drug testing, however, and Dixon (1998) indicated that the general principles can also be used in environmental applications. See also Blackwelder (1998), Diletti, Hauschke, and Steinijans (1992), and Chow and Liu (1999) for biostatistical applications, and see Friede and Kieser (2003) for considerations that should be made when an internal pilot study is used in conjunction with equivalence and noninferiority testing. O'Quigley and Baudoin (1988) is a paper on general approaches to bioequivalence and Zhang (2003) gave a simple formula for sample size calculation in bioequivalence studies. See also Ganju, Izu, and Anemona (2008). Readers interested in the derivation of sample size formulas for equivalence testing as well as for tests of equality, noninferiority, and superiority are referred, in particular, to Chow, Shao, and Wang (2002, 2008). See Pocock (2003) for a discussion of the pros and cons of noninferiority trials.

■ **EXAMPLE 2.2**

To illustrate the computation of sample size for equivalence testing, consider Example 2.1 but now let's assume that a process yield of 105 from a new process that requires less manual attention is "equivalent" to a process yield of (at most) 100. Perhaps the (daily) process yield in excess of 102 could not be easily utilized. That is, there is more or less a target for process yield. The null hypothesis might be set up so that the difference is greater than 2, with the alternative hypothesis being that the difference is at most 2. Thus, we would want to reject the null hypothesis.

We will assume, as in Example 2.1, that 3.77 is our estimate of σ and that the power is to be .80, with $\alpha = .05$. The necessary sample size would be computed as follows (see Chow, Shao, and Wang, 2008, p. 57), using a normal approximation approach.

$$n = \frac{(Z_{\alpha/2} + Z_\beta)^2 \sigma^2}{\delta^2}$$

with δ denoting the equivalence limit, which here is 2. Thus,

$$n = \frac{(1.645 + 0.84)^2 (3.77)^2}{(2)^2} = 21.94$$

so that $n = 22$ would be used. Note that this is a one-sample test whereas it was stated earlier in this section that equivalence testing was developed for testing the equivalence of two means or proportions. It can also be used for one-sample problems, as illustrated in this SAS Software documentation (http://support.sas.com/documentation/cdl/en/anlystug/58352/HTML/default/viewer.htm#chap12_sect4.htm). ∎

See also a simple method for sample size determination that was given by Zhang (2003). For additional information on equivalence testing, see Wellek (2010).

2.11 SOFTWARE AND APPLETS

Although sample size determination and power computation formulas are available for hand computation, if desired, it is preferable to use either commercial software or Java applets (i.e., freeware), or a combination of the two. Therefore, in subsequent chapters the formulas are given, where appropriate, but there is also considerable discussion of available software (and their strengths), as well as applets. Sample size determination software and applets vary greatly in terms of overall capabilities. For example, some software offer an option for a continuity correction when a normal approximation is applied to a discrete random variable, whereas other software do not.

Although there is considerable software discussion (and some illustration) in the succeeding chapters, the discussion is limited to a relatively small number of software and a few applets. A broader discussion of software is given by Dattalo (2008), which includes recommendations of which software to use for each type of test that is presented. It is obvious that Dattalo (2008) has a preference for freeware, which is evidenced by the statement (p. 13): "Readers should be aware that, whenever possible, the approach recommended here is to estimate sample size with GPower, which is a free power analysis program."

Certainly freeware and Java applets do have a role to play, especially in education. This is discussed in some detail by Anderson-Cook and Dorai-Raj (2003), who have a link to a nice applet (http://www.amstat.org/publications/jse/v11n3/java/Power/Power3Applet.html) that can be used to see with dynamic graphics the relationship between power and the value specified for the alternative hypothesis for one-sample and two-sample tests of means and proportions. Lenth's applet (http://www.cs.uiowa.edu/~rlenth/Power) is the most popular and best known general purpose applet for sample size determination and power. The Web page http://statpages.org/#Power also has considerable capabilities and note the long list of Web pages at http://www.webstatschecker.com/stats/keyword/sample_size_calculation_power. Applets are great for students and people engaged in self-study who may not have access to software for sample size determination.

Regarding the software PASS that was mentioned in Section 2.1, Dattalo (2008, p. 13) stated: "For researchers who prefer a comprehensive statistical package, PASS is recommended. PASS is capable of providing a wide range of sample size calculations."

In addition to PASS, Power and Precision, nQuery, and SiZ will be discussed and illustrated in subsequent chapters, and there will also be references to other software, including Stata and SAS Software. Users of the latter who want to employ it for sample size determination may want to start with the overview at http://support.sas.com/documentation/cdl/en/statug/63347/HTML/default/viewer.htm#intropss_toc.htm. The sample size determination capabilities of SAS Software are somewhat limited compared to the capabilities of certain software that is solely for sample size determination and power, so users will need to write short SAS Software programs to match those capabilities. There is some discussion of this in subsequent chapters. See http://support.sas.com/documentation/cdl/en/statug/63347/HTML/default/viewer.htm#statug_clientpss_sect002.htm for a list of the sample size and power capabilities of Version 9.22 using the SAS Power and Sample Size (PSS) application, and also see Watson (2008). See also Zhao and Li (2011), who illustrated how to determine sample size using simulations in SAS Software for models that are more complicated than the models that are handled by the POWER procedure in SAS Software.

Stata also has sample size determination, primarily with its sampsi command and also with the stpower command, which computes power and sample size for survival analysis (see Chapter 9). Unlike MINITAB, however, Stata has limited sample size determination capability and does not have a menu mode option, whereas MINITAB does have such an option.

Regarding freeware, probably the best-known and most often used freeware for sample size computations is Lenth's applet (http://www.cs.uiowa.edu/~rlenth/Power/), although Dattalo (2008, p. 13) expresses a preference for G*Power (http://www.psycho.uni-duesseldorf.de/abteilungen/aap/gpower3). See also Faul, Erdfelder, Lang, and Buchner (2007). Users of R may be interested in the code for sample size determination given in Cohen and Cohen (2008).

Although G*Power does have considerable capabilities, especially for freeware, PASS 11 can do much more. In particular, PASS has capability for sample size determination in quality control; such capability is not available in any other software. This is discussed further in Chapter 8.

2.12 SUMMARY

Determining sample size will generally be difficult because of the necessity of having to specify values for unknown parameters, such as σ, or having to specify the change that an experimenter wishes to detect in standard deviation units when it is more natural for an experimenter to think in terms of the unit of measurement. As when any statistical tool is used, the results will be only as good as the assumptions that are made.

These types of problems do not render sample size determination useless, but experimenters should keep in mind that the specified power used in sample size determination is not going to be the actual power that a study has. (There is always uncertainty in statistics because random variables are involved.)

REFERENCES

Adcock, C. J. (1988). A Bayesian approach to calculating sample sizes. *The Statistician*, **37**, 433–439.

Adcock, C. J. (1997). Sample size determination: A review. *The Statistician*, **46**(2), 261–283.

Altman, D. (1980). Statistics and ethics in medical research, III: How large a sample. *British Medical Journal*, **281**, 1336–1338.

Anderson, K. M. (2006). Adaptive designs. Sample size-reestmation: A review and recommendations. Slide presentation in the FDA/Industry Statistics Workshop, PhRMA Adaptive Designs Working Group, Philadelphia, October 27. (www.amstatphilly.org/events/fall/2006/KeavenSSR.ppt)

Anderson-Cook, C. M. and S. Dorai-Raj (2003). Making the concepts of power and sample size relevant and accessible to students in introductory statistics using applets. *Journal of Statistics Education*, **11** (electronic journal).

Ariola, M. M. (2006). *Principles and Methods of Research*. Manila, Phillipines: Rex Book Store, Inc.

Bacchetti, P. (2010). Current sample size conventions: Flaws, harms, and alternatives. *BMC Medicine,* **8**, 17. Rejoinder: Good intentions versus CONSORT's actual effect.

Bacchetti, P., S. G. Deeks, and J. M. McCune (2011). Breaking free of sample size dogma to perform innovative translational research. *Science Translational Medicine,* **3**(87), 24.

Bacchetti, P., C. E. McCulloch, and M. R. Segal (2008). Simple, defensible sample sizes based on cost efficiency. *Biometrics,* **64**, 577–585.

Bacchetti, P., L. E. Wolf, M. R. Segal, and C. E. McCulloch (2005). Ethics and sample size. *American Journal of Epidemiology,* **161**(2), 105–110. Discussion: pp. 111–113.

Berg, N. (2006). A simple Bayesian procedure for sample size determination in an audit of property value appraisals. *Real Estate Economics,* **34**, 133–155.

Betensky, R. A. and C. Tierney (1997). An examination of methods for sample size recalculation during an experiment. *Statistics in Medicine,* **16**(22), 2587–2598.

Binkett, M. A. and S. J. Day (1994). Internal pilot studies for estimating sample size. *Statistics in Medicine,* **13**, 2455–2463.

Blackwelder, W. C. (1998). Equivalence Trials. In *Encyclopedia of Biostatistics,* Vol. 2. New York: Wiley, pp. 1367–1372.

Bland, J. M. (2009). The tyranny of power: Is there a better way to calculate sample size? *British Medical Journal,* **339**, 1133–1135.

Bland, J. M. and D. G. Altman (1994). One- and two-sided tests of significance. *British Medical Journal,* **309**, 248. Response as Letters to the Editor by R. Wolterbeen and M. W. Enkin, with response by Bland and Altman, **309**, 873–874. (This is free to registered users; see http://www.bmj.eom/cgi/content/full/309/6958/873/a.)

Boos, D. D. and J. M. Hughes-Oliver (2000). How large does n have to be for Z and t intervals? *The American Statistician,* **54**(2), 121–128.

Bristol, D. R. (1989). Sample sizes for constructing confidence intervals and testing hypotheses. *Statistics in Medicine,* **8**, 803–811.

Browne, R. H. (1995). On the use of a pilot sample for sample size determination. *Statistics in Medicine,* **14**, 1933–1940.

Brush, G. G. (1988). *How to Choose the Proper Sample Size.* Volume 12: The ASQC Basic References in Quality Control: Statistical Techniques (J. A. Cornell and S. S. Shapiro, eds.). Milwaukee, WI: American Society for Quality Control.

Chalmers, T. C., H. Levin, H. S. Sacks, D. Reitman, J. Berrier, and R. Nagalingham (1987). Meta-analysis of clinical trials as a scientific discipline, I: Control of bias and comparison with large co-operative trials. *Statistics in Medicine,* **6**, 315–328.

Chow, S. C. and J. P. Liu (1999). *Design and Analysis of Bioavailability and Bioequivalence Studies.* New York: Marcel Dekker.

Chow, S.-C, J. Shao, and H. Wang (2002). A note on sample size calculations for mean comparisons based on noncentral t-statistics. *Journal of Biopharmaceutical Statistics,* **12**, 441–456.

Chow, S.-C, J. Shao, and H. Wang (2008). *Sample Size Calculations in Clinical Research,* 2nd edition. Boca Raton, FL: Chapman and Hall/CRC.

Coffey, C. S. and K. E. Muller (1999). Exact test size and power of a Gaussian error linear model for an internal pilot study. *Statistics in Medicine,* **18**(1), 1199–1214.

Coffey, C. S. and K. E. Muller (2001). Controlling test size while gaining the benefits of an internal pilot study. *Biometrics,* **57**, 625–631.

Cohen, J. (1988). *Statistical Power Analysis for the Behavioral Sciences*, 2nd edition. Mahwah, NJ: Lawrence Erlbaum.

Cohen, Y. and J. Y. Cohen (2008). *Statistics and Data with R: An Applied Approach Through Examples*. Hoboken, NJ: Wiley.

Dattalo, P. (2008). *Determining Sample Size: Balancing Power, Precision, and Practicality*. New York: Oxford University Press.

Day, S. (2000). Operational difficulties with internal pilot studies to update sample size. *Drug Information Journal*, **34**, 461–468.

De Santis, F. (2004). Statistical evidence and sample size determination for Bayesian hypothesis testing. *Journal of Statistical Planning and Inference*, **124**(1), 121–144.

De Santis, F. (2006). Sample size determination for robust Bayesian analysis. *Journal of the American Statistical Association*, **101**(473), 278–291.

De Santis, F. (2007). Using historical data for Bayesian sample size determination. *Journal of the Royal Statistical Society, Series A: Statistics in Society*, **170**, 95–113.

Dendukuri, N., E. Rahme, P. Bélisle, and L. Joseph (2004). Bayesian sample size determination for prevalence and diagnostic test studies in the absence of a gold standard test. *Biometrics*, **60**, 388–397. (Note that software is available for the methodology in the paper; see http://www.medicine.mcgill.ca/epidemiology/joseph/Bayesian-Software-Bayesian-Sample-Size.html and see on that page other software available corresponding to other papers.)

Denne, J. S. and C. Jennison (1999). Estimating the sample size for a *t*-test using an internal pilot. *Statistics in Medicine*, **18**(13), 1575–1585.

Diletti, E., D. Hauschke, and V. W. Steinijans (1992). Sample size determination for bioequivalence assessment by means of confidence intervals. *International Journal of Clinical Pharmacology, Therapy, and Toxicology*, **30**, 1–8.

Dixon, P. M. (1998). Assessing effect and no effect with equivalence tests.Chapter 12 in *Risk Assessment: Logic and Measurement* (M. C. Newman and C. L. Strojan, eds.). Ann Arbor, MI: Ann Arbor Press.

Dudewicz, E. J. (1972). Confidence intervals for power with special reference to medical trials. *Australian Journal of Statistics*, **14**, 211–216.

Faul, F., E. Erdfelder, A.-G. Lang, and A. Buchner (2007). G*Power 3: A flexible statistical power analysis program for the social, behavioral, and biomedical sciences. *Behavior Research Methods*, **39**(2), 175–191.

Fox, D. R., Y. Ben-Haim, K. R. Hayes, M. A. McCarthy, B. Wintle, and P. Dunstan (2007). An info-gap approach to power and sample size calculations. *EnvironMetrics*, **18**, 189–203.

Freiman, J. A., T. C. Chalmers, H. Smith, Jr., and R. R. Kuebler (1978). The importance of beta, the type II error and sample design in the design and interpretation of the randomized control trial: Survey of 71 "negative" trials. *New England Journal of Medicine*, **299**, 690–694.

Friede, T. and M. Kieser (2003). Blinded sample size reassessment in non-inferiority and equivalence trials. *Statistics in Medicine*, **22**, 995–1007.

Ganju, J., A. Izu, and A. Anemona (2008). Sample size for equivalence trials: A case study from a vaccine lot consistency trial. *Statistics in Medicine*, **27** (19), 3743–3754; Discussion, **28**, 175–179.

Garrett, K. A. (1997). Use of statistical tests of equivalence (bioequivalence tests) in plant pathology (Letter to the Editor). *Phytopathology*, **87**(4), 372–374.

Gauch, H. G. Jr. (2006). Winning the accuracy game. *American Scientist*, **94**(2), 133–141.

Glick, H. A. (2011a). Sample size and power for cost-effectiveness analysis (part 1). *Pharmacoeconomics*, **29**(3), 189–198.

Glick, H. A. (2011b). Sample size and power for cost-effectiveness analysis (part 2): The effect of maximum willingness to pay. *Pharmacoeconomics*, **29**(4), 287–296.

Goldstein, M. (1981). A Bayesian criterion for sample size. *Annals of Statistics*, **9**, 670–672.

Greenland, S. (1987). On sample-size and power calculations for studies using confidence intervals. *American Journal of Epidemiology*, **128**(1), 231–237.

Guenther, W. C. (1965). *Concepts of Statistical Inference*. New York: McGraw-Hill.

Guo, J. H., H. J. Chen, and W. M. Luh (2011). Sample size planning with the cost constraint for testing superiority and equivalence of two independent groups. *The British Journal of Mathematical and Statistical Psychology*, **64**(3), 439–461.

Gustafson, P. (2006). Sample size implications when biases are modelled rather than ignored. *Journal of the Royal Statistical Society, Series A: Statistics in Society*, **169**, 865–881.

Halpern, S. D., J. H. T. Karlawish, and J. A. Berlin (2002). The continuing unethical conduct of underpowered clinical trials. *Journal of the American Medical Association*, **288**, 358–362.

Halpern, S. D., J. H. T. Karlawish, and J. A. Berlin (2005). Comment on "Ethics, and sample size" by Bacchetti, Wolf, Segal, et al. *American Journal of Epidemiology*, **162**, 195–196.

Hare, L. B. (2008). Statistics Roundtable: There is no such thing as parity. *Quality Progress* (January), 78–79.

Inoue L. Y. T., D. A. Berry, and G. Parmigiani (2005). Relationship between Bayesian and frequentist sample size determination. *The American Statistician*, **59**(1), 79–87.

Jiroutek, M.R., K. E. Muller, L. L. Kupper, and P. W. Stewart (2003). A new method for choosing sample size for confidence interval-based inferences. *Biometrics*, **59**, 580–590.

Joseph, L. and P. Bélisle (1997). Bayesian sample size determination for normal means and differences between normal means. *The Statistician*, **46**(2), 209–226.

Joseph, L., R. du Berger, and P. Bélisle (1997). Bayesian and mixed Bayesian/likelihood criteria for sample size determination. *Statistics in Medicine*, **16**, 769–781.

Julious, S. A. (2010). *Sample Sizes for Clinical Trials*. Boca Raton, FL: Chapman and Hall/CRC.

Kieser, M. and T. Friede (2000). Re-calculating the sample size in internal pilot study designs with control of the type I error rate. *Statistics in Medicine*, **19**, 901–911.

Knottnerus, J. A. and L. M. Bouter (2001). The ethics of sample size: Two-sided testing and one-sided thinking. *Journal of Clinical Epidemiology*, **54**, 109–110.

Kraemer, H. C, J. Mintz, A. Noda, J. Tinklenberg, and Y. A. Yesavage (2006). Caution regarding the use of pilot studies to guide power calculations for study proposals. *Archives of General Psychiatry*, **63**, 484–489.

Kupper, L. L. and K. B. Hafner (1989). How appropriate are popular sample size formulas? *The American Statistician*, **43**(2), 101–105.

Lancaster, G. A., S. Dodd, and P. R. Williamson (2004). Design and analysis of pilot studies: Recommendations for good practice. *Journal of Evaluation in Clinical Practice*, **10**(2), 307–312.

Lautoche, A. and R. Porcher (2007). Sample size calculations in the presence of competing risks. *Statistics in Medicine*, **26**, 5370–5380.

Lenth, R. V. (2001). Some practical guidelines for effective sample size determination. *The American Statistician*, **55**(3), 187–193.

Lenth, R. V. (2006–2009). Java applets for power and sample size (computer software). (Available at http://www.cs.uiowa.edu/~rlenth/Power.)

Lindley, D. V. (1997). The choice of sample size. *The Statistician*, **46**(2), 129–138.

Lohr, S. L. (1999). *Sampling: Design and Analysis*. North Scituate, MA: Duxbury.

Machin, D. and M. J. Campbell (2005). *The Design of Studies for Medical Research*. Hoboken, NJ: Wiley.

Matthews, J. N. S. (1995). Small clinical trials—are they all bad? *Statistics in Medicine*, **14**, 115–126.

Maxwell, S. E. (2004). The persistence of underpowered studies in psychological research: Causes, consequences, and remedies. *Psychological Methods*, **9**(2), 147–163.

Maxwell, S. E., K. Kelley, and J. R. Rausch (2008). Sample size planning for statistical power and accuracy in parameter estimation. *Annual Review of Psychology*, **59**, 537–563.

Moyé, L. A. and A. T. N. Tita (2002). Defending the rational for the two-tailed test in clinical research. *Circulation*, **105**, 3062–3065. (Available at http://circ.aha journals.org/cgi/content/full/105/25/3062.)

Noordzij, M., F. W. Dekker, C. Zoccali, and K. J. Jager (2011). Sample size calculations. *Nephron Clinical Practice*, **118**, 319–323.

O'Quigley, J. and C. Baudoin (1988). General approaches to the problem of bioequivalence. *The Statistician*, **37**, 51–58.

Parker, R. A. and N. G. Berman (2003). Sample size: More than calculations. *The American Statistician*, **57**(3), 166–170.

Pezeshk, H. (2003). Bayesian techniques for sample size determination in clinical trials: A review. *Statistical Methods in Medical Research*, **12**, 489–504.

Pezeshk, H, N. Nematollahi, V. Maroufy, and J. Gittins (2009). The choice of sample size: A mixed Bayesian/frequentist approach. *Statistical Methods in Medical Research*, **18**, 183–194.

Pham-Gia, T. and A. Bekker (2005). Sample size determination using Bayesian decision criteria under absolute value loss function. *American Journal of Mathematical and Management Sciences*, **25**(3/4), 259–291.

Phillips, K. F. (1990). Power of two-one-sided tests procedure in bioequivalence.*Journal of Pharmacokinetics and Biopharmaceutics*, **18**(2), 137–144.

Pocock, S. J. (2003). The pros and cons of noninferiority trials. *Fundamental and Clinical Pharmacology*, **17**, 483–490.

Posch, M. and P. Bauer (2000). Interim analysis and sample size reassessment. *Biometrics*, **56**, 1170–1176.

Rahardja, D. and Y. D. Zhao (2009). Unified sample size calculations using the competing probability. *Statistics in Biopharmaceutical Research*, **1**(3), 323–327.

Ryan, T. P. (2011). *Statistical Methods for Quality Improvement*, 3rd edition. Hoboken, NJ: Wiley.

Sahu, S. K. and T. M. F. Smith (2006). A Bayesian method of sample size determination with practical applications. *Journal of the Royal Statistical Society, Series A: Statistics in Society*, **169**, 235–253.

Schulz, K. F. and D. A. Grimes (2005). Sample size calculations in randomised trials: Mandatory and mystical. *Lancet*, **365**, 1348–1353.

Schulz, K., D. Moher, and D. G. Altman (2010). A fundamental misinterpretation of CONSORT. Comment on Bacchetti (2010). *BMC Medicine*, **8** (online journal; http://www.biomedcentral.eom/1741-7015/8/17/comments#414700).

Sedlmeier, P. and G. Gigerenzer (1989). Do studies of statistical power have an effect on the power of studies? *Psychological Bulletin*, **105**, 309–316.

Shao, J. and S.-C. Chow (2002). Reproducibility probability in clinical trials.*Statistics in Medicine*, **21**(12), 1727–1742.

Shih, W. J. (2001). Sample size re-estimation — journey for a decade. *Statistics in Medicine*, **20**, 515–518.

Simon, S. (2008). Too much power and precision? (Web page: http://www.pmean .com/08/TooMuchPower.html.)

Sims, M., D. A. Elston, M. P. Harris, and S. Wanless (2007). Incorporating variance uncertainty into a power analysis of monitoring designs. *Journal of Agricultural, Biological, and Environmental Statistics*, **12**(2), 236–249.

Stein, C. (1945). A two-sample test for a linear hypothesis whose power is independent of the variance. *Annals of Mathematical Statistics*, **24**, 243–258.

Strug, L. J., C. A. Rohde, and P. N. Corey (2007). An introduction to evidential sample size calculations. *The American Statistician*, **61**, 207–212.

Stüger, H. P. (2006). Asymmetric loss functions and sample size determination: A Bayesian approach. *Austrian Journal of Statistics*, **35**, 57–66.

Sutton, A. J., N. J. Cooper, D. R. Jones, P. C. Lambert, J. R. Thompson, and K. R. Abrams (2007). Evidence-based sample size calculations based upon updated meta-analysis. *Statistics in Medicine*, **26**, 2479–2500.

Taylor, D. J. and K. E. Muller (1995). Computing confidence bounds for power and sample size of the general linear model. *The American Statistician*, **49**(1), 43–47.

Thomas, S. (1999). Retrospective power analysis. *Conservation Biology*, **11**, 276–280.

van Belle, G. (2008). *Statistical Rules of Thumb*, 2nd edition. Hoboken, NJ: Wiley.

Vickens, A. J. (2003). Underpowering in randomized trials reporting a sample size calculation. *Journal of Clinical Epidemiology*, **56**, 719–720.

Walker, S. G. (2003). How many samples? A Bayesian nonparametric approach. *The Statistician*, **52**, 475–482.

Wang, F. and A. E. Gelfand (2002). A simulation-based approach to Bayesian sample size determination for performance under a given model and for separating models. *Statistical Science*, **17**(2), 193–208.

Wang, J. and J. D. Stamey (2010). A Bayesian algorithm for sample size determination for equivalence and non-inferiority test. *Journal of Applied Statistics*, **37**, 1749–1759.

Watson, W. (2008). Updates to SAS power and sample size software in SAS/STAT 9.2. Paper 368-2008.

Webb, R. Y., P. J. Smith and A. Firag (2010). On the probability of improved accuracy with increased sample size. *The American Statistician*, **64**, 257–262.

Weiss, R. (1997). Bayesian sample size calculations for hypothesis testing. *The Statistician*, **46**(2), 185–191.

Wellek, S. (2010). *Testing Statistical Hypotheses of Equivalence and Noninferiority*, 2nd editon. Boca Raton, FL: CRC Press.

Wilburn, A. J. (1984). *Practical Statistical Sampling for Auditors*. Boca Raton, FL: CRC Press.

Wittes, J. and E. Brittain (1990). The role of internal pilot studies in increasing the efficiency of clinical trials. *Statistics in Medicine*, **9**, 65–72.

Wittes, J., O. Schabenberger, D. Zucker, E. Brittain, and M. Proschan (1999). Internal pilot studies I: Type 1 error rate of the naive *t*-test. *Statistics in Medicine*, **18**(24), 3481–3491.

Yin, K., P. K. Choudhary, D. Varghese, and S. R. Goodman (2008). A Bayesian approach for sample size determination in method comparison studies. *Statistics in Medicine*, **27**, 2273–2289.

Zhang, P. (2003). A simple formula for sample size determination in equivalence studies. *Journal of Biopharmaceutical Statistics*, **13**(3), 529–538.

Zhao, W. and A. X. Li (2011). Estimating sample size through simulations. PharmaSUG2011, Paper SP08.

Zucker, D. M., J. T. Wittes, O. Schabenberger, and E. Brittain (1999). Internal pilot studies II: Comparison of various procedures. *Statistics in Medicine*, **18**, 3493–3509.

EXERCISES

2.1. Assume a $N(\mu, \sigma^2)$ distribution, with $\mu = \sigma^2 = 16$. Solve for n such that the maximum possible error of estimation of μ is to be 2 with probability .95. Then generate 10,000 samples of size n, with the value of n being what you solved for. What percentage of observations is within 2 units of μ? (Obviously a computer program will have to be written to generate the 10,000 samples and to determine the percentage.) What have you demonstrated?

2.2. Explain how a study could have "too much power." How could this be prevented?

2.3. The following request was (tersely) made on a Web blog some years ago: "Alpha .05, Power 0.8. What is the sample size to detect an outcome difference of .20 versus .30 for an adverse event. Thank you." This was used as a lead-in to the author's mention of websites that will do this type of calculation. If you were a consultant and you received such a request, would you refer the person asking the question to a website or two, or would you react differently? Explain.

2.4. As explained in Section 2.2, there is no reason why designed studies should always focus on a power of .80. There is some dialogue from an episode of the television show *Walker, Texas Ranger* that can be used to dramatize this point. A mobster will soon be on trial and his attorney states: "I've run some simulations and there is an 83% chance that you will be acquitted. I must say those are excellent odds." The mobster then replies: "Oh, really. That's like 5 out of 6, isn't it?" The attorney replies "Yes sir." The mobster then puts a bullet in a gun, points the gun at the attorney and states: "One bullet, one chamber. If I spin the chamber and fire the gun, there is an 83% chance that I won't blow you away. Do you still think those are excellent odds?" The attorney then replies "No sir." Similarly, if you are conducting a study whose results might greatly benefit humankind, do you want to have an 80% chance of making such an important discovery, or would you want the odds to be more in your favor?

2.5. Assume that a study was performed and approximate normality was a reasonable assumption for the population of observations. The standard deviation was unknown but values below 10 or above 70 are rarely observed. Without giving any regard to power, an experimenter insists on using 100 observations and is interested in detecting a five-unit increase in the population mean with probability .90, using a one-tailed test with $\alpha = .05$. What was the power of the test? Would you recommend that the experimenter use a larger or a smaller sample size in a future study involving the same population? Explain your recommendation.

2.6. Explain why the assumed power for a study will almost certainly not be the actual power.

2.7. An experimenter wants to determine the sample size for a 95% confidence interval for μ that will be used to test the null hypothesis that $\mu = 50$ and have a probability of .95 of rejecting the null hypothesis when the true mean exceeds 50 by one standard deviation of the mean. Can this be accomplished? Explain.

2.8. Often the planned sample size will not be the actual sample size because circumstances may prevent the number of subjects being available that was originally proposed (people can drop out of a study, data can be lost, etc.). Assume that the sample size of 75 was determined to provide a power of .90 but a sample size of only 68 subjects could be used. Does this automatically mean that the *actual* power of the study was less than .90? Explain.

2.9. If some of the participants in a study subsequently withdraw, will the power of the study increase or decrease? Explain.

2.10. If, after a study has been initiated, a scientist decides that it is more important to detect a smaller effect than the effect stated when the sample size for the study was computed, if that sample size is used and everything else remains the same, will the power for detecting this smaller effect be larger or smaller than the power that was originally specified? Explain.

2.11. Assume that a sample size was determined for an upper one-tailed test but there was a miscommunication and the test to be used will actually be a lower one-sided test, with the difference to be detected from the hypothesized mean being the same in absolute value as it would have been if the upper one-tailed test had been used. If nothing else changes, will it be necessary to recompute the sample size or will it be the same? Explain.

CHAPTER 3

Means and Variances

In this chapter we consider power and sample size determination for a mean for a single population and means for two populations, for both independent and dependent samples, and also cover sample size for testing a single variance and for testing the equality of two variances. We also briefly discuss the case of more than two means, with this covered fully in Chapter 6 in the context of experimental designs.

The emphasis in this chapter and in subsequent chapters is on hypothesis testing because that is what is emphasized in the literature and in software. Sample size determination for confidence intervals is also covered since it is also important and has been covered in the literature in articles such as those by Kelley and Rausch (2006), Jiroutek, Muller, Kupper, and Stewart (2003), Bristol (1989), and Beal (1989). See also Grieve (1991), who examined the suggestion of Beal (1989).

It is highly desirable for researchers to indicate how they obtained the sample sizes that they used in their studies because various assumptions must be made in the calculation of sample sizes, including parameter values, which will almost always be unknown. Nevertheless, Nayak (2010) cited the study of Moher, Dulberg, and Wells (1994), who found that sample size calculations were given in only 32% of studies that did *not* result in statistical significance. This could have occurred in some studies because the study was underpowered and/or unrealistic assumptions were made, such as bad inputs for parameter values. The reader of research articles needs enough information to be able to determine if the study was not well designed, so both the sample size and the manner in which it was determined should be provided in research articles.

Sample Size Determination and Power, First Edition. Thomas P. Ryan.
© 2013 John Wiley & Sons, Inc. Published 2013 by John Wiley & Sons, Inc.

3.1   ONE MEAN, NORMALITY, AND KNOWN STANDARD DEVIATION

Example 2.1 was used partly to show how one could obtain an initial estimate of σ, which is necessary for sample size determination and power computation, without obtaining the estimate from sample data, such as in a pilot study, although the desirability of using an internal pilot study was emphasized in Chapter 2. (Note that software is available to aid in the planning of pilot studies, including Lenth's applet, as was discussed and illustrated in Section 2.1.)

In this section, we discuss designing a study for testing a single mean in more detail than was given in Example 2.1. The expression for n was given in that example for a one-sided hypothesis test. The general expression given in Eq. (2.3) for a one-sided test is

$$n = \left[\frac{(Z_\alpha + Z_\beta)\sigma}{\mu - \mu_0} \right]^2 \tag{3.1}$$

which, among other things, shows that a sample size necessary to detect a small departure from μ_0 requires, for fixed α, β, and σ, a larger sample size than when the departure is not small. For a fixed difference, $\mu - \mu_0$, with μ_0 denoting the hypothesized mean and μ denoting the mean value that one wishes to detect with the stated power, the sample size is increased if either α or β is decreased, or if σ is increased. This should be intuitive because decreasing β means that the power, $1 - \beta$, is increased, and a more powerful test requires, other things being equal, an increased sample size. Although the power or n can be changed and the other one will also change in the same direction, α is chosen independently of n and β. In "modern" hypothesis testing, α might not be specified before the data are collected and analyzed; instead, a decision would be reached based on the magnitude of the p-value. A benchmark value for the p-value must be used, however, because the experimenter must decide if the p-value is small enough to reject the null hypothesis. That decision is certainly going to depend on the field of application and the type of study that has been conducted.

In general, the smaller the value of α, the less area under the curve for the actual distribution will lie in the rejection region, as can be seen from Figure 3.1.

Therefore, decreasing α (i.e., increasing Z_α) will decrease power (increase β, which will decrease Z_β). These changes will be somewhat offsetting in Eq. (3.1). Consequently, sample size is most straightforwardly viewed as being most strongly influenced by the difference between the parameter value that an experimenter wishes to detect and the hypothesized parameter value. (Of course, σ will also have an effect on the sample size and it will also strongly affect the power for a given sample size if a bad estimate of σ is used as input.)

The expression for n is slightly more involved when a two-sided test is used, which would be used if the experimenter simply wanted to detect a difference

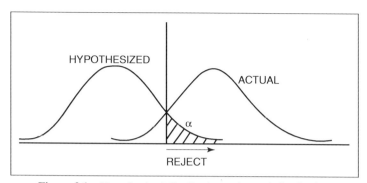

Figure 3.1 Hypothesized distribution and actual distribution.

from the hypothesized parameter value, without having a preconceived notion of the direction of the departure.

As an approximation that should usually work reasonably well (which of course would be unnecessary if software were used), we could simply replace Z_α by $Z_{\alpha/2}$ in Eq. (3.1). If we did so, we would be acting as if the test was actually a one-sided test using a significance level of $\alpha/2$ rather than a two-sided test with significance level α. Although this might seem improper, we need to take a commonsense approach to determining sample size and computing power for a two-sided test. Specifically, if the true value of a population parameter is greater than the hypothesized value, should the information about the assumed distribution on the side opposite the true value have any influence on sample size determination and power? For example, assume that $\mu_0 = 50$ and $\mu = 51$. If there is a small difference between the hypothesized value and the true value, relative to σ, a value of the sample mean below 50 could result, and the value of the test statistic could be negative and fall in the rejection region on the low (opposite) end. Should that possibility influence sample size determination? It should probably not because if, say, the sample mean were 48 and the value of the test statistic was in the rejection region, we would not logically conclude that the mean was some value in excess of 50. We would simply conclude that the mean was not 50. When we calculate power, however, we can't calculate it for something like "not 50"; we have to specify a value. Therefore, one could argue that it is logical to simply replace Z_α by $Z_{\alpha/2}$ in Eq. (3.1) and use that expression to solve for the sample size. We will see later that this will often give the correct result, although it is not necessarily recommended as a routine procedure. Of course, we should also keep in mind that we are "approximating" anyway because σ is never known. (See the discussion in Section 3.2 of a way to address the problem of σ being unknown.)

Note: For the examples that follow in this chapter and throughout the remainder of the book, it is important to recognize the difference between *assumed power* and *actual power*, as well as *target power*, as used by some software. The assumed power is what the power would be (i.e., the actual power) if the true values for all "nuisance parameters" (such as sigma when sample size is being determined for testing a population mean) are equal to the values that are entered into software. Since this will hardly ever happen, we should think of the assumed power as almost always incorrect and not equal to the actual power. Certain software, such as MINITAB, will show "target power" and "actual power" in juxtaposition in output when a discrete random variable is involved, as then there is a difference between target power and assumed power since target power cannot be achieved, in general, even if nuisance parameter values were known, because of jumps in cumulative probabilities between successive possible values of the random variable. Thus, for example, the assumed power might jump from .884 to .918 and bypass .900. Such output labeling is actually incorrect because what is being called actual power in the output is really retrospective power, and as explained in Section 1.4, it doesn't make any sense to use that term.

■ EXAMPLE 3.1

To illustrate the use of Eq. (3.1) and its modification, we will assume $\alpha = .05$, power $= .80$, $\sigma = 3$, $\mu_0 = 50$, and $\mu = 52$. For a one-sided test, Eq. (3.1) applies directly and we obtain $n = 13.91$, so $n = 14$ would be used. When software such as PASS, Power and Precision, or MINITAB is used, $n = 14$ results with actual power of .802.

As implied in Section 2.5 and by Parker and Berman (2003), the user may be interested in more than a specific difference $(\mu - \mu_0)$ and the corresponding power, so the power curve in Figure 3.2, produced by MINITAB, can be useful.

We generally won't be able to hit the desired power exactly simply because sample size is, of course, discrete, so there will be jumps in the power value per unit change in the sample size, and the power will not generally be a round number. Here the power is slightly greater than .80 because 14 is slightly greater than 13.91. Curiously, Power and Precision gives the two-sided confidence interval when the user specifies that sample size is to be determined for a one-sided hypothesis test. (The confidence interval limits are computed using the entered value of σ and value of μ specified in the alternative hypothesis. That is, assumed parameter values are used, which is not the way that orthodox confidence intervals are constructed.)

For a two-sided test, substituting $Z_{\alpha/2}$ for Z_α in Eq. (3.1) results in $n = 17.66$. When software such as MINITAB or Power and Precision is used, $n = 18$ results with actual power of .807. The corresponding power curve then contains the portion shown in Figure 3.2 plus the mirror image of that curve, with the full curve symmetric about 0.   ■

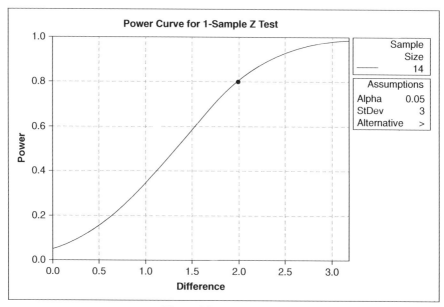

Figure 3.2   Power curve.

It was stated in Section 3.1 that using either .95 or .99 for power could, depending on the value of the standard error, require such a large sample size as to be impractical. For example, if the desired power in Example 3.1 had been .95 or .99 instead of .80, the necessary sample size would have been 25 for power of .95 (actually .9543), and 36 for power of .99. Although the latter sample size is not large, it is almost three times the sample size that is needed for a power of .80.

Although there is agreement between the use of

$$n = \left[\frac{(Z_{\alpha/2} + Z_\beta)\sigma}{\mu - \mu_0} \right]^2 \tag{3.2}$$

for a two-sided test and the result obtained using software for this example, that won't always be the case. We can see what is happening if we consider the expression that is used as the starting point in solving for n in the two-sided case:

$$1 - \Phi\left(Z_{\alpha/2} + \frac{\mu_0 - \mu}{\sigma/\sqrt{n}}\right) + \Phi\left(-Z_{\alpha/2} + \frac{\mu_0 - \mu}{\sigma/\sqrt{n}}\right) = 1 - \beta \tag{3.3}$$

which is derived in the chapter Appendix. The first two terms on the left side are the same as those used in deriving the sample size for an upper one-sided test, except that Z_α is used instead of $Z_{\alpha/2}$ (with the third term, using Z_α, used for a lower one-sided test), so if the third term is essentially zero for the computed sample size, then the third term is not having any effect on the determination of the sample size. If the third term is not very close to zero, however, as could happen if μ_0 was greater than μ, and the difference was small such that the sum of the first two terms in Eq. (3.3) is not approximately zero, then Eq. (3.2) will only approximate the sample size. Since a closed-form expression for n cannot be obtained because Φ^{-1} is not a linear operator, the use of software is highly desirable. [Of course, Eq. (3.3) is easy to solve numerically for n.]

In general, Eq. (3.2) would give a sample size that is off slightly whenever $(\mu_0 - \mu)/(\sigma/\sqrt{n})$ is small because then neither the third term nor the sum of the first two terms in Eq. (3.1) would be close to zero. Fortunately, however, the fraction really can't be very small because a large value of n is needed to detect a small difference $(\mu_0 - \mu)$, and if n is large, the denominator of the fraction will be small. Of course, the fraction could be small if σ is quite large, but we would expect the difference $(\mu_0 - \mu)$ to be related to σ, such as perhaps being equal to σ. So these effects would be offsetting.

To illustrate, if $\mu = 50.8$, Eq. (3.2) gives $n = 111$, which agrees with the result obtained using software including MINITAB, Power and Precision, and PASS if we select the "variance known" option of Power and Precision and the "known standard deviation" option of PASS so that a z-test is assumed, with such specification unnecessary using MINITAB since the 1-sample Z routine assumes a known standard deviation. (Note that such an option is not available with Lenth's applet, as it assumes the use of a t-test. This results in $n = 113$, so the difference is only slight, and it can be shown that the difference is also slight, and virtually constant, for similar values of $|\mu_0 - \mu|$.)

Similarly, if $\mu = 50.6$, $n = 197$ by Eq. (3.2) and by MINITAB, PASS, and Power and Precision. In the first case, $(\mu_0 - \mu)/(\sigma/\sqrt{n}) = 2.80951$ (using $n = 111$) and 2.821 in the second case—almost the same. Even when $\mu = 50.2$, so that $n = 1766$, the ratio is 2.802, which differs very little from the other two values. Of course, we would expect the fraction to be essentially constant at about 2.8 because the first term is essentially 1.0 when the fraction is about 2.8, since $\Phi(4.76) \approx 1$ and thus

$$1 - \Phi\left(Z_{\alpha/2} + \frac{\mu_0 - \mu}{\sigma/\sqrt{n}}\right)$$

is not going to make a contribution to the desired power value of .80, and $\Phi(-1.96 + 2.8) = \Phi(.84) = .80$.

In essence, a huge sample size shrinks the distribution of $\bar{X}$ so much that there is hardly any spread of values. The area under the curve for the distribution with assumed mean $= 50.1$ that is in the nonrejection region for the distribution with the hypothesized mean is .20, as can be seen in Figure 3.3. Therefore, the power is .80.

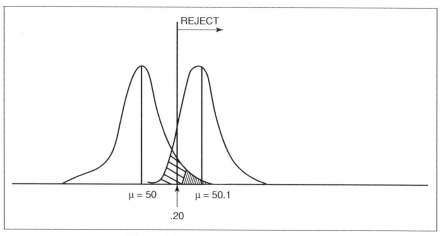

Figure 3.3 Effect of huge sample size.

Using software to obtain sample sizes renders unnecessary the need for simple approximations, unless a user does not have access to software or does not want to use formulas that might be viewed as complicated. Van Belle (2008, Chapter 2) gave a simplified formula for the one-sample case and a two-sided hypothesis test, which is $n = 8/\Delta^2$, with $\Delta = [(\mu - \mu_0)/\sigma]^2$, with μ denoting the true population mean and μ_0 denoting the hypothesized mean value. This will provide a reasonable approximation only if $\alpha = .05$ and power $= .80$, however, as then the two Z-values in Eq. (3.2) are 1.96 and 0.8416, respectively, the sum of which is 2.8016 and the square of that sum is 7.85—close to 8.0. Since a user would generally not be interested in detecting a small difference from the hypothesized value, Δ^2 probably won't be very small, so the approximation will usually be reasonably good. If a user preferred to have power $\geq .90$, however, the approximation would likely be poor since $(1.96 + 1.28)^2 = 10.50$ for power $= .90$. Thus, the approximation could be applied only when the test is two-sided with $\alpha = .05$ and power $= .80$ for detecting the effect size Δ.

■ **EXAMPLE 3.2**

In illustrating applications in orthodontics, Newcombe (2001) focused attention on determining sample size so as to give a confidence interval for a population mean with a specified width. (Recall the discussion of this in Section 2.4.) The objective was to estimate the mean toothbrushing force before the attachment of an orthodontic appliance. Newcombe (2001) used as an estimate of σ the sample standard deviation from a similar study described by Heasman, MacGregor, Wilson, and Kelly (1998). That study, which had an objective of determining whether or not toothbrushing forces were affected by wearing fixed orthodontic appliances, had a sample standard deviation of 124, with 30 children (10 males and 20 females, ages 10–15) used in the study.

There are some questions that should have been addressed regarding the use of that estimate of σ, one of which would seem to be the spread of the ages of children for the study in Newcombe (2001) relative to the spread of the ages of the children in the Heasman et al. (1998) study, as this would probably be related to the standard deviation. This issue was not addressed by Newcombe (2001), however. The use of a standard deviation from a study performed by different investigators is potentially shaky regarding the comparability of the two sets of subjects. When comparability cannot be assessed, it seems almost imperative to use the upper limit of a confidence interval for σ rather than using simply the standard deviation from the other study.

Indeed, using the upper limit of an 80% confidence interval has been proposed in the literature, as Browne (1995) showed by the use of simulations that using a $100(1 - \alpha)\%$ upper one-sided confidence limit on σ will provide a sample size that is sufficient to achieve the desired power $100(1 - \alpha)\%$ of the time. This idea is discussed further in Section 3.3. Kieser and Wassmer (1996) provided some analytical insights into Browne's proposal.

We can see how this would affect the sample size for the Newcombe (2001) study. No distributional assumption was made for the latter although approximate normality was tacitly assumed by the assumption that a 95% confidence interval for the mean is approximately $\bar{x} \pm 2\hat{\sigma}/\sqrt{n}$ when n is large. The initial objective was to select n so that $2\hat{\sigma}/\sqrt{n} = 30$ (i.e., the confidence interval width would be 60). Solving for n produces $n = (2\hat{\sigma}/30)^2 = [2(124)/30]^2 = 68.34$, so $n = 68$ or 69 could be used. Newcombe (2001) used $n = 68$ and since the multiplier "2" is being used as an approximation (instead of, say, 1.96), there is not strong motivation for rounding up, as is done in hypothesis testing.

If we assume normality, following Browne (1995), we could use at least an 80% one-sided upper confidence bound for σ. Since a standard deviation is being used from a study performed by different investigators and the two sets of subjects may differ in important ways, a 95% upper confidence bound may be preferable. The upper bound is obtained as

$$\hat{\sigma}\sqrt{\frac{n - 1}{\chi^2_{1-\alpha, n-1}}} = 124\sqrt{\frac{29}{17.7084}} = 158.68$$

Using the latter in place of 124 produces a sample size of $[2(158.68)/30]^2 = 111.9$, so $n = 112$ would be used. This would be a much safer, albeit also more costly, sample size.

Newcombe (2001) stated that it might be decided that a confidence interval of $\bar{x} \pm 30$ could be deemed too wide to be informative. If 30 is replaced by 15, however, the required sample size will be four times the original sample size, which we can see without doing any calculations since $15 = 30/2$ and the 2 will be squared in performing the computation. Newcombe (2001) indicated that this would require a sample size of 273, whereas using the upper confidence bound for σ would result in a sample size of 448. Both 448 and 273 may be impractical or even impossible for the new study, however. At the very least, the cost would be greatly increased.

Could software be used for this problem to determine sample size? The answer is "yes" although slightly fewer options exist since software for sample size determination emphasizes hypothesis tests with less attention devoted to confidence intervals. PASS is one software that can be used for this problem and it does have moderately extensive capability for confidence intervals. The user would select "Confidence intervals" from the main menu and then select "Means." It is necessary to enter .9544 for the confidence level since that corresponds to the 2σ limits used by Newcombe (2001). Doing so and entering 30 for the "Distance from Mean to Limits," then checking "Known Standard Deviation," indicating a two-sided interval and entering 124 for σ results in a sample size of 69, in general agreement with the hand computation result of 68.34. Similarly, using 158.68 as the upper bound estimate of σ results in $n = 112$, in agreement with the hand computation result of 111.9. These results are also obtained using nQuery, which has overall confidence interval capabilities similar to that of PASS.

These results can also be produced using MINITAB (Release 16 or later). Specifically, the user selects "Power and Sample Size" from the main menu, then selects "Sample Size for Estimation" and then "Mean (Normal)" from the options that are available. Then entering 124 for the standard deviation, 30 for the margin of error, indicating that the standard deviation is known, and specifying 95.44 for the degree of confidence produces $n = 69$. Similarly, when 158.68 is used for the assumed known value of σ, $n = 112$ is produced, with both of these results in agreement with the results given by PASS and nQuery. Finally, with Lenth's software it is not possible to specify a 95.44% confidence interval so the user would have to settle for a 95% confidence interval. Entering the same inputs as when the other software was used produces $n = 68.06$ and $n = 109.9$, respectively, for the two inputted values of σ. Thus, there are some small differences, especially for the larger inputted value of σ, which is due to the fact that the degree of confidence is not matched exactly. ∎

3.1.1 Using the Coefficient of Variation

Van Belle and Martin (1993) pointed out that the information provided by a consulting client will often be in terms of the percentage change expected from a treatment, the percentage change that would be clinically significant, and the "percentage variability" in the data. Of course, the latter is rather vague but the authors stated that this can be a lead-in to estimating a coefficient of variation (*CV*). (The population *CV* is defined as μ/σ and the sample *CV* defined as $\bar{X}/s$.) Furthermore, the client may be interested in a percentage change in the mean.

Van Belle (2008, p. 34) pointed out that we can define a percentage change using either the current mean or the mean to be detected in the denominator, which of course is obvious. Van Belle uses the average of the two means in the denominator, however, and defines the percentage change, PC, as

$$PC = \frac{\mu_0 - \mu_1}{\mu}$$

and then, apparently assuming $\alpha = .05$ and power $= .80$, states that the sample size is "estimated remarkably accurately" by

$$n = \frac{16(CV)^2}{(PC)^2}$$

Since a coefficient of variation of 35% is apparently quite common in biological systems (van Belle, 2008, p. 34), a rule-of-thumb for the sample size in such applications is then

$$n = \frac{2}{(PC)^2}$$

since $16(0.35)^2 = 1.96$.

I am not aware of any software that can be used for sample size determination when the value of a coefficient of variation is used as input, so hand computation is apparently necessary. As should be apparent, the computation is quite simple, especially if the van Belle rule-of-thumb is used. It should be kept in mind, however, that this is indeed just a simple rule-of-thumb.

3.2   ONE MEAN, STANDARD DEVIATION UNKNOWN, NORMALITY ASSUMED

When σ is unknown (the usual scenario), the sample size formula for n is, as we logically expect, obtained by substituting $t_{\alpha, n-1}$ for Z_α in Eq. (3.1) and substituting $t_{\beta, n-1}$ for Z_β. Of course, this does not produce a simple expression that can be used to solve for n directly since the two t-variates are each a function of n. Thus, n must be solved for using iteration. We can, however, assuming a one-sided test and $\hat{\sigma}$ being some estimate of σ, use the expression

$$n = \left[\frac{\left(t_{\alpha, n-1} + t_{\beta, n-1}\right)\hat{\sigma}}{\mu - \mu_0} \right]^2 \tag{3.4}$$

to obtain the same value of n that is obtained using software, thus illustrating the formula computation.

To illustrate, assume that $\alpha = .05$, power $= .80$, $\hat{\sigma} = 3$, $\mu_0 = 50$, and $\mu = 52$, and the test is one-sided. If we assume that $\sigma = 3$ and use Eq. (3.1), we obtain $n = 13.91$, so $n = 14$ would be used. We would expect a slightly larger value of n to result from the assumption that σ is unknown. Although we can't use Eq. (3.4) to solve for n directly, we can use it to verify the solution obtained from software. That solution is $n = 16$, which gives a power value of .8156. Thus, when we use $n = 16$ in Eq. (3.4), we would expect to obtain a solution that is closer to 15 than 16 since the power for $n = 15$ is .7908. That is what happens as the computed value is 15.44.

Thus, the assumption of an unknown σ has resulted in a sample size that is two units larger. In both cases, however, we had to input a value of σ, thus showing the artificiality of the computation for the case of σ unknown. Early work on sample size determination for t-tests included Guenther (1981).

3.3 CONFIDENCE INTERVALS ON POWER AND/OR SAMPLE SIZE

Confidence intervals on power are not generally computed and are not available in sample size determination software. The potential usefulness of such an interval should be apparent, however, since it is important to recognize that power is rarely known because it partially depends on σ, which is unknown and must be estimated. Such estimation, however it is performed, causes the assumed power to actually be estimated power and to be a random variable if the estimate is obtained using historical data, which might be data from a pilot study.

For a one-sample t-test, we would expect, for a fixed sample size and significance level, the width of a confidence interval on power to be directly related to the width of a confidence interval on σ, if such an interval were constructed. Under the assumption of normality of the individual observations, a $100(1-\alpha)\%$ confidence interval for σ is given by

$$\text{Lower Limit: } s\sqrt{\frac{n-1}{\chi^2_{a/2,\,n-1}}} \qquad \text{Upper Limit: } s\sqrt{\frac{n-1}{\chi^2_{1-a/2,\,n-1}}}$$

(Note that subscripts on χ^2 are typically written, as is done here, such that $\alpha/2$ designates the cumulative area, not the area in the right tail.) Thus, the width depends on the sample size and the value of the estimate of σ, which in turn would logically be related to the magnitude of σ.

Dudewicz (1972) suggested substituting exact confidence bounds for $\hat{\sigma}$ into the power calculations for a t-test. This would have the effect of producing approximate confidence limits on the power of the test and would be more realistic. Of course, this could easily be performed with software as the endpoints of the interval could be entered, in turn, in the t-test routine, fixing the value of n at perhaps the value that resulted from the use of a point estimate of σ.

The limits would be only approximate because the general form of the limits is based on the assumption that σ is known. Substituting a value for σ into an expression developed for σ known is not the same as using the appropriate expression constructed under the assumption that σ is unknown and is being estimated. Therefore, it is highly desirable to determine the worth of the approximate limits. Dudewicz (1972), however, did not, as indicated by Taylor and Muller (1995), note that this was only an approximate approach and thus did not provide any asymptotic or simulation results indicating the extent to which these limits can be expected to deviate from the correct limits, and apparently this has not been investigated to any extent.

Recognizing the need to numerically investigate the Dudewicz approach, Taylor and Muller (1995) used simulation to examine the method for one-way analysis of variance and found that the results support use of the method, which were in general agreement with the asymptotic result given by Clark (1987) that the method provides asymptotically unbiased confidence intervals for power. They recommended that a one-sided (lower) confidence bound be used for power since there is generally interest in having power at least equal to a target value. They also recommended an upper confidence bound on the sample size and gave the methodology for obtaining the upper bound, which requires the iterative solution of two equations. They also proposed the use of simultaneous confidence bounds for power and sample size and suggested the use of graphs that show exact confidence limits on power.

■ **EXAMPLE 3.3**

Taylor and Muller (1995) illustrated their methodology by applying it to a research problem involving deteriorating renal function that was addressed by Falk, Hogan, Muller, and Jeannette (1992). The latter defined a clinically significant improvement in renal function as a doubling of reciprocal serum creatinine level. Thirteen patients were randomly assigned to each treatment in a clinical trial and the use of a variance estimate of 0.68 resulted in a power estimate of .92. Taylor and Muller (1995) addressed the uncertainty in that number and obtained a 95% confidence interval on power as [.688, .999]. Of course, that is a very wide interval, with the upper limit being overkill and the lower limit being a value that most researchers would probably consider unacceptable. They stated that increasing the number of patients assigned to each treatment from 13 to 17.95 (i.e., 18) would ensure with probability .975 a lower bound on power of .90. Thus, for this study, the actual power may have been much lower than the assumed power, so an increase in the number of patients assigned to each group would have been desirable. If there was a considerable per-patient cost involved, the researchers might have settled for 16 or 17 patients per group since they might have been willing to accept a lower bound on power of slightly less than .90, but the need for providing researchers with such a confidence bound should be obvious. ■

In related and more recent work, Wong (2010) explained how to obtain a confidence interval on the power of the one-sample t-test, with the alternative hypothesis presumed to be $\mu = \mu_0 + k\sigma$, with μ_0 denoting the mean under the null hypothesis. Sample size could also be determined as a by-product, but this would require an iterative solution. Consequently, it is not likely to be used by practitioners unless it is incorporated into the software most frequently used for sample size determination. (The authors did state that R code is available on request.)

As stated by Wong (2010), Lehmann (1959) proved that the probability of committing a Type II error for a one-sided, one-sample t-test with significance level α is given by

$$\beta = G_{n-1, k\sqrt{n}}(t_{n-1,1-\alpha}) \tag{3.5}$$

with $G_{v, a}(\cdot)$ denoting the cumulative distribution function of the noncentral t-distribution with v degrees of freedom, noncentrality parameter, a, and $k = (\mu - \mu_0)/\sigma$. Of course, n is unknown but could be solved for numerically using Eq. (3.5) for a selected value of power $= 1 - \beta$ and thus β.

Certainly σ is also generally unknown and would have to be estimated unless one wishes to bypass that issue by specifying a value for k, which represents the effect size. If that approach were taken, a point estimate of power and a confidence interval for it could be computed before data are obtained, thus avoiding the type of criticism that has been leveled at retrospective power, but incurring the type of criticism that Lenth (2001) stated for dealing directly with effect sizes.

Deviating from the methodology given by Wong (2010), let's assume that this was not done, but rather that σ was estimated using prior information and *then* the effect size was computed. Similarly, we will specify upper and lower bounds on σ (without data), and we will need to specify a tentative sample size for the confidence interval on power. (Of course, σ might be estimated from data in a small pilot study; this will be illustrated later.)

Unfortunately, such methods are not available in sample size determination software and it seems unlikely that they will be available in the foreseeable future.

In general, it would be desirable for the methodology advocated by Dudewicz (1972) to be extended to other types of tests, with simulation results, preferably, or at least asymptotic results indicating how well the method performs. This has apparently not been discussed in the literature, however, but the extension would be reasonably straightforward when only a single parameter had to be estimated, such as in simple linear regression when testing the slope parameter, as a confidence interval for σ^2_{error} would be needed, although a value for the spread of the regressor values would also be required. At the other extreme, it would be very complex and perhaps even intractable when confidence bounds (or a joint confidence region) must be developed for handling multiple unknown parameters, as when an entire variance–covariance matrix must be estimated. Consequently, what some discerning readers might call a naive approach of substituting values for unknown parameters will continue to be used throughout this book because that is simply all that is available—both in the literature and in software, although of course software could be used with confidence limits on σ^2 simply by using the appropriate routine twice, using the lower limit and then the upper limit on σ^2.

If there is any faith at all in the value of σ that is inputted for use with the t-statistic, then the t-statistic should not necessarily be used, as that utilizes the sample standard deviation, computed after the sample has been taken. Assuming normality, the sample standard deviation is biased, with the amount of bias a function of the sample size, as is Var(s). If E(s) is approximately equal to the value of σ that is inputted and software gives a large value of n, then using the t-statistic approach is not particularly bad, but we would nevertheless generally use a z-statistic if we strongly believe that we have an excellent estimate of σ that is inputted. Remember that there is very little difference between the values of t-variates and the corresponding z-variates for large sample sizes.

3.4 ONE MEAN, STANDARD DEVIATION UNKNOWN, NONNORMALITY ASSUMED

The t-test for a single mean is not undermined by slight-to-moderate nonnormality. However, when there is considerable nonnormality, a t-test should not be used. Assumptions are tested with data, but if an experimenter is at the stage of trying to determine the sample size, the data have not yet been obtained. So there is a problem unless data are available from a prior study. Subject matter knowledge might at least suggest the general shape of the distribution, and that knowledge might be used along with a book on distributions that shows the shape of each distribution for various combinations of parameter values. Evans, Hastings, Peacock, and Forbes (2010) is one such book.

For example, a t-distribution has heavier tails than a normal distribution, and the difference will be considerable for a t-distribution with a small number of degrees of freedom. So if the individual values have approximately such a distribution rather than a normal distribution, the values of α, power, and sample size will be off considerably from what they should be under the assumption of normality.

Mahnken (2009) discussed the determination of power and sample size when the distribution is unknown and provided a quasi-likelihood approach for use when the variance as a function of the mean is known, or at least can be assumed. Of course, such sample size determination cannot be done exactly and the proposed methodology is based on asymptotic properties. Consequently, the estimates of sample size and power could be poor for small study designs, except, as the author points out, when the underlying distribution is normal.

3.5 ONE MEAN, EXPONENTIAL DISTRIBUTION

PASS has a routine for testing the mean of an exponential distribution and is the only major sample size determination software package that has this feature. It is perhaps also the only software or applet of any type with this capability. The exponential distribution has only one parameter, θ which is the mean of the distribution, so the null hypothesis would be a stated value of θ and the objective would be to determine the sample size for detecting a different value of θ that is considered important to detect.

To illustrate, let $\theta_0 = 2$ and $\theta_1 = 3$, with desired power of .90 and $\alpha = .05$ for a one-sided test. PASS gives various test criteria, including specifying a threshold value for $\hat{\theta}$, which is just the sample mean. The algorithm uses the theoretical result that $2n\bar{X}/\theta_0 \sim \chi^2_{2n}$ (Epstein, 1960), with "$\sim$" read "is distributed as," followed by the statistical distribution. It follows that $\bar{X} \sim (\theta_0/2n)\, \chi^2_{2n}$. This result will be used in allowing us to see the threshold value. The software gives $n = 51$. With $2n = 102$, $\chi^2_{102,.05} = 126.74$, and $\theta_0/2n = 2/102 = 1/51$, it follows that $(\theta_0/2n)\, \chi^2_{2n,.05} = 126.74/51 = 2.48$, and the software gives 2.5. Thus, $\theta_0 = 2$ is rejected when $\theta_1 = 3$ using the reject criterion of $\hat{\theta} > 2.5$, with sampling without replacement and a fixed duration time of at least 12 time units, such that the study is terminated when that time has been reached. (By comparison, if the study duration time had been one unit, the necessary sample size would have been $n = 156$.)

3.6 TWO MEANS, KNOWN STANDARD DEVIATIONS—INDEPENDENT SAMPLES

As is the case for other tests covered in this chapter, there is an incongruity with some software in testing for the equality of two means with independent samples, as standard deviations of the two populations must be entered into software, but if the standard deviations were known, then the appropriate test would be the two-sample z-test, not the independent-sample t-test that some software assumes.

There are also some other problems with certain software, as when an independent-sample t-test is selected from the menu for the Power and Precision software but when the "variance is known" option is selected, the software indicates the selection with the message "z-test for two independent samples with common variance" at the top of the screen. There is no such test as it isn't necessary for the two variances to be equal when the z-test is used.

Initially, it is not possible to enter two different values for σ_1 and σ_2 with that software, although it is possible to override it.

The form of the test statistic when Z is used is

$$Z = \frac{(\bar{x}_1 - \bar{x}_2) - (\mu_1 - \mu_2)}{\sqrt{\dfrac{\sigma_1^2}{n_1} + \dfrac{\sigma_2^2}{n_2}}}$$

with $\mu_1 - \mu_2$ usually equal to zero under the null hypothesis. For a one-sided test, assuming the use of $n_1 = n_2 = n$, the expression for n derived in the chapter Appendix, is

$$n = \frac{\left(\sigma_1^2 + \sigma_2^2\right) \left(Z_\alpha + Z_\beta\right)^2}{(\Delta - \Delta_0)^2} \tag{3.6}$$

with Δ denoting the difference, $\mu_1 - \mu_2$, that one wishes to detect, and Δ_0 is the difference under the null hypothesis, with Δ_0 usually but not necessarily being zero. For a two-sided test, Z_α is replaced by $Z_{\alpha/2}$. Although this simple formula modification will generally work, it won't necessarily work for the same reason that it won't work in the one-sample case, as discussed in Section 3.1.

For example, assume that $\sigma_1 = \sigma_2 = 1$, a two-sided test of $H_0: \mu_1 = \mu_2$ is to be performed with $\alpha = .05$, power $= .80$, and $\Delta = 1$. The computed value of n is 15.7, so $n = 16$ would be used for each sample size. This is the same solution that is obtained using PASS. If a one-sided test were used, with the same value of α and everything else also the same, then $n = 13$ for each group, which is what PASS gives. (Note that no solution is produced if the PASS user inadvertently selects the wrong side for the one-sided test, which would correspond to $\Delta = -1$ in this example.)

In this "variances known" case, we would hope that σ_1^2 and σ_2^2 are each estimated from a very large amount of data, which would justify the use of Z instead of t.

Simplified formulas are often given to industrial personnel to minimize the statistical expertise that is needed by the user. Kohavi and Longbotham (2001) gave the sample size formula

$$n = \frac{16\sigma^2}{\Delta^2} \tag{3.7}$$

for a t-test against a control, with σ^2 denoting the variance of the "overall evaluation criterion," and 16 is the number chosen to give power of .80, with $\alpha = .05$.

There is no indication how the 16 is obtained, however, and also no mention of a significance level. The authors indicated that replacing 16 by 21 will increase the power to .90. Again, no explanation, but the article reflects an obvious attempt to avoid technical details and give a simplified presentation. We can verify the 16 and 21 numbers if we let $\sigma_1^2 = \sigma_2^2 = \sigma^2$ in Eq. (3.6) and replace Z_α by $Z_{\alpha/2}$ for a two-sided test. Then the constants are 15.68, which would round to 16, and 21.015, which would round to 21. The latter is calculated as $(1^2 + 1^2)(1.95996 + 1.28155)^2 = 21.0148$. (The calculation of 15.68 is shown later.) This formula was indicated by Kohavi, Longbotham, Sommerfield, and Henne (2009) as being from van Belle (2008), who gave it as a rule-of-thumb that can be found in Chapter 2.

Kohavi et al. (2009) also mentioned the "more conservative" portable power formula of Wheeler (1974), which is $n = (4 \, r\sigma/\Delta)^2$, with r denoting, in general, the number of levels of a factor in experimental design, so $r = 2$ here because there are two populations involved. Wheeler (1974) assumed the use of $\alpha = .05$ and power $= .90$, presumably for a two-sided test, although Wheeler did not indicate whether it is for a one-sided test or a two-sided test. It is obvious that Wheeler intended the power to be used in experimental design since there is only a single standard deviation symbol in the formula, whereas there are two such terms in Eq. (3.6). The following quote from Wheeler (1974, p. 193) is rather illuminating.

> We do not, however, think it always desirable to use the precise formulas because 1) their precision is in part illusionary due to poorly known parameter values, and 2) their richness produces client-consulting dialogues which are counter-productive: e.g., should the power be 0.90, 0.95, or 0.99?

Undoubtedly many statisticians and others would disagree with that position. A counterargument would be that it is preferable to start with the correct sample size expression and then show what the sample size would be for different parameter values. (This is illustrated in Section 3.11.) Furthermore, consultant–client relationships are best when the client has a reasonable knowledge of statistics, or at least a good aptitude for it. (I speak from the position of someone with many years of consulting experience.)

Wheeler's sample size formula was used by Kohavi, Henne, and Sommerfield (2007), with the authors pointing out that the sample size could be overestimated by 25% for large n. (Of course, an approximation error of that magnitude is generally unacceptable.) The formula was also criticized by Bowman and Kastenbaum (1974), which motivated a rejoinder by Wheeler (1975).

The approximation formula given by Lehr (1992) is essentially the same as the one later proposed by Kohavi and Longbotham (2001). The former is $n = 16 \, s^2/d^2$, with s designating an estimate of the standard deviation, and d corresponding to Δ in Eqs. (3.6) and (3.7). As in the explanation of the Kohavi and Longbotham

(2001) formula, the "16" results from the fact that, if we assume $\sigma_1^2 = \sigma_2^2 = \sigma^2$ and assume use of a two-sided test with $\alpha = .05$ and power $= .80$, $2(1.96 + 0.84)^2 = 15.68$, with $Z_{\alpha/2} = 1.96$ and $Z_{.20} = 0.84$. So 15.68 is rounded to 16.

Thus, the approximation formula of Lehr (1992) can essentially be justified, but the Wheeler (1974) formula cannot be justified if it is used for a test of the equality of two means, as the constant is then 64 [obtained from $(4*2)^2$], which is much too large.

It is worth noting that although the use of these approximation formulas does simplify matters for scientists, they won't necessarily be satisfied with power of .80, nor should they be. So simplification does have a price.

3.6.1 Unequal Sample Sizes

Although equal sample sizes would be used in most applications, in some applications it might not be possible or practical to do so. Consider the example given in Section 3.6 but this time we won't assume that $n_1 = n_2 = n$. If two distinct sample sizes are to be used, a relationship must be specified since they can't be solved for individually, which wouldn't make any sense. We will enter $n_2 / n_1 = 1.4$, and see how that affects the results. When PASS is used, the sample sizes obtained are 14 and 20 and the power is given as .8185. To obtain this solution in Power and Precision it is necessary to "link" the sample sizes. Accessing the option "N-cases" and then entering 10 and 14, respectively (so that the ratio is 1.4), in "Enter cases in ratio," results in the same solution as given by PASS. (Neither nQuery nor Lenth's applet has a procedure for testing two means with known standard deviations.)

It is worth noting the discussion in Campbell, Julious, and Altman (1995), who pointed out that if the sample size is computed under the assumption that $n_1 = n_2$ will be used but an unequal allocation is actually used, there will be a loss of power. They stated that the loss in power is only about 5% if the allocation ratio is actually 2:1, but drops off considerably beyond that point, with the loss being about 25% if the ratio is 5:1.

3.7 TWO MEANS, UNKNOWN BUT EQUAL STANDARD DEVIATIONS—INDEPENDENT SAMPLES

Technically, this case actually cannot be handled because power has to be computed with all necessary parameter values specified, including σ_1 and σ_2. If either they are not known or values are not assumed for them, then power cannot be computed. (Of course, parameter values are generally unknown, whether we assume known values for the purpose of determining sample sizes or not.)

When software is used, however, such as Power and Precision, one of the options is "t-test for independent samples with common variance." A standard deviation must be entered for one of the populations, with the standard deviations linked so that the same standard deviation is used for the other population, as required for the test. The sample sizes are also linked, so that the use of equal sample sizes is assumed. There is an obvious problem with doing this because if the standard deviations were known, a z-test would be used rather than a t-test, but sample size cannot be computed without specifying the standard deviations. Of course, the same thing happens with other software but PASS does allow the user to specify a range of values for the standard deviations with the output showing what the sample size would be for each value of $\sigma = \sigma_1 = \sigma_2$. (This would have to be done manually in Power and Precision, after the user has specified the increment size for σ. nQuery does not have the capability for providing results for multiple values of σ without the user having to enter each value individually and then running the program.)

Using multiple values of σ is somewhat more realistic than specifying a single value of $\sigma = \sigma_1 = \sigma_2$ and using the sample size that the software gives since the software is determining the sample size for the t-test that is based on the assumption that the common standard deviation is unknown. This option is available in SAS Software for this test. As shown in the documentation at `http://supp ort.sas.com/documentation/cdl/en/statug/63347/HTML/default/ viewer.htm#statug_power_a0000000970.htm`, there is the wording "you conjecture two scenarios for the common group standard deviation." This is the type of wording that is preferable for all sample size determination software that determines sample size under the assumption that a t-test will be used.

To see the effect of assuming the use of a t-test rather than the z-test that was assumed for the example that was used at the beginning of Section 3.6, let's return to that example. The objective was to detect a difference of one in the population means, with $\alpha = .05$, power $= .80$, and $\sigma_1 = \sigma_2 = 1$ for a two-sided test. The common sample size that was obtained was 16. For the t-test, the sample size that is obtained is 17, so there is a very slight increase in the sample size.

Of course, the assumptions that underlie the t-test should be met approximately before the test is used. This is another motivation for the use of an internal pilot study because the data from such a study could be used to test those assumptions. Should the assumptions appear to not be approximately met, the experimenter could then pursue a new direction, such as determining the sample size for the corresponding nonparametric test. Rasch, Kubinger, and Moder (2011) contended, however, that the assumptions should *not* be tested as doing so on the same data that will be used for the test alters the Type I and Type II errors in an unknown way. Instead, they recommended routinely using the Welch (nonparametric) test.

That is not a strong reason to avoid testing the assumptions, however, especially since the amount of contamination is unknown but would likely be slight, especially if an internal pilot study was less than half of the total study.

3.7.1 Unequal Sample Sizes

Although equal sample sizes are generally desirable, that isn't always possible or practical, as illustrated by the following example.

■ EXAMPLE 3.4

Newcombe (2001) referred to a study by Heasman et al. (1998) in which they found that the mean toothbrushing force at baseline was 220 grams for boys and 181 grams for girls. Motivated somewhat by this study, Newcombe (2001) stated: "Suppose we decided that in a new study, we want an 80 percent power to detect a difference of 30 grams as statistically significant at the 5 percent level. Based on the existing study, it seems reasonable to assume a SD of 130g. Suppose that, as in the published study, we expect to recruit twice as many girls as boys."

The anticipated difference in sample sizes can easily be handled by most sample size determination software. Using PASS and assuming a common standard deviation of 130, $\alpha = .05$ for a two-sided test, desired power = .80, an expected difference of 30 grams, and a 2:1 ratio for sample sizes, PASS gives 223 and 446 for the two sample sizes with power = .8017, whereas both nQuery and Power and Precision give 222 and 444 for the sample sizes. When these sample sizes are entered in nQuery, the latter displays power = .8004. The power value given by Power and Precision is almost identical, as the output shows power = .8005. (MINITAB does not have a two-sample Z-test and does not permit unequal sample sizes in solving for sample size with its two-sample t-test.)

Newcombe (2001) used a rather crude approach to arrive at 221 and 442 for the two sample sizes, which used an initial guess for the sample sizes (obtaining 100 and 200), computing the value of the t-statistic if those sample sizes had been used (1.88), then multiplying the 100 and 200 by $(2.80/1.88)^2$ Although not explained in the article, the $2.80 = 1.96 + 0.84 = Z_{\alpha/2} + Z_{\beta}$—a large-sample approximation since the use of a t-test is being assumed, not a Z-test. Actually, Newcombe (2001) should have given the smaller sample size as 222 instead of 221 since the computed value is 221.077 and the sample size is always rounded up to the next integer. The 223 given by PASS is due to the search procedure employed by PASS, which ensures that the power is at least equal to the desired power. With 222 and 444 as the sample sizes, PASS gives the power as .79994, which of course is essentially .80, although technically it is less than .80. The power jumps to .8017 for sample sizes of 223 and 446. Thus, we can think of either pair of sample sizes as being "correct."

The bottom line is that the two-stage approach of Newcombe (2001) does work, although it is unnecessary now and also then since software can be used to obtain the sample sizes with less effort. Of course, we might question why a two-sided test was being assumed since the example was motivated by a study that showed results in a particular direction.

Other software that can be used when it is desired to use unequal sample sizes includes PASS, which gives the same solution as nQuery. The latter does not give the actual power in its sample size determination output, but the power can be obtained after the sample sizes are determined by entering those sample sizes in addition to the other required input. Doing so results in nQuery giving the power as .8195. This differs slightly from the power given by PASS, which is .8185. Power and Precision does not permit the direct determination of the sample sizes unless n_2/n_1 is a specified ratio. The user can manipulate the two sample sizes individually, however, and see what effect that has on power. Specifying $n_1 = 15$ and $n_2 = 21$ gives .8195 for the power, in agreement with nQuery. Lenth's applet gives the same value for power for this combination of sample sizes. ∎

3.8 TWO MEANS, UNEQUAL VARIANCES AND SAMPLE SIZES—INDEPENDENT SAMPLES

Schouten (1999) proposed a method for determining sample sizes in testing the equality of two means for unequal variances and unequal sample sizes that the experimenter wishes to use. Such a method will often be needed because unequal sample sizes exacerbate the effect of unequal variances. The sample size formula is

$$n_2 = (Z_{\alpha/2} + Z_\beta)^2 \frac{(\tau + \gamma)\sigma_2^2}{\gamma(\mu_2 - \mu_1)} + \frac{(\tau^2 + \gamma^3)Z_{\alpha/2}^2}{2\gamma(\tau + \tau)^2}$$

$$n_1 = \gamma n_2$$

$$n = n_2 + n_1$$

with γ denoting the ratio of the sample size from population 1 to the sample size from population 2, τ is the ratio of the population 1 variance to the population 2 variance, and σ_2^2 is the population 2 variance. Note that Z is used, which means that approximate normality is assumed. The need for a method such as given by Schouten (1999) is not as great when the sample sizes are equal, although Schouten's method might still be used.

3.9 TWO MEANS, UNKNOWN AND UNEQUAL STANDARD DEVIATIONS—INDEPENDENT SAMPLES

The obvious question is: "If we assume that the standard deviations are unknown, how do we know that they are unequal?" The answer to this apparent conundrum is that the assumption of unknown standard deviations (which technically is always the case, regardless of what we assume) results in the t-test being used by software, but the hypothesis of equality of the variances should be tested, as illustrated in Section 3.11.

3.10   TWO MEANS, KNOWN AND UNKNOWN STANDARD DEVIATIONS—DEPENDENT SAMPLES

Even though computationally the sample from each of two populations is collapsed into a single set of differences between each pair when the data are paired, the sample size to be used and the power associated with the selected sample size should logically depend on the variability of the data in each of the populations and the correlation between the random variables being used for each of the two populations.

This can be seen by examining the denominator of the test statistic. For simplicity, we will initially assume that the two populations each have a normal distribution and that the population standard deviations are known. We will let d_i represent the ith difference in a set of n paired differences. The test statistic is then

$$Z = \frac{\bar{d}}{\sigma_d}$$

If we let the observations from the first population be represented by y_1 and the observations from the second population be represented by y_2, then $d = y_1 - y_2$ and $\sigma_d = \sigma_{y_1 - y_2}$. Since

$$\sigma_{y_1-y_2} = \sqrt{\sigma_{y_1}^2 + \sigma_{y_2}^2 - 2\sigma_{y_1 y_2}} = \sqrt{\sigma_{y_1}^2 + \sigma_{y_2}^2 - 2\rho_{y_1 y_2}\sigma_{y_1}\sigma_{y_2}}$$

with $\sigma_{y_1 y_2}$ and $\rho_{y_1 y_2}$ denoting the covariance and correlation, respectively, between y_1 and y_2, it is obvious that the variability of each population and the correlation between the two random variables will influence the power of the test since they determine the denominator of the test statistic.

We can see this more formally if we derive the sample size expression, proceeding analogous to what was done for a one-sample mean. That is, we will assume that the null hypothesis is $\mu_d = 0$ and that the alternative hypothesis is $\mu_d = \mu^* > 0$. Then, still assuming known values for the population variances, covariance, and correlation, the development of the expression for n would have been exactly the same as the development in Example 2.1, resulting in Eq. (2.3), so that will not be repeated here. The end result is

$$n = \left[\frac{(Z_\alpha + Z_\beta)\sigma_d}{\mu_d} \right]^2$$

■ **EXAMPLE 3.5**

To illustrate, let's assume that the data are paired because the same people are going to be used for "before" and "after" readings, with "after" perhaps being readings after some type of treatment program. With $d = y_1 - y_2$ and the null hypothesis being that $\mu_d = 0$, assume that we wish to detect $\mu_d = 1$. We will let $\alpha = .05$, assume that the alternative hypothesis is $\mu_d > 0$, and use the customary .80 as the selected power value. We will also assume $\sigma_{y_1} = \sigma_{y_2} = 5$ and $\rho_{y_1 y_2} = .80$. Then $\sigma_d = \sqrt{25 + 25 - 2(.80)(25)} = \sqrt{10} = 3.162$. Thus,

$$n = \left[\frac{(1.645 + 0.84)\sqrt{10}}{1} \right]^2 = 61.75 \text{ (round to 62)}$$

■

When PASS is used, the user must input the 3.162 for the standard deviation and check "known standard deviation." When this is done, the output gives $n = 62$, in agreement with the above calculation. When the standard deviation is not assumed to be known, PASS gives the sample size as 64. (MINITAB does not give an option regarding the standard deviation being known or not and simply gives the sample size as 64.) The larger sample size is due to the fact that t would be used rather than z. The sample size is thus computed as

$$n = \left[\frac{(t_{\alpha, n-1} + t_{\beta, n-1})\hat{\sigma}_d}{\mu_d} \right]^2$$

$$= \left[\frac{(t_{\alpha, 64-1} + t_{\beta, 64-1})\hat{\sigma}_d}{\mu_d} \right]^2$$

$$= \left[\frac{(1.6694 + 0.847364)\, 3.162}{1} \right]^2$$

$$= 63.33$$

so $n = 64$ would be used. (Of course, here the known solution for n is being used to obtain that solution; this is simply for illustration.)

In this example, the two standard deviations and the correlation were assumed to be known. Generally, they won't be known and will have to be estimated in some manner. For before and after measurements, especially the latter, and for other types of paired data, it may not be possible to estimate standard deviations. An experimenter may have to assume that the "after" variability will be the same as the "before" variability, with any change being only a change in the mean. Depending on the nature of the experiment, this could be a very shaky assumption. Furthermore, how does one estimate the correlation between "before" and "after" when "after" hasn't even occurred? The assumption of only a mean change (at most) and no change in variability implies a correlation of 1.0 between the before and after measurements, which could also be a very shaky assumption. (If the variability does change, then that will be reflected in the variability of the differences when they are formed and the value of the test statistic is computed.)

Thus, some very shaky assumptions could be made when sample size is determined for a paired-t test, which the test would have in common with other statistical methods when sample size is determined.

When variances are assumed to be unknown, software such as Power and Precision, MINITAB (Release 16), and Lenth's applet tacitly assume that the standard deviations and correlation *have been estimated* from the same number of pairs as the algorithm computes, as the sample size is computed as if a paired-t test was being used with the degrees of freedom for the t-statistic being that which results from the computed sample size. For example, for the previous example, the Power and Precision software gave $n = 64$ as the solution for n, as does MINITAB. Similarly, when Lenth's applet is used (for which the user must compute an estimate of σ_d and enter that), the solution is $n = 64$ and the power is given as .8038. It is clear from the menu that the sample size is being computed for a t-test. If we do the hand computation using the "known" value of n to obtain the t-values, we would obtain $n = (1.6694 + 0.847364)^2(10) = 63.34$, so $n = 64$ would be used.

Of course, it is unrealistic to assume that the variances have already been estimated from two paired samples each of size $n = 64$. It would be even more unrealistic to assume that after the experiment has been performed, s_d will be equal to the value that we have assumed for σ_d.

In this example, the difference between $n = 62$ and $n = 64$ is apt to be inconsequential, but strictly speaking, the sample size should be computed based on how the standard deviations and correlation are estimated. If we assume that the difference, d, has a normal distribution and the standard deviations and correlation are estimated (perhaps poorly) without the use of data, the appropriate statistic is Z, not t.

Unfortunately, a "z-test" for paired data, as available in MINITAB and Lenth's applet, doesn't seem to be an option in some software. Although it is not part of the menu and thus might be easily overlooked, the Power and Precision software does have an option for each of its t-tests to convert the test to a z-test with the assumption of known variance(s), just as it does in the one-sample case. For the current example, if the option of a known σ_d is selected and 3.162 is entered for the assumed known value, the software gives $n = 62$, in agreement with the value obtained by hand computation for this example.

For all practical purposes, this distinction between "known" and "unknown" population standard deviations is a superficial one at best because population parameters are never really known. When the standard deviations are assumed unknown, values for them must still be entered for the algorithm to be able to compute sample size. When values must be entered into an algorithm for the purpose of determining the necessary sample size, the parameter values are being guessed, both for the "known" case and the "unknown" case. If such guesses are being made based on, say, a very large amount of data accumulated over time, then a *t*-test would be inappropriate.

In teaching an online sample size determination and power course a few years ago, I encountered a student who was interested in not just a confidence interval on the mean difference for treatment minus control, but also wanted separate confidence intervals for treatment and control. Such analyses are generally not done but under certain conditions separate confidence intervals could provide important information. For example, although no mean value for "control" is assumed when a paired-*t* test is performed, such a value is assumed in determining the sample size to use. Perhaps that assumed value is incorrect/unrealistic. A confidence interval constructed for the mean might just barely contain the assumed mean, which would cast some doubt on the latter. If there is some evidence that the control mean is greater than the assumed control mean, the paired-*t* test might not give a significant result even though a confidence interval for the treatment mean may suggest that the treatment is very beneficial.

A power analysis for a paired-*t* test using SAS can be performed using PROC Power, with the code given and the analysis illustrated at http://www .ats.ucla.edu/stat/sas/dae/t_test_power3.htm.

3.11 BAYESIAN METHODS FOR COMPARING MEANS

There are various articles in the literature on Bayesian methods of sample size determination for testing hypotheses about means. This is a natural consideration because some information regarding population parameters must be used as input when sample sizes are determined using software. Furthermore, it is almost essential to first use a pilot study to obtain some data for parameter estimation, so some type of prior information is essential.

Wang, Chow, and Chen (2005) proposed a very simple Bayesian approach for sample size determination in comparing two means. Since their method was proposed for clinical research, it is discussed in Section 7.8. Joseph and Bèlisle (1997) provided Bayesian sample size determination methods for population means and differences between means for normal distributions.

3.12 ONE VARIANCE OR STANDARD DEVIATION

There is often interest in testing a variance or standard deviation, hoping to see if there has been a reduction since reduced variability is desirable for virtually anything that is measured, especially a process characteristic in manufacturing.

There might seem to be a major problem in trying to test a hypothesis on σ^2 or construct a confidence interval for it, however, because when normality is assumed, $\mathrm{Var}(s^2)$ is a function of σ^4. Thus, a practitioner would seem to need a good estimate of σ or σ^2 in order to determine the sample size.

That isn't the case, however, as can be seen with the following example. Assume that we want to test $H_0: \sigma^2 = 2$ vs. $H_0: \sigma^2 < 2$, using $\alpha = .05$. We want the power to be .90 if $\sigma^2 = 1$. Using PASS, if we enter these numbers, the output has $n = 39$ as the sample size, which gives power $= .90423$. We can verify this as follows. $(n - 1) s^2/\sigma^2$ has a chi-square distribution with $(n - 1)$ degrees of freedom. Let $X = (n - 1) s^2/2$. Then $X \sim \chi^2_{n-1}$. We may show using statistical software $\chi^2_{38, .05} = 24.8839$. Reducing σ^2 to 1 has the effect of doubling the value of X. Since $2X \sim 2\chi^2_{n-1}$, we thus want $P(X < 2\chi^2_{38, .05}) = .90$. It can be shown that $P(X < 2x^2{}_{38, .05} = 2(24.8839) = 49.7678) = .90423$, which is the value that PASS gives for the power.

So the solution can easily be seen and verified as correct, but a straightforward derivation is not possible because the distribution of the test statistic depends on the sample size, which is what we are trying to determine! Consequently, an exact expression for the sample size cannot be obtained and an iterative solution is necessary.

Approximations have been proposed, which might appeal to practitioners who don't have access to sample size determination software and don't need an exact solution for the sample size. Bonett and Al-Sunduqchi (1994) examined the performance of an approximation given by Duncan (1986, p. 401) and found that it worked well only when $\alpha = \beta$. Since values of α greater than .05 are seldom used, and similarly power values of at least .95 are typically not used, this requirement generally will not be met. They gave the following approximation:

$$n = \left(\frac{Z_{\alpha/2} + Z_\beta}{Z_{p1}} \right)^2$$

with $Z_{p1} = (|\ln(\sigma^2) - \ln(k)|)/2^{1/2}$ and $Z_{\alpha/2}$ replaced by Z_α for a one-sided test. Here k denotes the hypothesized value of σ^2, with σ^2 in the expression for Z_{p_1} denoting the actual variance, and $Z_{\alpha/2}$ and Z_β are as defined in Section 2.1. Applying this approximation to the current example (and using Z_α in place of $Z_{\alpha/2}$ since it is a one-sided test), we obtain

$$n = \left(\frac{1.645 + 1.28}{0.4901} \right)^2$$

$$= 35.6$$

so $n = 36$ would be used, differing from the solution of $n = 39$ obtained using PASS. Bonett and Al-Sunduqchi (1994) recommended the sample size obtained with this approximation be averaged with the sample size obtained using the Duncan approximation. The latter is

$$n = \left(\frac{k^{1/2} Z_{\alpha/2} + \sigma Z_\beta}{Z_{p2}} \right)^2$$

with $Z_{p2} = 2^{1/2}| k^{1/2} - \sigma |$. After again replacing $Z_{\alpha/2}$ by Z_α, we obtain a sample size of 37.9, so 38 would be used.

As stated, Bonett and Al-Sunduqchi (1994) recommended averaging the sample size obtained using this approximation with the value obtained using Duncan's approximation. If we average 35.6 and 37.9, we obtain 36.75, so 37 would be used, slightly less than the 39 obtained using PASS. So the recommended approximation is a bit lacking for this example but certainly adequate if only a ballpark figure is needed.

If the objective is to simply estimate a standard deviation as a percentage of its true value, Greenwood and Sandomire (1950) addressed the determination of sample size for this purpose.

3.13 TWO VARIANCES

It is often necessary to test the equality of two variances, as procedures such as the independent-sample t-test assume that the two variances are equal. Therefore, equality of the two variances should be tested before the t-test is used. There are also many scenarios when a t-test will not be used for which it is desirable to test equality of variances, such as when a supposedly improved manufacturing process has been installed and there is a desire to see if this has resulted in more uniform manufactured products being produced (i.e., smaller variance).

Since two variances will hardly ever be equal, there is the obvious question of what departure from equality should the experimenter attempt to detect. If equal sample sizes will be used and normality can be assumed, there can be a moderate difference in two variances without causing any problems with the t-test. Markowski and Markowski (1990) stated: "Specifically, for equal sample sizes, the t test is generally robust and hence no preliminary test is needed. Boneau (1960) reported exceptions to this robustness, such as with one-tailed alternatives when sampling from skewed distributions or with very small significance levels." Thus, if the use of equal sample sizes is planned, most of the time it won't be necessary to test the equality of variances assumption, but it would still be a good idea to try to gain insight into the shape of the distributions for the two populations, as severe nonnormality could create a problem.

Let's assume equal sample sizes and slight-to-moderate nonnormality for the following example. Recognizing that the appropriate sample size will be determined by the ratio of the two variances, not their individual values, let's consider ratios of 3:1, 5:1, 7:1, and 9:1, as in 10 for the first population variance and 30, 50, 70, and 90 for the second population variance. Using $\alpha = .05$ for a two-sided test and desired power of .90, PASS gives the sample sizes from each population as 37, 19, 14, and 11, respectively. This assumes use of an F-test, however, which is very sensitive to departures from normality, as was first noted by George Box, who also noted the t-test is robust to nonnormality. Unfortunately, software developers have generally not provided an option for determining sample size using something other than the F-test, with no option provided by PASS or G*Power, and no test of any kind is available in Power and Precision or nQuery. MINITAB does, however, have Levene's test as an option. The corresponding sample sizes produced by MINITAB when the Levene test option is selected are 46, 25, 19, and 16, respectively, which can be seen to differ considerably from the sample sizes for the F-test under the assumption of normality. It is generally better to use a test of the equality of two variances that does not assume normality. So here it would be wise to be guided by the sample sizes needed for Levene's test. [See Gibbons (2000) for the determination of sample sizes for Levene's test.] Markowski and Markowski (1990) discouraged the use of an F-test even under normality, stating: "However, our study has shown that even when sampling from a normal distribution, the F test is unlikely to detect many situations where the t test should be avoided. In conclusion, we feel the F test is flawed as a preliminary test."

Although a test for equality of variances is typically performed when the two samples are independent, Pitman (1939) proposed a test for equality of variances for paired, normally distributed data that was based on the correlation between the sums and differences within the pairs. Bogle and Hsu (2002) proposed three methods for testing two population variances with paired data and illustrated the method with the highest power in an example involving bilirubin tests.

3.14 MORE THAN TWO VARIANCES

There is often a need to test for the equality of more than two variances, such as when Analysis of Variance (ANOVA) is used with unequal sample sizes. Wludyka, Nelson, and Silva (2001) provided power curves for the Analysis of Means (ANOM) for variances, which, as they stated, can be helpful in determining sample size when ANOM for Variances is used to test for homogeneity of variances. Table B.5 and Appendix A in Nelson, Wludyka, and Copeland (2005) can also be used for determining sample size and corresponding power.

3.15 CONFIDENCE INTERVALS

Determining sample size for a confidence interval for a single mean was discussed in detail and illustrated in Section 2.4, and also illustrated in Example 3.2. Since most sample size determination software is focused primarily on hypothesis tests, there is slightly less software to choose from for determining sample size for confidence intervals, as indicated previously. MINITAB does have that capability, however, as does PASS.

To illustrate, in Section 2.4 the sample size was determined for a 95% confidence interval for μ, assuming $\sigma = 2$, and E (the maximum error of estimation) $= 1$. Both hand computation and the use of PASS resulted in $n = 16$. When MINITAB is used and the same information is inputted, $n = 16$ is the output. Since σ is unknown, it is a good idea to input multiple values of σ and see what n is for each value. So for this example 1.5, 2.0, and 2.5 might be used and when this is done in PASS, the sample sizes are 9, 16, and 25, respectively. Of course, as discussed in Section 2.2, there are ways to estimate σ without data and PASS and nQuery, in particular, can be useful in this regard.

This is not possible in MINITAB, however, except for individually solving for n for each desired value of σ, but it is possible to input multiple values of E at one time. PASS does allow both to be inputted at one time, however, so if three values are inputted for σ and three values inputted for E, the output will show nine sample sizes—one for each combination.

3.15.1 Adaptive Confidence Intervals

The term "adaptive confidence intervals" has been used in the literature, such as in Hartung and Knapp (2010). This refers to a multistage approach, such as when an internal pilot study is used. Hartung and Knapp (2010) pointed out that this is an old problem, with Stein (1945) having provided a two-stage procedure, with the sample size for the second stage based on the results from the first stage. Seelbinder (1953) showed how to select the sample size for the second stage when there is some prior information on σ^2.

3.15.2 One Mean, Standard Deviation Unknown—With Tolerance Probability

When σ is unknown and approximate normality is assumed, the t-distribution is used. Of course, a value for σ must be entered and, as in every sample size determination situation, the inputted value will almost certainly not be the same as the true value. Both PASS and nQuery have two routines for determining sample size for μ with σ unknown—one that accounts for the variability in the estimate of σ and one that does not. The former is called a "coverage correction" by nQuery and a "tolerance probability" by PASS, with nQuery recommending use of a coverage correction (probability) of .80. PASS does not give a specific recommendation but the default value is .90. When this option is not used, the sample size that is determined is valid only if σ is not greater than the assumed value. If it is greater, then the sample size that has been computed will be too small.

If σ is being estimated from a previous sample, the adjustment, as given originally by Harris, Horvitz, and Mood (1948), produces

$$n = \left(\frac{t_{\alpha/2,n-1}\hat{\sigma}}{E}\right)^2 F_{1-\gamma,n-1,m-1} \tag{3.8}$$

with $1 - \gamma$ denoting the probability that the distance from the mean to the $100(1 -\alpha)\%$ two-sided confidence limits, E, will be less than the specified value, and m is the size of the previous sample used in estimating σ.

When no previous sample is used for estimation, the sample size expression, as given by Kupper and Hafner (1989), for example, is

$$n = \left(\frac{t_{\alpha/2,\,n-1}\sigma^*}{E}\right)^2 \left(\frac{\chi^2_{1-\gamma,\,n-1}}{n-1}\right) \tag{3.9}$$

with $1 - \gamma$ and E having the same representation as in the previous formula and $\hat{\sigma}$ assumed to be the population value. The first fraction in Eq. (3.9) results from modifying the sample size expression given in Eq. (2.7) by replacing $Z_{\alpha/2}$ by $t_{\alpha/2,\,n-1}$ (since σ is unknown) and replacing σ by s^*, the upper $100(1-\gamma)\%$ prediction bound for s, the sample standard deviation for the future sample whose sample size is being determined. This gives

$$n = \left(\frac{t_{\alpha/2,\,n-1}s^*}{E}\right)^2 \tag{3.10}$$

The second fraction is obtained from the upper limit of a $100(1-\gamma)\%$ prediction bound for s, which is

$$s^* = \sigma^* \left(\frac{\chi^2_{1-\gamma,\,n-1}}{n-1}\right)^{1/2}$$

with σ^* denoting the true value of σ. Substituting this expression for s^* in Eq. (3.10) then produces Eq. (3.9).

Of course neither Eq. (3.8) nor Eq. (3.9) is a closed-form expression since n is on the right side of each formula. Thus, each one must be solved numerically. This would serve as an impediment to the use of coverage probability if this option were not available in software, but as indicated earlier in this section, it is available in software.

■ **EXAMPLE 3.6**

To illustrate, consider again a 95% confidence interval for μ with $E = 1$ and this time assume that, using a previous sample of size $m = 40$, $\hat{\sigma} = 2$. Using the default coverage probability in PASS of .90, the software gives $n = 27$. If we had (numerically) calculated the sample size using Eq. (3.8), we would have obtained

$$
n = \left(\frac{t_{\alpha/2,n-1}\hat{\sigma}}{E}\right)^2 F_{1-\gamma,n-1,m-1}
$$

$$
= \left(\frac{(2.05553)(2)}{1}\right)^2 (1.5660)
$$

$$
= 26.4667
$$

so $n = 27$ would be used. (Note that here I am using the known result from PASS of $n = 27$ to show that the formula gives that result.) Note also that we round up to the next integer value just as we do when a hypothesis is being tested, but for a different reason. We want the difference to be at most equal to the target value, just as we want the power to be at least equal to the target value for the hypothesis test. We usually won't be able to hit the target value exactly, however, so we have to decide whether we prefer a sample size that is slightly under the target value or slightly over the target value, with the former generally preferred.

The sample size is relatively insensitive to the size of the previous sample, provided it is large, as $m = 1000$ gives $n = 24$.

When the distribution of σ is assumed to have a mean of 2 (note that this is not the same as assuming that σ is known, as in that case all of the probability would be at the known value), $n = 24$, which is the same solution obtained using nQuery. Using Eq. (3.9) and still assuming a 95% confidence interval with $1 - \gamma = .90$ and $E = 1$, we obtain

$$
n = \left(\frac{t_{\alpha/2,n-1}\hat{\sigma}}{E}\right)^2 \left(\frac{x_{1-\gamma,n-1}^2}{n-1}\right)
$$

$$
= \left(\frac{(2.06866)(2)}{1}\right)^2 \left(\frac{32.0069}{23}\right)
$$

$$
= 23.8207
$$

so $n = 24$ would be used (again using the known result to illustrate the formula). (Note that although n appears in the denominator of the second fraction, there is no point in trying to write the sample size formula in a cleaner fashion since *n* also appears in the numerator of that fraction and the numerator of the other fraction.) ∎

3.15.3   Difference Between Two Independent Means, Standard Deviations Known and Unknown—With and Without Tolerance Probability

If we consider the simplest case of constructing a confidence interval for $\mu_1 - \mu_2$ with σ_1 and σ_2 assumed known and equal sample sizes, n, to be used, the sample size expression is obtained by using the expression for the Z-statistic given in Section 3.5. Specifically, the expression for the halfwidth of a $100(1-\alpha)\%$ confidence interval, with equal sample sizes, is

$$Z_{\alpha/2}\sqrt{\frac{\sigma_1^2 + \sigma_2^2}{n}} = E$$

Solving this expression for n gives

$$n = \frac{Z_{\alpha/2}^2 \left(\sigma_1^2 + \sigma_2^2\right)}{E^2}$$

For example, if $\sigma_1^2 = 9$, $\sigma_2^2 = 16$, $E = 2$, and a 95% confidence interval is to be constructed,

$$n = \frac{(1.96)^2 (9 + 16)}{2^2}$$
$$= 24.01$$

Somewhat oddly, neither PASS nor nQuery has the capability to solve for the sample size in this the simplest of the two-sample mean cases.

If we assume that both standard deviations are unknown, but equal, we would then use a pooled-*t* test if we could assume approximate normality for the two populations. For the sake of comparison with the preceding example, we will use 3 and 4 as estimates of σ_1 and σ_2, respectively, and again use $E = 2$. We would expect the common sample size to be somewhat larger than 24 and, using PASS, the result is $n = 26$.

Thus,

$$E = t_{\alpha/2,2n-2}s_p\sqrt{\frac{2}{n}}$$

with s_p denoting the pooled standard deviation, which here is $\sqrt{(9+16)/2}$. Therefore,

$$
\begin{aligned}
n &= \frac{2t_{\alpha/2,2n-2}^2 s_p^2}{E^2} \\
&= \frac{2(2.00856)^2(12.5)}{2^2} \\
&= 25.2145
\end{aligned}
$$

so $n = 26$ would be used, as given by PASS. When nQuery is used, however, the solution given is $n = 25$. (MINITAB cannot be used for this since its capability for determining sample sizes for confidence intervals does not extend to two means.)

Both PASS and nQuery have the capability for a confidence interval for the difference of two means with a coverage probability. As in the one-sample case, there is a choice to be made between the common standard deviation being estimated from a prior pair of samples or not. Thus, the relevant equations are extensions of Eqs. (3.8) and (3.9) to the two-sample case.

First, if we use the same information as in the preceding example and specify a coverage probability of .90 with σ *not* estimated from a previous pair of samples, nQuery and PASS each give the sample size as $n = 32$. Of course, we expect the common sample size to be larger than in the case where the uncertainty in the estimates of the common standard deviation was not factored in, and we would expect the sample size to be larger than 32 if we assume that a prior pair of samples were used. Making that specification, and assuming 30 for each of the two prior sample sizes, PASS gives $n = 35$ but nQuery does not have this sample size capability, just as it does not in the one-sample case. (Of course, the sample size that PASS gives will approach 32 if we let the prior sample sizes be larger.)

For the case of standard deviations unknown with coverage probability, if a previous sample from each population is used to estimate each standard deviation and we assume both those samples and the samples to be taken from each population are equal, the sample size formula is

$$
n = \frac{2t_{\alpha/2,2n-2}^2 s_p^2 F_{1-\gamma,2n-2,2m-2}}{E^2} \tag{3.11}
$$

with $1-\gamma$, s_P, and E as previously defined, and similarly for n and m. If a previous sample from each population is not available, then

$$
n = \frac{t_{\alpha/2,2n-2}^2 s_p^2 x_{1-\gamma,2n-2}^2}{E^2(n-1)} \tag{3.12}
$$

To illustrate Eq. (3.11), PASS gives $n = 35$ as the sample size when a previous sample of size 30 has been obtained from each population. Making the appropriate substitutions in Eq. (3.11), we obtain

$$n = \frac{2t_{\alpha/2, 2n-2}^2 s_p^2 F_{1-\gamma, 2n-2, 2m-2}}{E^2}$$

$$= \frac{2(1.99167)^2 (12.5)(1.38113)}{4}$$

$$= 34.24$$

so $n = 35$ would be used, as given by PASS.

As indicated, both PASS and nQuery give $n = 32$ when σ is *not* estimated from a sample taken from each population. To illustrate how the sample size would be computed using Eq. (3.12), we have

$$n = \frac{t_{\alpha/2, 2n-2}^2 s_p^2 x_{1-\gamma, 2n-2}^2}{E^2 (n-1)}$$

$$= \frac{(1.99897)^2 (12.5)(76.6302)}{4(31)}$$

$$= 30.8675$$

so $n = 31$ would be used. Thus, the computed sample size is one unit less than the solution given by PASS and nQuery, but the PASS output shows that the actual value of E using $n = 32$ is 1.964 rather than the desired value of 2.0, compared to $E = 1.98517$ when $n = 31$ is used. That is, both PASS and nQuery give a solution with a smaller error of estimation than requested, which means a narrower confidence interval than requested and a narrower confidence interval than would result from the use of $n = 31$. For a given degree of confidence and a given coverage probability, the narrower the interval the better, but the slightly narrower interval that would result from using the PASS and nQuery results comes at the expense of a larger sample size.

3.15.4 Difference Between Two Paired Means

The hypothesis test for two paired means was discussed in Section 3.9. The form of a $100(1-\alpha)\%$ confidence interval for μ_d is, again assuming that σ_d is known, $\bar{d} \pm Z_{\alpha/2}\sigma_d/\sqrt{n}$, with n denoting the number of differences, d, and, equivalently, the common size of each paired observation in the paired samples.

Then D, the halfwidth of the interval, is $D Z_{\alpha/2}\sigma_d/\sqrt{n}$. Solving for n gives $n = Z_{\alpha/2}^2 \sigma_d^2 / D^2$. To illustrate, if $\sigma_d = 4$ and $D = 1$ and we want a 95% confidence for μ_d, we obtain $n = (1.96)^2 (4)^2 / 1^2 = 61.4656$, so $n = 62$ would be used, which is the solution given by PASS. If σ_d is not assumed to be known, but is estimated from a pilot study or some type of previous study or estimate, the formula is $n = t_{\alpha/2,n-1}^2 \sigma_d^2/D^2$, which would have to be solved numerically, as is the case whenever the sample size expression is a function of a t-value. PASS gives $n = 64$ and using the formula with this known result we have $n = (1.99962)^2(16)/1 = 63.9757$, so $n = 64$ would be used.

If sample size is to be determined with a coverage probability of .90 with the same information as in the previous example, except that σ_d is estimated to be 4 from a previous sample of size $m = 30$, PASS gives $n = 96$. Since a paired-t test becomes effectively a one-sample t-test once the differences, d, have been formed, Eq. (3.8) applies when σ_d has been estimated from a prior sample, as in this case. Therefore,

$$
n = \left(\frac{t_{\alpha/2,n-1}\hat{\sigma}}{D}\right)^2 F_{1-\gamma,n-1,m-1}
$$
$$
= [(1.98525)(4)]^2(1.51937)
$$
$$
= 95.8107
$$

so $n = 96$ would be used, in agreement with PASS. If a previous sample is not used and the user is willing to assume that future samples will have a standard deviation of 4 (a possibly unreasonable assumption), PASS gives $n = 77$ as the solution. Here Eq. (3.9) applies so that

$$
n = \left(\frac{t_{\alpha/2,n-1}\sigma^*}{D}\right)^2 \left(\frac{x_{1-\gamma,n-1}^2}{n-1}\right)
$$
$$
= [(1.98525)(4)]^2 \left(\frac{92.1662}{76}\right)
$$
$$
= 76.4731
$$

so $n = 77$ would be used, in agreement with PASS.

3.15.5 One Variance

The expression for a two-sided confidence interval for σ^2 is obtained starting from

$$
P\left(x_{n-1,\alpha/2}^2 \le \frac{(n-1)S^2}{\sigma^2} \le x_{n-1,1-\alpha/2}^2\right) = 1 - \alpha
$$

From this starting point we simply need to manipulate the form so that σ^2 will be in the middle of the double inequality. Doing the appropriate algebra produces

$$P\left(\frac{(n-1)S^2}{\chi^2_{n-1,\alpha/2}} \le \sigma^2 \le \frac{(n-1)S^2}{\chi^2_{n-1,1-\alpha/2}}\right) = 1 - \alpha \qquad (3.13)$$

with the lower limit of the $100(1-\alpha)\%$ confidence interval being on the left side of the double inequality and the upper limit being on the right side of the double inequality.

This is an example of an asymmetric confidence interval because the distances from the sample variance, S^2, to each confidence limit are unequal. Therefore, it wouldn't make any sense to use a value for D, as with the preceding confidence intervals. Accordingly, with PASS the user specifies the width, W, of the confidence interval, which is the upper limit minus the lower limit.

Assume that we want the width of a 99% confidence interval to be $W = 8$ and we will assume that future samples will have $S^2 = 10$. PASS gives $n = 95$ as the solution. Taking the difference between the two limits in Eq. (3.13) and performing the necessary algebra, we obtain

$$n = 1 + \frac{W\,\chi^2_{n-1,1-\alpha/2}\,\chi^2_{n-1,\alpha/2}}{S^2\left(\chi^2_{n-1,1-\alpha/2} - \chi^2_{n-1,\alpha/2}\right)}$$

$$= 1 + \frac{8\,(133.059)\,(62.4370)}{10\,(133.059 - 62.4370)}$$

$$= 95.11$$

Here we would not round up because with $n = 95$ the actual width of the interval is 7.991, as reported by PASS, whereas if we had used $n = 96$, the width would have been 7.943, which is further away from the target width than when $n = 95$ is used. We round up for hypothesis testing so that the power is at least equal to the desired power, but of course there is no power involved in confidence intervals, so our objective is different. If we wanted the confidence interval to have at least the target width and use the smallest sample size that would provide that width, we would use $n = 94$ and the width would be 8.039.

3.15.6 One-Sided Confidence Bounds

In some applications, a one-sided confidence bound is more appropriate than a two-sided confidence interval. Sample size can also be computed for one-sided confidence bounds (not "intervals"), although the software for accomplishing this is somewhat limited. MINITAB has this capability for each type of two-sided confidence interval for which sample size can be determined, with the user specifying either an upper bound or a lower bound. For example, referring to the example discussed in Section 3.12, for which the sample size for the two-sided interval was 16, if we use the same inputs but specify that the sample size is to be determined for a 95% one-sided confidence bound, MINITAB gives the sample size as $n = 11$. (Of course, the sample size is the same regardless of whether a lower bound or upper bound is specified.) Why is the sample size less than in the two-sample case? The expression for, say, a 95% lower bound is: Lower Bound $= \bar{X} - Z_\alpha \sigma / \sqrt{n}$, with the error of estimation, E, equal to $\bar{X} -$ Lower Bound. So, $E = Z_\alpha \sigma / \sqrt{n}$ and thus $n = Z_\alpha^2 \sigma^2 / E^2 = (1.645)^2 (2)^2 / 1^2 = 10.82$, so $n = 11$ would be used. The smaller sample size results from the fact that $Z_\alpha < Z_{\alpha/2}$, as is always the case.

Other software that can be used for one-sided confidence bounds includes PASS and nQuery. Although Power and Precision does give confidence interval results, there is no option to select a confidence interval rather than a hypothesis test; the user simply solves for sample size for a hypothesis test and the corresponding confidence interval is part of the output.

Among well-known applets, Lenth's applet can also be used to solve for sample size for two-sided confidence intervals, but that is for one mean or one proportion, so its capabilities for confidence intervals is very limited.

3.16 RELATIVE PRECISION

As discussed by, for example, Lohr (1999, p. 38), sometimes there is an objective to achieve a desired relative precision, with the latter defined for estimating a mean as

$$\left| \frac{\bar{y} - \mu}{\mu} \right|$$

Thus, relative to the maximum error of estimation discussed in Section 3.13, for which the relevant probability statement would be $P(|\bar{y} - \mu| \leq E) = 1 - \alpha$, the corresponding probability statement for relative precision is $P(|(\bar{y} - \mu)/\mu| \leq E) = 1 - \alpha$, or equivalently, $P(|\bar{y} - \mu| \leq \mu E) = 1 - \alpha$.

Sample size determination for a maximum error of estimation for μ was discussed and illustrated briefly in Section 2.4. The appropriate formula (not given in that section) is

$$Z_{\alpha/2} \sigma / \sqrt{n} \leq E$$

which leads to the sample size formula

$$n = \left(\frac{Z_{\alpha/2}\sigma}{E} \right)^2$$

The sample size formula for relative precision is obtained by substituting μE for E, which produces

$$n = \left(\frac{Z_{\alpha/2}\sigma}{\mu E} \right)^2$$

Since the population coefficient of variation (CV) was defined in Section 3.1.1 as σ/μ, we can thus write the formula as

$$n = \left(\frac{Z_{\alpha/2}CV}{E} \right)^2$$

[Note that this is *not* comparable to the sample size expression using CV given by van Belle (1993) and discussed in Section 3.1.1 because there is no assumption of a hypothesis test in this section.]

Thus, what is presented here is similar to the presentation for sample size using relative precision given in Lohr (1999, p. 40), with the exception that the latter assumes a finite population size and gives the formula using a finite population correction factor (fpc), as discussed in Section 2.3, although the fpc used by Lohr (1999) is $(N - n)/N$ rather than $(N - n)/(N - 1)$ that was given in Section 2.3.

3.17 COMPUTING AIDS

In addition to the software and applets that have been discussed and illustrated in this chapter and Chapter 2, Altman (1980) gave a nomogram that links power to sample size in comparing the means for two independent samples. This was also illustrated in Newcombe (2001). Nomograms for use in diagnostic studies were also given by Carley, Dosman, Jones, and Harrison (2005).

3.18 SOFTWARE

PASS, in particular, was used to compute sample sizes for various types of tests that were covered in this chapter, and nQuery, Power and Precision, MINITAB, Stata, and SAS were also mentioned. PASS has by far the broadest capability of the software that is specifically for sample size determination. Users do have a wide variety of options for the standard statistical tests given in this chapter, and it has capabilities for some tests that were not covered in this chapter, nor are they covered in succeeding chapters. The `sampsi` and `sampncti` commands in Stata can be used for sample size determination, with development of the `sampncti` command motivated by the fact that the `sampsi` command does not work particularly well for small sample sizes (see Harrison and Brady, 2004).

3.19 SUMMARY

Determining sample size to test one or two means is a very common application of sample size determination and these applications were covered in this chapter. It is important to recognize that the assumed power for hypothesis tests is almost certainly not the actual power, so confidence limits for power for a fixed sample size are important, at least a lower confidence limit. Similarly, if a researcher wants to specify power and view an interval on sample sizes to produce a desired power, this would be another option. The bottom line is that power is not "known" and this should be addressed in practical applications. Of course, that problem can be avoided by constructing a confidence interval rather than performing a hypothesis test, and there is much support in the literature for doing so, but this does not completely avoid problems caused by unknown parameter values.

The tests and confidence intervals presented in this chapter are based on a normal distribution. When there is pronounced nonnormality, a nonparametric approach (Chapter 10) can be used. Alternatively, if a particular nonnormal distribution is known to be an adequate population model, sample sizes can be determined for such distributions. For example, Ren, Chu, and Lai (2008) gave sample size and power computations for a left-truncated normal distribution. Problems may be encountered with the specification of a nonnormal distribution, however, and Singh, Singh, and Engelhardt (1999) discussed some problems with the lognormal distribution assumption and how they relate to sample size determination.

APPENDIX

Equation (3.3) can be derived using the same general approach that was used to derive Eq. (2.3). That is, we start with

$$P\left[(\bar{X}_1 - \bar{X}_2) > \Delta_0 + Z_\alpha \sqrt{\frac{\sigma_1^2 + \sigma_2^2}{n}} \,\middle|\, \mu_1 - \mu_2 = \Delta\right] = .80$$

with Δ_0 and Δ being the hypothesized and assumed values of $\mu_1 - \mu_2$, respectively. Then,

$$P\left[(\bar{X}_1 - \bar{X}_2) - \Delta > \Delta_0 - \Delta + Z_\alpha \sqrt{\frac{\sigma_1^2 + \sigma_2^2}{n}} \,\middle|\, \mu_1 - \mu_2 = \Delta\right] = .80$$

Dividing through by $\sqrt{(\sigma_1^2 + \sigma_2^2)/n}$ produces, under the assumption of normality,

$$1 - \Phi\left(Z_\alpha + \frac{\Delta_0 - \Delta}{\sqrt{(\sigma_1^2 + \sigma_2^2)/n}}\right) = .80$$

$$\Phi\left(Z_\alpha + \frac{\Delta_0 - \Delta}{\sqrt{(\sigma_1^2 + \sigma_2^2)/n}}\right) = .20$$

so

$$Z_\alpha + \frac{\Delta_0 - \Delta}{\sqrt{(\sigma_1^2 + \sigma_2^2)/n}} = -Z_\beta$$

Solving this last equation gives

$$n = \frac{\left(\sigma_1^2 + \sigma_2^2\right)\left(Z_\alpha + Z_\beta\right)^2}{(\Delta - \Delta_0)^2}$$

REFERENCES

Altman, D. (1980). Statistics and ethics in medical research, III: How large a sample? *British Medical Journal*, **281**, 1336–1338.

Beal, S. L. (1989). Sample size determination for confidence intervals on the population mean and on the difference between two population means. *Biometrics*, **45**, 969–977.

Bogle, W. and Y. S. Hsu (2002). Sample size determination in comparing two population variances with paired data: Application to bilirubin tests. *Biometrical Journal*, **44**, 594–602.

Boneau, C. A. (1960). The effects of violations of the assumptions underlying the *t*-test. *Psychological Bulletin*, **57**, 49–64.

Bonett, D. G. and M. S. Al-Sunduqchi (1994). Approximating sample size requirements for s^2 charts. *Journal of Applied Statistics*, **21**(5), 425–429

Bowman, K. O. and M. A. Kastenbaum (1974). Potential pitfalls of portable power. *Technometrics*, **16**(3), 349–353.

Box, G. E. P. (1953). Non-normality and tests on variances. *Biometrika*, **40**, 318–355.

Bristol, D. R. (1989). Sample sizes for constructing confidence intervals and testing hypotheses. *Statistics in Medicine*, **8**, 803–811.

Browne, R. H. (1995). On the use of a pilot sample for sample size determination. *Statistics in Medicine*, **14**(17), 1933–1940.

Campbell, M. J., S. A. Julious, and D. G. Altman (1995). Estimating sample sizes for binary, ordered categorical, and continuous outcomes in two group comparisons. *British Medical Journal*, **311**, 1145–1148. (Available at www.bmj.com/content/311/7013/1145.full.)

Carley, S., S. Dosman, S. R. Jones, and M. Harrison (2005). Simple nomograms to calculate sample size in diagnostic studies. *Journal of Emergency Medicine*, **22**, 180–181.

Clark, A. (1987). Approximate confidence bounds for estimated power in testing the general linear hypothesis. M. S. thesis, Department of Biostatistics, University of North Carolina, Chapel Hill.

Dudewicz, E. J. (1972). Confidence intervals for power with special reference to medical trials. *Australian Journal of Statistics*, **14**, 211–216.

Duncan, A. J. (1986). *Quality Control and Industrial Statistics*, 5th edition. Homewood, IL: Irwin.

Epstein, B. (1960). Statistical life test acceptance procedures. *Technometrics*, **2**(4), 435–446.

Evans, M., N. Hastings, J. B. Peacock, and C. Forbes (2010). *Statistical Distributions*, 4th edition. Hoboken, NJ: Wiley.

Falk, R. J., S. L. Hogan, K. E. Muller, and J. C. Jennette (1992). Treatment of progressive membrane glomerulopathy. *Annals of Internal Medicine*, **6**, 438–445.

Gibbons, C. (2000). *Determination of Power and Sample Size for Levene's Test*. Master's thesis submitted to The University of Colorado.

Greenwood, J. A. and M. M. Sandomire (1950). Sample size required for estimating the standard deviation as a per cent of its true value. *Journal of the American Statistical Association*, **45**(250), 257–260.

Grieve, A. P. (1991). Confidence intervals and sample sizes. *Biometrics*, **47**, 1597–1603.

Guenther, W. C. (1981). Sample size formulas for normal theory T tests. *The American Statistician*, **35**(4), 243–244.

Harris, M., D. J. Horvitz, and A. M. Mood (1948). On the determination of sample sizes in designing experiments. *Journal of the American Statistical Association*, **43**(243), 391–402.

Harrison, D. A. and A. R. Brady (2004). Sample size and power calculations using the noncentral t-distribution. *The Stata Journal*, **4**(2), 142–153.

Hartung, J. and G. Knapp (2010). Adaptive confidence intervals of desired length and power for normal means. *Journal of Statistical Planning and Inference*, **140**, 3317–3325.

Heasman, P. A., I. D. M. MacGregor, Z. Wilson, and P. J. Kelly (1998). Toothbrushing forces in children with fixed orthodontic appliances. *British Journal of Orthodontics*, **27**, 270–272.

Jiroutek, M. R., K. E. Muller, L. L. Kupper, and P. W. Stewart (2003). A new method for choosing sample size for confidence interval-based inferences. *Biometrics*, **59**, 580–590.

Joseph, L. and P. Bélisle (1997). Bayesian sample size determination for normal means and differences between normal means. *The Statistician*, **46**(2), 209–226.

Kelley, K. and J. R. Rausch (2006). Sample size planning for the standardized mean difference: Accuracy in parameter estimation via narrow confidence intervals. *Psychological Methods*, **11**(4), 363–385.

Kieser, M. and G. Wassmer (1996). On the use of the upper confidence limit for the variance from a pilot sample for sample size determination. *Biometrical Journal*, **38**(8), 941–949.

Kohavi, R. and R. Longbotham (2007). Online experiments: Lessons learned. *IEEE Computer*, 40(9), 103–105. (Available at http://exp-platform.com/Documents/ IEEEComputer2007OnlineExperiments.pdf.)

Kohavi, R., R. M. Henne, and D. Sommerfield (2007). Practical guide to controlled experiments on the Web: Listen to your customers not to the hippo. Paper presented at KDD2007.

Kohavi, R., R. Longbotham, D. Sommerfield, and R. M. Henne (2009). Controlled experiments on the Web: Survey and practical guide. *Data Mining and Knowledge Discovery*, **18**, 140–181.

Kupper, L. L. and K. B. Hafner (1989). How appropriate are popular sample size formulas? *The American Statistician*, **43**(2), 101–105.

Lehmann, E. L. (1959). *Statistical Hypotheses*. New York: Wiley.

Lehr, R (1992). Sixteen *s* squared over *d* squared: A relation for crude sample size estimates. *Statistics in Medicine*, **11**, 1099–1102.

Lenth, R. V. (2001). Some practical guidelines for effective sample size determination. *The American Statistician*, **55** 187–193.

Lohr, S. L. (1999). *Sampling Design and Analysis*. Pacific Grove, CA: Duxbury. (The current edition is the 2nd edition.)

Mahnken, J. D. (2009). Power and sample size calculations for models from unknown distributions. *Statistics in Biopharmaceutical Research*, **1**(3), 328–336.

Markowski, C. A. and E. P. Markowski (1990). Conditions for the effectiveness of a preliminary test of variance. *The American Statistician*, **44**(4), 322–326.

Moher, D., C. S. Dulberg, and G. A. Wells (1994). Statistical power, sample size, and their reporting in randomized controlled trials. *Journal of the American Medical Association*, **272**, 122–124.

Nayak, B. K. (2010). Understanding the relevance of sample size calculation. *Indian Journal of Ophthalmology*, **58**, 469–470.

Nelson, P. R., P. S. Wludyka, and K. A. F. Copeland (2005). *The Analysis of Means : A Graphical Method for Comparing Means, Rates and Proportions*. ASA-SIAM Series on Statistics and Applied Probability. Philadelphia, PA: Society for Industrial and Applied Mathematics.

Newcombe, R. G. (2001). Statistical applications in orthodontics, part III: How large a study is needed? *Journal of Orthodontics*, **28**(2), 169–172.

Parker, R. A. and N. G. Berman (2003). Sample size: More than calculations. *The American Statistician*, **57**(3), 166–170.

Pitman, E. J. G. (1939). A note on normal correlation. *Biometrika*, **31**(1,2), 9–12.

Rasch, D., K. D. Kubinger, and K. Moder (2011). The two-sample *t* test: Pre-testing its assumptions does not pay off. *Statistical Papers*, **52**, 219–231.

Ren, S., H. Chu, and S. Lai (2008). Sample size and power calculations for left-truncated normal distribution. *Communications in Statistics—Theory and Methods*, **37**(6), 847–860.

Schouten, H. J. A. (1999). Sample size formula with a continuous outcome for unequal group sizes and unequal variances. *Statistics in Medicine*, **18**, 87–91.

Seelbinder, B. M. (1953). On Stein's two-stage sampling scheme. *Annals of Mathematical Statistics*, **24**, 640–649.

Singh, A. K., A. Singh, and M. Engelhardt (1999). Some practical aspects of sample size and power computations for estimating the mean of positively skewed distributions in environmental applications. United States Environmental Protection Agency, Office of Research and Development, Office of Solid Waste and Emergency Response, EPA/600/s-99/006.

Stein, C. (1945). A two-sample test for a linear hypothesis whose power is independent of the variance. *Annals of Mathematical Statistics*, **24**, 243–258.

Taylor, D. J. and K. E. Muller (1995). Computing confidence bounds for power and sample size of the general linear model. *The American Statistician*, **49**(1), 43–47.

van Belle, G. (2008). *Statistical Rules of Thumb*, 2nd edition. Hoboken, NJ: Wiley.

van Belle, G. and D. C. Martin (1993). Sample size as a function of coefficient of variation and ratio of means. *The American Statistician*, **47**(3), 165–167.

Wang, H., S.-C. Chow, and M. Chen (2005). A Bayesian approach on sample size calculation for comparing means. *Journal of Biopharmaceutical Statistics*, **15**, 799–807.

Wheeler, R. E. (1974). Portable power. *Technometrics*, **16**, 193–201.

Wheeler, R. E. (1975). The validity of portable power. *Technometrics*, **17**, 177–179.

Wludyka, P. S., P. R. Nelson, and P. R. Silva (2001). Power curves for the analysis of means for variances. *Journal of Quality Technology*, **33**(1), 60–65.

Wong, A. (2010). A note on confidence interval for the power of the one-sample t-test. *Journal of Probability and Statistics*. Open access journal, article ID 139856.

EXERCISES

3.1. Assume that $\sigma = 3$ and it is desired to detect with a one-tailed upper test, power of at least .80 when $\mu = 36$ and the null hypothesis is $\mu = 35$. Also assuming normality, what is the minimum sample size that will accomplish this? If the experimenter is set on using $n = 100$, what power will this provide?

3.2. Explain why it is not very logical to use an expression like Eq. (3.4) to solve for a sample size, even if the computation is performed by software but is based on Eq. (3.4).

3.3. Suppose we want to estimate the mean systolic blood pressure of men who are more than 25% above their ideal maximum body weight as indicated by body fat index charts. How many men should be sampled to estimate the mean with a 95% confidence interval of width 10 units? You will need to estimate σ from the range of blood pressures of men who are considerably overweight, perhaps searching the Internet for such information.

3.4. Kohavi, Longbotham, Sommerfield, and Henne (2009) gave a sample size determination example. An e-commerce site was assumed to exist such that 5% of the users who visited the site made some purchase, spending about $75. The average amount spent over all visitors was thus assumed to be $3.75, with the standard deviation assumed to be $30. They stated that if a 5% change in revenue is to be detected with 80% power, over 409,000 site visitors would be needed. Although that might not be an exorbitant number for a popular website, they indicated that the number would be computed using the formula given in this chapter as Eq. (3.7).

   (a) What is the actual number of site visitors that would be needed?

   (b) If such a sample size is considered impractical, is there any action that the site owners might take to reduce the sample size and still have power of at least .80? Explain.

3.5. A clinical dietitian wants to compare the effectiveness of two different diets, A and B, for diabetic patients. She intends to obtain a random sample of diabetic patients from a very large group of patients and randomly assign them to each diet such that there will be an equal number of patients for each diet. The experiment will last 3 months, at the end of which a fasting blood glucose test will be administered to each patient. She doesn't know which diet will likely be shown to be the better one, but she is interested in detecting an average difference of 10 milligrams per deciliter between the diets, as she believes that is adequate for claiming superiority. In the absence of any prior information, she is willing to assume that the standard deviations for the two diets should be approximately equal, and from similar studies that she has read about in the literature, she estimates that the assumed common standard deviation should be about 15. She believes that the two populations should be approximately normal. How many observations should she have for each group if she uses a significance level of .05 and she wants the power to be .90?

3.6. Data from the now-famous Framingham study (www.framinghamheart study.org) permit a comparison of initial serum cholesterol levels for two populations of males: those who go on to develop heart disease and those who do not. The mean serum cholesterol level of men who did *not* develop heart disease is $\mu = 219$ milligrams per deciliter (mg/dL), with a standard deviation of 41 mg/dL. Assume that you wish to conduct a study of those men who *did* develop heart disease and you believe that their serum cholesterol level must have been at least 20 milligrams higher, and this is the minimum difference that you want to detect. You are willing to assume that the standard deviation for this group is approximately the same as for the other group. If $\alpha = .05$ and the power is to be .90, how many men should be in the study of men who did develop heart disease?

3.7. Consider the example in Section 3.6 with $\alpha = .05$, power $= .80$, $\Delta = 1$ and the assumption that $\sigma_1 = \sigma_2 = 1$ for a one-sided test of H_0: $\mu_1 = \mu_2$. For that example the solution was $n = 13$ for each group. Now assume, as in Example 3.4, that we want to have $n_2/n_1 = 2$. What sample sizes should be used? Note that $n_1 + n_2$ differs noticeably from $2(13) = 26$. Comment.

3.8. If the power for detecting a difference of 3.0 between two population means is .80, will the power be less than .80 or greater than .80 for detecting an actual difference of 2.0? Explain.

CHAPTER 4

Proportions and Rates

The need frequently arises to test the equality of two or more proportions, in addition to working with rates.

For example, the proportion of nonconforming units of a new, and purported improved manufacturing process might be compared with the proportion conforming under the standard process. The sample size could be determined so as to detect a certain minimum level of improvement.

The parameter λ of the Poisson distribution is frequently a rate, such as the rate at which some event occurs during a specified time period, such as the rate of arrivals of United Parcel Service trucks per hour at a particular UPS loading dock. There is also frequently interest in comparing two rates, such as incidence rates (e.g., exposure vs. no exposure to a toxin).

We will first consider proportions, noting that the software PASS lists a staggering number (81) of procedures that it has for proportions (one proportion, two proportions; independent proportions, correlated proportions; equivalence tests, noninferiority tests, etc). Many of these procedures are discussed and illustrated throughout the chapter.

4.1 ONE PROPORTION

We will first consider the case of a single proportion, with p_0 denoting the value of p under the null hypothesis, and p_1 denoting the true value. For a one-sided test, the usual textbook test statistic (but not necessarily the best approach), which is based on the assumed adequacy of the normal approximation to the binomial distribution is

$$Z = \frac{\hat{p} - p_0}{\sqrt{\dfrac{p_0(1 - p_0)}{n}}} \tag{4.1}$$

Sample Size Determination and Power, First Edition. Thomas P. Ryan.
© 2013 John Wiley & Sons, Inc. Published 2013 by John Wiley & Sons, Inc.

The test statistic is appropriate when both $\hat{p}$ and p_0 do not differ greatly from 0.5 when n is large and are close to 0.5 when n is not large. When this requirement is not met, an arcsin transformation should be used. One form of the transformation is $p* = 2 \arcsin \sqrt{\hat{p}}$. The reason for the "2" is that $\text{Var}(p*) = 1/n$, which is easier to work with than $1/4n$. When this transformation is used, it can easily be shown that the required sample size for a two-sided test with significance level α and power $1 - \beta$ is

$$n = \left(\frac{z_\beta + z_{\alpha/2}}{\arcsin(\sqrt{p_0}) - \arcsin(\sqrt{p_1})} \right)^2 \tag{4.2}$$

with p_0 and p_1 denoting the null hypothesis value of the population proportion and the value that the experimenter wishes to detect, respectively. As with sample size formulas in previous chapters, $z_{\alpha/2}$ would be replaced by z_α for a one-sided test. Note that the use of the z terms means that a normal approximation is being used; the proportions are simply being transformed before the normal approximation is applied.

To illustrate, if $p_0 = .2$, $p_1 = .1$, and a one-sided test is to be performed with $\alpha = .05$ and power $= .90$,

$$n = \left(\frac{z_\beta + z_\alpha}{2\arcsin\left(\sqrt{p_0}\right) - 2\arcsin\left(\sqrt{p_1}\right)} \right)^2$$

$$= \left(\frac{1.28155 + 1.64485}{0.927295 - 0.643502} \right)^2$$

$$= 106.332$$

so $n = 107$ would be used. One software package that uses this transformation in determining sample size is Power and Precision, as the only other option is to use the exact binomial distribution approach. Power and Precision does give $n = 107$ as the sample size for this example.

This transformation will often be needed because, for example, if we are looking at performance measures of a company measured by proportions, we would expect proportions to be not far from 0 or 1, depending on whether what is being measured is good or bad, and thus a proportion near 0.5 could be uncommon.

The transformation can also be used when there are two proportions; this is illustrated and discussed in Section 4.2.

Of course, a major disadvantage of transformations is that a transformed proportion generally won't have any practical meaning. For confidence intervals, there is some evidence (Vollset, 1993; Newcombe, 1998) that the Score method with continuity correction may provide the best results when p is very small ($\leq .01$).

Another option is to use the binomial distribution directly, and to determine sample size for confidence intervals using the "exact" approach, which the software PASS terms the "Exact (Clopper–Pearson)" option, following Clopper and Pearson (1934). Samuels and Lu (1992) provided guidelines, expressed as a percentage of the length of the Clopper–Pearson interval, for when the normal approximation confidence interval $\left(\hat{p} \pm z_{\alpha/2}\sqrt{\hat{p}(1-\hat{p})/n}\right)$ is an adequate substitute for the Clopper–Pearson interval. Tobi, van den Berg, and de Jong-van den Berg (2005) concluded from their study that the best method to use in reporting confidence intervals when p is less than or equal to .01 is to use either the Exact method or the Score method with continuity correction.

To illustrate the Exact method, Clopper and Pearson (1934) gave an example for which a crude measure of quality for a particular manufacturing process has been the percentage of articles that must pass a certain test. The percentage has fluctuated around $p = .60$ but an intensive effort is to be undertaken to improve quality and thus increase the percentage. After completion of that effort, a sample is to be undertaken to see if there is evidence of improvement and the objective is to determine how large a sample should be obtained such that a 95% confidence interval for p will have a width of .05. Clopper and Pearson (1934) gave confidence belts for p for various sample sizes, but those figures could not be used to solve for the exact, or even approximate, value of n. So the best that they could do was to say that the sample size must exceed 1000, based on .60 as an estimate for p. The sample size can be obtained using PASS and selecting the "Exact (Clopper–Pearson)" confidence interval method in the "Confidence Intervals for One Proportion" procedure. Doing so produces $n = 1513$, which is indeed (much) greater than 1000. This solution can easily be checked, if desired, by using software that gives binomial distribution probabilities. For example, using MINITAB, the (approximate) 97.5 percentile of the binomial distribution when $p = .60$ and $n = 1513$ is $X = 945$, with X being the binomial random variable. The approximate 2.5 percentile is 870. Since $870/1513 = 0.575$ and $945/1513 = 0.625$, to three decimal places, the confidence interval about 0.60 thus has width 0.05, as desired.

One objection to this approach might be that the necessary sample size is determined assuming that the proportion is being estimated without error. Gould (1983) gave a method for determining sample size for a proportion that incorporates estimation uncertainty explicitly in the form of joint confidence distributions obtained from a pilot study or from prior information.

When the test statistic given in Eq. (4.1) is used, *one possible* expression for n (derived in the chapter Appendix, but note the discussion there, especially in regard to software) is

$$n = \left[\frac{z_\alpha\sqrt{p_0(1-p_0)} + z_\beta\sqrt{p'(1-p')}}{p' - p_0}\right]^2 \qquad (4.3)$$

■ **EXAMPLE 4.1**

To illustrate, assume a one-sided test and that $p_0 = .5$, $p' = .6$, the desired value of β is .80, and $\alpha = .05$. Then

$$n = \left[\frac{1.64485\sqrt{.5(1-.5)} + 0.841621\sqrt{.6(1-.6)}}{.6 - .5} \right]^2$$

$$= 152.457$$

so n is set equal to 153, with the resultant power then being slightly greater than .80 since the rounding is upward. It should be noted that whereas this is the solution obtained using MINITAB, Power and Precision, and nQuery, PASS uses this normal approximation approach as its starting point for the purpose of obtaining the critical value of the test statistic, but then uses a search procedure starting from a sample size of one and obtains $n = 146$. The power is .8059 and since this exceeds the target power of .80, one could contend that this is a better solution than $n = 153$ when the cost of sampling is considered.

If the test had been two-sided, the only change to Eq. (4.3) is that z_α would be replaced by $z_{\alpha/2}$. For this example, but with the test two-sided instead of one-sided with $z_{\alpha/2} = 1.96$, the sample size would be computed as $n = 193.852$ and rounded up to 194.

As in any sample size determination problem, it is desirable to conduct a sensitivity analysis, to see how power changes as the sample size changes. For a two-sided test of $p_0 = .5$ when the true value is $p' = .6$, the relationship between power and sample size is shown in Figure 4.1.

The curvilinear pattern is obvious, and a regression model fit with linear terms in n and n^2 provides almost an exact fit, as the sum of the squared residuals is 0.0002. Thus, the regression model $\hat{Y} = 0.046796 + 0.00567292\, n - 0.00000921\, n^2$ produces the power values almost exactly. (Such a fitted equation could be useful if there is some indecision or disagreement about the sample size to use in a particular application, as possible sample sizes and the corresponding power values could easily be compared.) From a practical standpoint, the convexity of the curve means that there are (slightly) diminishing increases in power for constant increases in the sample size for the range of sample sizes depicted in Figure 4.1.

Although this approach will often be satisfactory, an approximation based on the beta distribution will often be preferred, and an exact test based on the binomial distribution will frequently be better than both approximations (as we would guess), although exact tests do have some shortcomings. In particular, they have been criticized as being too conservative. Nevertheless, exact test results will be discussed later.

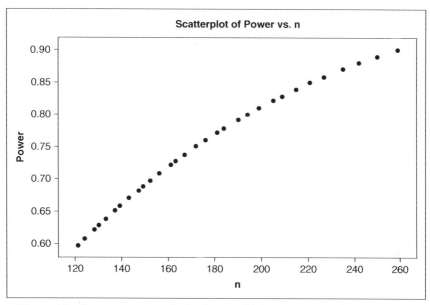

Figure 4.1 Power versus sample size for two-sided test: $p_0 = .5$, $p' = .6$, $\alpha = .05$.

As stated previously, there is nothing magical about a power value of .80. If more observations than are needed to give a power of .80 can be afforded and power of greater than .80 is desired, graphs such as Figure 4.1 can be helpful.

If the test had been one-sided, as in the original example, then Figure 4.2 shows the relationship between power and sample size.

As in Figure 4.1, the curvilinear relationship between power and sample size is obvious, and as before, a regression model with linear and quadratic terms in sample size provides an almost exact fit.

Since the true value of p is, of course, unknown, it may also be of interest to look at the sample size requirement for other values of p', such as .55, .65, and .70 or some subset of these numbers. A single graph using multiple values of p' can be constructed using software such as Power and Precision. ∎

4.1.1 One Proportion—With Continuity Correction

Although Eq. (4.3) is commonly used to determine sample size, Fleiss, Levin, and Paik (2003) recommended using the continuity correction $n^* = n + 1/\delta$, with n denoting the sample size before the correction and $\delta = z_\alpha \sqrt{p_0(1 - p_0)/n} + z_\beta \sqrt{p_1(1 - p_1)/n}$. For a two-sided test, z_α would be replaced by $z_{\alpha/2}$.

If we apply this to Example 4.1, we obtain $n^* = 155 + 1/.0998 = 165$. Thus, use of the continuity correction factor makes a noticeable difference, although use of the continuity correction for determining sample size is somewhat controversial,

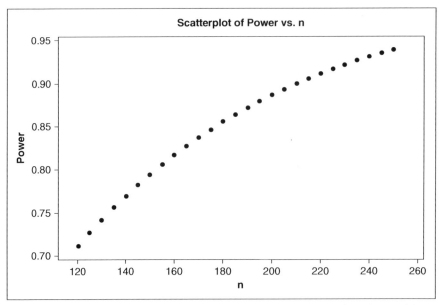

Figure 4.2   Power versus sample size for one-sided test: $p_0 = .5$, $p' = .6$, $\alpha = .05$.

as Gordon and Watson (1996) recommended that it *not* be used for inferences involving two proportions.

The corresponding hypothesis test with the continuity correction is

$$Z = \frac{\hat{p} - p_0 - c}{\sqrt{\dfrac{p_0(1 - p_0)}{n}}}$$

with the value of c dependent on the form of the alternative hypothesis and thus essentially dependent on the sign of $(\hat{p} - p_0)$. If the sign is positive, then $c = 1/2n$; if the sign is negative, $c = -1/2n$; with no adjustment made if $|\hat{p} - p_0| < 1/2n$. The logic behind these adjustments is the same as the logic behind the $\pm 1/2$ adjustment that is used when $X = n\hat{p}$ is used instead of $\hat{p}$. That is, since X is discrete and we are using a normal approximation (i.e., continuous), X is converted to the continuum $(X - 1/2, X + 1/2)$. It then follows that $X/n = \hat{p}$ would be converted to the continuum $(X/n - 1/2n, X/n + 1/2n)$.

4.1.2   Software Disagreement and Rectification

There is the potential for confusion when users try different sample size determination software and receive different answers for the same problem. This can especially be a problem involving proportions, as the reader should note. To illustrate, Chow, Shao, and Wand (2008, p. 87) gave an example of testing a single proportion, for which the null hypothesis is $p_0 = .3$, but after a particular treatment the proportion is expected to be around .5. So .5 is to be detected with power .80 and $\alpha = .05$ is used for a two-sided test. In deriving their expression for the power of the test using a normal approximation (i.e., using Z), the authors stated: "When n is large, the power of the test is approximately...." Thus, they did not derive the exact expression for the power of the test, which means that their expression for n is not exact for a normal approximation. We will see that their solution, $n = 49$, does not agree with the solution for *any* of the software discussed so far. If Eq. (4.3) is used, $n = 44$ is obtained, which is also the solution given by nQuery, SiZ, and Lenth's applet. MINITAB, PASS, and Power and Precision give $n = 47$, however. Why the difference? As stated in Section 4.1, Power and Precision uses an arcsin transformation of p, so the use of Eq. (4.1) should produce $n = 47$. Thus,

$$n = \left(\frac{z_\beta + z_\alpha}{2\arcsin\left(\sqrt{p_0}\right) - 2\arcsin\left(\sqrt{p_1}\right)} \right)^2$$

$$= \left(\frac{0.84 + 1.645}{2\arcsin\left(\sqrt{.3}\right) - 2\arcsin\left(\sqrt{.5}\right)} \right)^2$$

$$= 46.2957$$

so $n = 47$ would be used, in agreement with MINITAB, PASS, and Power and Precision.

Thus, although these software packages are using a normal approximation, there is an attempt to first normalize the sample proportion since a normal approximation does not do so. That is desirable when p is small and much less than .5, although here it is questionable whether or not an arcsin transformation is necessary. See also the discussion of an arcsin transformation for proportions data in Section 4.2.

4.1.3 Equivalence Tests and Noninferiority Tests for One Proportion

Recall that equivalence, noninferiority, and superiority testing were discussed briefly in Section 1.5. For proportions data, a single proportion might be considered "equivalent" to the hypothesized value if the difference is small enough to be deemed inconsequential.

Of the software mentioned previously, PASS is the only software that can be used for sample size determination for equivalence tests with a single proportion. To illustrate, let power $= .80$, $\alpha = .05$ for a two-sided test, and assume that $p = .60$ has been the standard proportion value and that this is expected to continue (i.e., p and p_0 are the same). We will use 0.2 as the equivalence value, meaning that all values in the interval (0.40, 0.80) are considered to be equally good. Chow et al. (2008, p. 88) gave $n = 52$. They used a large sample approximation in deriving the expression for power from whence came their expression for n, which is

$$n = \frac{\left(z_\alpha + z_{\beta/2}\right)^2 p\left(1 - p\right)}{\left(\delta - |p - p_0|\right)^2}$$

Thus, for this problem,

$$\begin{aligned} n &= \frac{\left(z_\alpha + z_{\beta/2}\right)^2 p\left(1 - p\right)}{\left(\delta - |p - p_0|\right)^2} \\ &= \frac{(1.645 + 1.28)^2(.6)(.4)}{(.2 - |.6 - .6|)^2} \\ &= 51.337 \end{aligned}$$

which is then rounded up to $n = 52$.

Notice that this solution is obtained despite the fact that $p = p_0$; that is, the true proportion and hypothesized proportion are assumed to be the same. Would this equality work when PASS is used? Yes, provided that the "Equivalence Tests for One Proportion (Differences)" is used. They give several options for the form of the test statistic and although their solutions do not agree with the Chow et al. (2008) solution, for some options the solution is $n = 53$, which differs by only one unit from the solution given by Chow et al. (2008). One source of difference is that the latter is based on hitting the desired power and significance levels exactly, which generally will not be possible with discrete data and distributions, with the PASS output giving the actual power and significance level, which differ somewhat from the target values. (The formula or approach that PASS uses is not indicated.) See also the discussion for sample size determination for equivalence testing of proportions given by Farrington and Manning (1990).

4.1.4   Confidence Interval and Error of Estimation

Since $\sigma_p = \sqrt{p(1 - p)/n}$, which is thus a function of the parameter that is to be estimated, it is not possible to obtain an exact expression for the sample size so as to give a confidence interval for p of a specified width since the (large-sample) $100(1 - \alpha)\%$ confidence interval is of the form

$$\hat{p} \pm z_{\alpha/2}\sqrt{\hat{p}(1 - \hat{p})/n} \qquad (4.4)$$

if a continuity correction is not used, with the width of the interval being $2z_{\alpha/2}\sqrt{\hat{p}(1-\hat{p})/n}$. If a continuity correction *is* used, it would be reasonable for the form of the confidence interval to correspond to the form of the hypothesis test when the continuity correction is used. This leads to the upper limit (*U.L.*) and lower limit (*L.L.*) given by

$$U.L. = \frac{\hat{p} + \dfrac{z_{\alpha/2}^2}{2n} + z_{\alpha/2}\sqrt{\dfrac{\hat{p}(1-\hat{p})}{n} + \dfrac{z_{\alpha/2}^2}{4n^2}}}{1 + z_{\alpha/2}^2/n}$$

$$L.L. = \frac{\hat{p} + \dfrac{z_{\alpha/2}^2}{2n} - z_{\alpha/2}\sqrt{\dfrac{\hat{p}(1-\hat{p})}{n} + \dfrac{z_{\alpha/2}^2}{4n^2}}}{1 + z_{\alpha/2}^2/n}$$

This form of the interval has been supported by various researchers, including Agresti and Coull (1998). See Ryan (2007, p. 159) for further discussion.

Like the hypothesis test, this approach is based on the assumed adequacy of the normal approximation to the binomial distribution, which will not necessarily work when p is small. [The value of p is more important than the products np and $n(1 - p)$ in determining whether or not the normal approximation should be adequate. See, for example, Schader and Schmid (1989).]

The maximum error of estimation of p is half the width of the confidence interval, with $\hat{p}$ being in the center of the interval. Specifically, since the width of the interval is Upper Limit $-$ Lower Limit $= \hat{p} + z_{\alpha/2}\sqrt{\hat{p}(1-\hat{p})/n} - (\hat{p} - z_{\alpha/2}\sqrt{\hat{p}(1-\hat{p})/n}) = 2z_{\alpha/2}\sqrt{\hat{p}(1-\hat{p})/n})$, the halfwidth is thus $z_{\alpha/2}\sqrt{\hat{p}(1-\hat{p})/n}$.

Since the halfwidth is the maximum error of estimation with probability α, we could set $z_{\alpha/2}\sqrt{\hat{p}(1-\hat{p})/n} = E$ and solve for n, after we substitute a value for $\hat{p}$. Before doing the latter, we have

$$n = \frac{z_{\alpha/2}^2 \hat{p}(1-\hat{p})}{E^2}$$

Of course, we don't have a value for $\hat{p}$ before a sample has been taken, and whatever value is substituted for $\hat{p}$ in solving for n would almost certainly not be the value of $\hat{p}$ that results when the sample is taken. One approach that has been used is to substitute 0.5 for $\hat{p}$, as this maximizes $\sigma_{\hat{p}}$, and thus maximizes the value of n that is obtained when solving for it for a specified confidence interval width.

Doing so gives $n = Z_{\alpha/2}^2/4E^2$. Thus, for example, if $E = .05$ and a 95% confidence interval is to be used, $n = 100(1.96)^2 = 384.2$, so $n = 385$ would be used. (This value for E was selected deliberately, as it is useful for Example 4.2.)

This is essentially an infinite population size formula, as it is not a function of the population size. Furthermore, one could argue that relative error is more important than absolute error when p is very small. An alternative formula, which is a function of both the population size, N, and the relative error, ϵ, was given by Levy and Lemeshow (1991). For a 95% confidence interval, the expression is

$$n = \frac{1.96^2 N p(1-p)}{(N-1)\epsilon^2 p^2 + 1.96^2 p(1-p)}$$

If the objective were to estimate the population total rather than the population proportion, the total, Np, would be estimated by $N\hat{p}$, but the applicable sample size formula would *not* be simply $N^2 \left(Z_{\alpha/2}^2/4E^2 \right)$ if absolute rather than relative error were used because E would obviously have to be redefined since a total would be estimated with greater absolute error than a proportion. Therefore, the sample size expression would be $n = N^2 \left[Z_{\alpha/2}^2/4(E^*)^2 \right]$ for a suitably chosen value of E^*, if the finite population correction factor, $1 - n/N$, were ignored. It would be quite reasonable to let $E^* = NE$ since the total is estimated by $N\hat{p}$ and E is the acceptable error for estimating p.

■ EXAMPLE 4.2

Motivated by his work as an expert witness in one particular court case, Afshartous (2008) proposed a new way of looking at sample size determination for determining a confidence interval for a binomial proportion, with the proportion of interest being the proportion of bills sent out by a company that included a "special service handling fee," with such bills alleged to be erroneous. The Defendant proposed a margin of error of .05, which of course wouldn't make any sense if the proportion were close to zero. In particular, the computed lower confidence limit could be negative, so there would then not be a lower limit.

Afshartous (2008) presented the sample size formula in an awkward way because it was given as $n = (1.96 Ns)^2/E^2$, with $s^2 = s_y^2$, the sample variance for the realization of each of the n Bernoulli trials that form the binomial experiment and this E different from the E used previously and not necessarily equal to E^*.

It is somewhat awkward to give a sample size formula in terms of a sample variance since the sample won't be taken until the sample size is determined. Afshartous (2008) stated that a value would have to be used for s, but selecting a value may be difficult and of course would just be an approximation. In arguing for the use of relative error, Afshartous (2008) stated that it would be difficult to specify a value for E since the total is unknown. Of course, the use of $E^* = NE$ would be reasonable if E were reasonable. As indicated previously, however, this won't work if p is small.

Because of these difficulties, Afshartous (2008) contended that it would be better to solve for n using the coefficient of variation. The population coefficient of variation for a random variable Y is defined as σ_Y/μ_Y, with the corresponding sample coefficient of variation given by $s_Y/\bar{y}$. Since the expected value of $\hat{p}$ equals p, the expected value of $N\hat{p}$ is Np. Since $\sigma_{\hat{p}} = \sqrt{p(1-p)/n}$, $\sigma_{N\hat{p}} = N\sqrt{p(1-p)/n}$. Then, $\sigma_{N\hat{p}}/\mu_{N\hat{p}} = (1/\sqrt{n})\sqrt{(1-p)/p}$.

This last expression could be set equal to a value for the coefficient of variation and n solved for, but selecting a desired value for the coefficient of variation is likely to be more difficult than selecting a value for either E or E^*. Since the Plaintiff's lawyers had trouble just understanding the concept of a "coefficient of variation," Afshartous instead used "margin of error," with this term obviously used to represent the halfwidth of a confidence interval. The author stated that the standard deviation is roughly one-half the margin of error. (This is obviously based on the use of $z = 1.96$ for a 95% confidence interval.) This led to Afshartous (2008) defining Accuracy = Margin of Error/True Parameter, using the author's notation. This could be written as $(1/\sqrt{n})\sqrt{(1-p)/p}=$ Accuracy/2, with a set of possible values of n then obtained by solving for n using various reasonable combinations of Accuracy and p. This in turn led to Table 2 in Afshartous (2008), which enabled the lawyers to better understand the results. The eventual sample size that was used was stated as being "rather large" but was not given for obvious reasons of confidentiality. The margin of error for the total was 12.2%, with the sampling done so as to provide a confidence interval to be used in mediation.

The "moral of the story," if there is one, is that everyone involved in the settling of a legal dispute needs to understand the statistical methodology that is being used. ∎

4.1.5 One Proportion—Exact Approach

Although most software assume the use of the normal approximation to the binomial distribution, without a continuity correction, some software give the user the option of using an exact approach: that is, using the probabilities for the binomial distribution, which has considerable intuitive appeal. To illustrate, consider again Example 4.1. Using PASS, we find the exact solution to be $n = 158$.

Exact tests are often computer intensive and are not easy to illustrate because the solution results from the use of a search algorithm rather than the solution of an equation. That is the case here but we can still gain insight into the solution, if not see how it is obtained. If we use software to produce the cumulative mass function for the binomial distribution for $n = 158$ and $p = .5$, we see that $P(X \geq 90) = .04724$, and this is the closest we can come to .05. Therefore, the null hypothesis will be rejected when $X \geq 90$. Power is then computed as $P(X \geq 90 | p = .6)$. Using MINITAB or other software, we can see that $P(X \geq 90 | p = .6) = .80565$.

The output from PASS is given below, rounded to four decimal places.

```
                   Power Analysis of One Proportion
Page/Date/Time          1   10/20/2009 5:52:59 AM

Numeric Results for testing H0: P = P0 versus H1: P > P0
Test Statistic: Exact Test

              Proportion  Proportion                   Reject  H0
              Given H0    Given H1    Target  Actual            If
Power    N    (P0)        (P1)        Alpha   Alpha   Beta    R>=This
0.8057  158   0.5000      0.6000      0.0500  0.0472  0.1943    90
```

Chernick and Liu (2002) illustrated a quirk of the exact approach as power can actually decrease as the sample size is increased. Thus, the relationship between power and sample size is not monotonic. This is not a software problem: whereas they obtained such nonintuitive results using nQuery Advisor, the same results are obtained using PASS and presumably any other software that has capability for the exact approach. For example, using the Chernick and Liu (2002) example of performing a one-sided test with $\alpha = .025$ of $p_0 = .07$ and assuming that $p_1 = .03$ is the true value, PASS gives the power as .8126 when $n = 240$ and .7995 when $n = 244$. When PASS is used to solve for n with the target power specified as .80, it gives the solution as 240, whereas nQuery Advisor does not permit sample size to be solved for with their exact test routine. Instead, n is entered and the value of power is produced. Of course, this could require at least a modest amount of trial and error if the user has no idea how large the sample size should be in a particular application in order to produce the desired power. Their sidebar states that power does not increase monotonically with sample size and refers to Chernick and Liu (2002).

Chernick and Liu (2002) showed that in general there is a sawtooth pattern when power is graphed against sample size. Why does this happen and should it be of any concern? These types of problems should be expected whenever a discrete random variable is involved, as noted by Cesana, Reina, and Marubini (2001), who also noted the sawtooth pattern in presenting their two-step procedure for determining sample size for testing a proportion against a reference value. The values of the binomial random variable that result in rejection of the null hypothesis are 9 for both $n = 240$ and $n = 244$. Since this is a lower-tailed test, the cumulative probability at that reject number for each sample size is of interest. Since the reject number does not increase as the sample size increases, there is less cumulative probability at that point with the larger sample size because the total probability of one is spread over a larger number of possible values of the random variable (245 versus 241). Therefore, with the reject number being the same, the power must be smaller with the larger sample size. Thus, any computer algorithm that seeks to come as close as possible to the target power but does not require that the target power be exceeded is going to exhibit this quirk.

Although not discussed by Chernick and Liu (2002), the significance level also jumps around for these two sample sizes, being the specified value of .025 for $n = 240$, but being considerably less at .0214 for 244.

Chernick and Liu (2002) raised the question of which sample size should be used since although the power is greater than .80 at $n = 240$ and that is the smallest sample size for which that occurs, the power dips below the required .80 at 244. The authors reported that a colleague suggested that $n = 277$ be used, as this is the smallest sample size for which the power exceeds .80 at all larger sample sizes. It seems unwise to think that way, however, because parameter values assumed in the null hypothesis aren't going to be equal to the hypothesized value, so this isn't truly going to be an "exact" calculation (i.e., null hypotheses are almost always false, as was discussed in Section 1.1). What if p_0 had been .072 instead of .070? Then the necessary sample size would have been 215, which is quite different from 240. Sample size determination is never going to be an exact science, so being overly concerned with "exactness" in certain ways seems inappropriate.

4.1.6 Bayesian Approaches

M'Lan, Joseph, and Wolfson (2008) discussed estimating binomial proportions using Bayesian techniques and provided tables for determining sample size for each of several methods that they presented. Their paper is long, detailed, and at an advanced level and a discussion of it would be beyond the level of this book. Readers who are interested in using Bayesian methods in estimating binomial proportions may find the paper useful, however. In earlier work by two of these three authors, Joseph, Wolfson, and du Berger (1995) considered the use of Bayesian approaches for binomial data and for higher-dimensional applications. Bayesian sample size determination with a focus on estimating the binomial parameter was also considered by Pham-Gia and Turkkan (1992) and since Bayesian approaches have not generally been incorporated into sample size determination software, it is worth noting that, even though this was two decades ago, the authors stated a computer program that "handles all computational complexities" was available upon request.

4.2 TWO PROPORTIONS

Often it is desirable to test for the equality of two proportions: are two competing drugs equally effective, do two surgical procedures give equivalent results, and so on. There are several ways of doing so, however, and the selection is a bit complex and not textbook-simple. The determination of the sample size(s) for the two populations will depend on which test method is used. Some software offer several options, but some leading software offers very few options.

Thus, $H_0: p_1 = p_2$ is tested, which of course is the same as testing $p_1 - p_2 = 0$. *One* way to test this hypothesis is to use the test statistic

$$Z = \frac{\hat{p}_1 - \hat{p}_2 - 0}{\sqrt{\dfrac{2\bar{p}(1 - \bar{p})}{n}}} \tag{4.5}$$

with $\bar{p} = (\hat{p}_1 + \hat{p}_2)/2$ assuming that $n_1 = n_2 = n$. This test statistic assumes the adequacy of the normal approximation to the binomial distribution and will work well when $\hat{p}_1$ and $\hat{p}_2$ are both close to .5. This will often not be the case, as in many applications, such as the percentage of people who have a reaction to a drug or the percentage of nonconforming units in a manufacturing process, the proportions will be much less than .5. Then it is necessary to apply an arcsin transformation to the proportions or to use software that will perform the transformation and then determine the required sample size, such as the Power and Precision software.

Although an arcsin transformation is typically applied to data, it could also be applied directly to proportions. As stated in Section 4.1, one form of the transformation is $2 \sin^{-1} \sqrt{p}$ and the transformed proportion would then be used in place of each proportion. Although the transformation should be used before a normal approximation approach is employed when proportions are small, it can make only a small percentage difference at times in the computed sample size.

To illustrate, assume that we wish to test the equality of two proportions but for the purpose of sample size determination we want to be able to reject the null hypothesis of equal proportions when $p_1 = .01$ and $p_2 = .02$. With $\alpha = .05$, power $= .80$, and a one-sided test, $n = 1826$ for each sample if the normal approximation *without* the arcsin transformation is used, and $n = 1776$ when the arcsin transformation is used, as given by Power and Precision. (The sample size formula using a normal approximation with no arcsin transformation is given later in this section.) The sample size for a one-sided test using the arcsin transformation is computed as

$$n = \frac{1}{2} \left(\frac{z_\beta + z_\alpha}{\arcsin(\sqrt{p_1}) - \arcsin(\sqrt{p_2})} \right)^2$$

$$= \frac{1}{2} \left(\frac{0.84 + 1.645}{\arcsin(\sqrt{.01}) - \arcsin(\sqrt{.02})} \right)^2$$

$$= \frac{1}{2} \left(\frac{0.841621 + 1.64485}{0.100167 - 0.141897} \right)^2$$

$$= 1775.17$$

so that $n = 1776$ would be used, in agreement with Power and Precision.

Thus, the percentage difference between the two sample sizes is small. This is because the sample sizes are so large, which results from the very small difference between the two population proportions. Now let $p_2 = .10$, so that the difference in the two proportions is not small. Now $n = 63$ when the arcsin transformation approach is used and $n = 79$ when the normal approximation approach is used. Now the percentage difference between the two sample sizes is not small, and that is because the percentage difference between the two proportions is not small. Here the arcsin transformation approach should definitely be used, not only because the proportions are small, which necessitates its use, but in this case it makes a sizable difference in the sample size.

In sample size determination, the objective in a test of equality would be to determine the (usually common) sample size such that a specified nonzero difference will be detected with a high probability. The formula for the common sample size using a normal approximation and assuming a one-sided test is

$$n = \left[\frac{z_\alpha \sqrt{(p_1 + p_2)(1 - p_1 + 1 - p_2)/2} + z_\beta \sqrt{p_1(1 - p_1) + p_2(1 - p_2)}}{p_1 - p_2} \right]^2$$

$$(4.6)$$

(This formula is also derived in the chapter Appendix.) If the test is two-sided, z_α would be replaced by $z_{\alpha/2}$.

To illustrate, if a difference of .1 between the two proportions is to be detected with p_1 assumed to be .55 and p_2 assumed to be .65, with an alternative hypothesis of $p_1 < p_2$ and a probability of .80 using a one-sided test with a significance level of .05, the common sample size would be 296, which would give a power of .80, as the reader is asked to show in Exercise 4.1. PASS also gives 296 as the solution, as does nQuery, MINITAB, Lenth's applet, Power and Precision, and G*Power. Note the software agreement for the case of two proportions whereas there was considerable disagreement for one proportion because of the different methods that were used.

If the test had been two-sided, the result would have been $n = 375.14$ (rounded up to 376), which will be used later in this section for comparison purposes.

Although approximate sample size formulas aren't necessary since Eq. (4.4) is known and software are available, Campbell, Julious, and Altman (1995) gave an approximation formula that is simpler than Eq. (4.4). Specifically, for a power of .80 and a significance level of .05 for a two-tailed test, they gave $n = 16\bar{p}(1 - \bar{p})/(p_1 - p_2)^2$, with $\bar{p} = (p_1 + p_2)/2$, although they stated that this does slightly overestimate the sample size. (They did not discuss a one-tailed test.)

Another approximation was given by Fleiss, Tytun, and Ury (1980) and Fleiss, Levin, and Paik (2003, p. 73) which is, *in their notation,*

$$n = n' + \frac{2}{|P_2 - P_1|} \qquad (4.7)$$

with their n' the same as the n in Eq. (4.6). They indicated that this should be used when $n' |P_2 - P_1| \geq 4$ and stated that Eq. (4.7) is useful both in quickly estimating required sample sizes and in estimating power. They stated that the corresponding power can be obtained by inverting Eq. (4.6) and Eq. (4.7) to obtain

$$z_\beta = \frac{|P_2 - P_1| \sqrt{n - \dfrac{2}{|P_2 - P_1|}} - z_{\alpha/2} \sqrt{2 \bar{P} \bar{Q}}}{\sqrt{P_1 Q_1 + P_2 Q_2}}$$

with the power then easily obtainable from Z_β.

To illustrate the Campbell et al. (1995) approximation, if we assume, as in the previous example, that $p_1 = .55$ and $p_2 = .65$, with an alternative hypothesis of $p_1 < p_2$ and desired power of .80 using a one-sided test with a significance level of .05, their approximation gives a sample size of $n = 16\bar{p}(1 - \bar{p})/(p_1 - p_2)^2 = 16(.6)(.4)/(.55 - .65)^2 = 384$, which is, as expected, slightly larger than $n = 376$ obtained using Eq. (4.4). The solution using the Fleiss et al. (1980) approximation is $n = 396$, as can be seen from Eq. (4.7) combined with the solution from Eq. (4.6).

So which of the three solutions should a practitioner use? The question of sample size for testing the equality of two proportions will be addressed more broadly after considering the exact test discussed later in this section and the use of a continuity correction discussed in Section 4.2.1, but the touted "remarkable accuracy" (Fleiss et al., 2003, p. 73) of the Fleiss et al. (1980) approximation can be questioned, at least for this example, since the Campbell et al. (1995) approximation generally overestimates the necessary sample size but for this example the Fleiss et al. (1980) approximation gives an even larger sample size than does the Campbell et al. (1995) approximation!

Another commonly used test for testing the equality of two independent proportions against an inequality alternative is a chi-square test. It can be shown with the appropriate algebra that the chi-square test (using a 2×2 contingency table) without a continuity correction is equivalent to the Z-test with no continuity correction. (This result should not be surprising since the square of a standard normal random variable is a chi-square random variable with one degree of freedom.) See Suissa and Shuster (1985), who gave sample size methods for the chi-square test with the 2×2 contingency table, and compare these results with the sample sizes obtained using other tests.

We will label the entries in the two-way table and the marginal totals as follows.

	Sample 1	Sample 2	Totals
Success	a	b	s
Failure	c	d	f
Totals	m	n	N

The chi-square statistic for general usage is typically written as

$$\chi^2 = \sum_{i=1}^{4} \frac{(O_i - E_i)^2}{E_i}$$

with, in this case, 4 denoting the number of cells in the 2×2 table, O_i denotes the observed value in the ith cell and E_i denotes the corresponding expected value, computed under the assumption that the proportions are equal. It can be shown (see, e.g., Conover, 1980, p. 145) that for the 2×2 table the chi-square statistic can be written as

$$\chi^2 = \frac{N(ad - bc)^2}{(a + b)(c + d)(a + c)(b + d)} \tag{4.8}$$

It can be shown by appropriately inserting these letters in Eq. (4.5) that the square of the Z-statistic in Eq. (4.5) is equal to χ^2 in Eq. (4.8), as the reader is asked to do in Exercise 4.6. This should not be surprising because a random variable that has a chi-square distribution results from squaring a random variable that has a standard normal distribution, whereas the use of a Z-statistic implies either normality or a normal approximation.

Thus, the same conclusion will be reached with each test, which implies that the sample size computed for each test will be the same.

We will examine the other options for testing two proportions in Sections 4.2.1 and 4.2.2 and then try to draw a conclusion about what approach should be used by practitioners.

4.2.1 Two Proportions—With Continuity Correction

Although the formula in Eq. (4.6) is commonly used, and is what is given in introductory level textbooks, it might seem preferable to use the formula that incorporates a continuity correction, just as in the single proportion case.

With two proportions there is the obvious question of how the continuity correction should be used and should there be a correction for each proportion. If the alternative hypothesis is $p_1 > p_2$, one might assume that using $\hat{p}_1 + 1/2n_1$ and $\hat{p}_2 + 1/2n_2$ in the test statistic would be appropriate because this would be most favorable to that hypothesis (with the signs reversed for $p_1 < p_2$) but of course there should be justification for whatever continuity correction is used.

Levin and Chen (1999) examined the approximation of Casagrande, Pike, and Smith (1978a) and explained why it has "remarkable accuracy," which is because it is a valid approximation to the exact hypergeometric test procedure [as explained by Fleiss et al. (2003, p. 73)].

For a one-sided test, the sample size formula with the continuity correction is

$$n^* = \frac{n}{4} \left(1 + \sqrt{1 + \frac{4}{n \, |p_2 - p_1|}} \right)^2 \tag{4.9}$$

with n denoting the sample size from Eq. (4.6) without the continuity correction, with n assumed to be the same for the two populations. [See, for example, Fleiss et al. (2003, p. 72), Ury and Fleiss (1980), or Casagrande, Pike, and Smith (1978a,b).] Note that the formula is given slightly differently in Levin and Chen (1999) since they assume that the alternative hypothesis is $p_1 > p_2$, rather than giving the form applicable for either one-sided test. (The general form for a one-sided test simply entails using $|p_2 - p_1|$, rather than using either $p_1 - p_2$ or $p_2 - p_1$.)

If unequal sample sizes are desired, as can occur due to relative costs, the desire for more precise estimates from one population, to minimize the variance of the difference of two sample proportions or their ratio (Brittain and Schlesselman, 1982), or other factors (Walter, 1977), the sample size formula with the correction factor becomes

$$n_1^* = \frac{n^*}{4} \left(1 + \sqrt{1 + \frac{2(r+1)}{nr \, |p_2 - p_1|}} \right)^2 \tag{4.10}$$

with $n_2^* = rn_1^*$ and r denoting the desired ratio of the sample sizes, n_2^*/n_1^*, with n^* given by

$$n^* = \left[\frac{z_\alpha \sqrt{(r+1)(\bar{p}\bar{q})} + z_\beta \sqrt{rp_1(1-p_1) + p_2(1-p_2)}}{r^{1/2}(p_1 - p_2)} \right]^2 \tag{4.11}$$

with $\bar{p} = (p_1 + rp_2)/(r+1)$ and $\bar{q} = 1 - \bar{p}$ (Fleiss et al. 2003, p. 76). It should be noted that Gordon and Watson (1996) questioned the utility of n_1^*, however.

If a two-sided test is to be used, the expression for n^* still applies except that now n is defined not quite as in Eq. (4.6) but is defined with z_α replaced by $z_{\alpha/2}$, as was done in Section 4.2 for the uncorrected sample size expression when a two-sided test is used.

[The reader can verify that the use of Eq. (4.9) in conjunction with $n = 296$ from Eq. (4.6) and $|p_2 - p_1| = .1$ from the current example gives $n^* = 316$.

PASS gives the same solution, as does Lenth's applet and nQuery. MINITAB, Power and Precision, and SiZ do not have a continuity correction option for testing the equality of two proportions. It can also be shown, such as by using an applet or the appropriate equation in the chapter Appendix, that the power is .8007.]

We can see from Eq. (4.8) that $n*$ will always be larger than n, with the percentage difference being large when $n|p_2 - p_1|$ is small.

Another important point is that the "remarkable accuracy" stated by Levin and Chen (1999) is relative to the sample size for Fisher's exact size. That is not entirely relevant, however, because the latter will generally not be applicable. This is because one of the assumptions of the test is that all of the marginal totals are fixed. That is, the number of subjects who are sampled from each population are fixed, as are the total number of responses for each of the two categories, such as "yes" and "no." The first of these requirements is no problem; the second one is a big problem! For this reason, papers have been written that have dispraised Fisher's exact test, including at least one that had almost that wording in the title of the paper: Berkson (1978). The point is that we would generally prefer to use an unconditional test but Fisher's exact test is a conditional test that is conditional on the four marginal totals.

D'Agostino, Chase, and Belanger (1988) considered the appropriateness of some of the commonly used tests for testing the equality of two independent binomial proportions, including Fisher's exact test. In referring to an earlier study of Upton (1982), they stated: "We confirm Upton's results that both the Fisher exact and Yates continuity correction chi-squared tests are extremely conservative and inappropriate." They demonstrated that the chi-square test *without* the continuity correction and the independent sample t-test with pooled variance have actual levels of significance that are, in most situations, close to or smaller than the nominal levels. Similarly, Gordon and Watson (1996) also advised against continuity-corrected sample size formulas.

We don't normally think about using a t-test for proportions data. It is not presented in textbooks and, indeed, D'Agostino et al. (1988) stated that "readers may be surprised by the inclusion of the t-test in an article testing binomial data."

We obtain the form of a t-test if we let a "failure" be denoted by a zero and a "success" be denoted by a one, and compute the average for each sample, which is of course also the proportion for each sample. They further stated, however, that the computation for the t-test is very close to the computation for the (uncorrected) chi-square test, which is undoubtedly due largely to the fact that the sample average is also the sample proportion.

4.2.2 Two Proportions—Fisher's Exact Test

Some software that can be used for sample size determination (including Lenth's applet and Stata) do not provide the user with the option to do an exact test for two proportions, although this is part of the standard output of certain other software, including MINITAB. The exact test is Fisher's exact test but that test is, strictly speaking, not valid unless the four marginal totals are fixed: the sample size for population 1, the sample size from population 2, $n_1\hat{p}_1 + n_2\hat{p}_2$, and $n_1(1 - \hat{p}_1) + n_2(1 - \hat{p}_2)$. Whereas the first two will of course be fixed since the sample size from each population is being solved for, the last two will not. That is, the sum of the items from the two samples that possess a certain characteristic (e.g., lung cancer) will generally be random, not fixed.

The requirement for the fixed marginal totals results from the fact that the p-value for Fisher's exact test is obtained by computing the probability of each configuration of possible counts in the four cells of the two-way table (two samples and a "yes" or "no" categorization of each item in each sample) which is more extreme, relative to the alternative hypothesis, than what was observed. It wouldn't make any sense to do this if the marginal totals were not fixed.

Therefore, although the option for determining each sample size for the exact test is available in Power and Precision and PASS, for example, as well as other sample size determination software, the test will often be inappropriate.

If, for the sake of illustration, we assume that the test is appropriate for the example given in Section 4.2 for which $p_1 = .55$ and $p_2 = .65$, PASS shows the required common sample size to be 316, with the power being .8007.

4.2.3   What Approach Is Recommended?

D'Agostino et al. (1988) recommended the use of the t-test but also stated that "at a minimum" either the Z-test or equivalently the chi-square test should be used, without a continuity correction. Of the major sample size determination software, only PASS offers capability for a t-test. If we accept the advice of D'Agostino et al. (1988) and Gordon and Watson (1996), we will eschew approaches that employ a continuity correction and either use the sample size formula for the normal approximation in Eq. (4.6), which would indirectly also give the sample size if a chi-square test is used, or use the sample size that results from use of a t-test. For the example with p_1 assumed to be .55 and P_2 assumed to be .65, PASS gives the required sample size as $n = 296$ for use with the t-test, in agreement with the result given by PASS and certain other software for the normal approximation sample size for Eq. (4.6).

There is going to be a problem with virtually all of these approaches when population proportions are extremely small, however, such as $p = .00001$ or even less than .000001. Such proportions are encountered in low-prevalence epidemiological applications, such as those mentioned by Williams, Ebel, and Wagner (2007). They examined several sample size formulas, including those given here in Eqs. (4.9) and (4.11), and recommended a Monte Carlo approach for determining sample size "such that the achieved power of the test closely matches the nominal value." They also pointed out that such an approach can "reduce the overall sample size by hundreds to thousands of samples while still meeting the study objectives."

4.2.4 Correlated Proportions

A paired t-test is used when there is a pairing of observations made on subjects, such as when two observations (measurements) are made, under different conditions, on each person, as covered in Section 3.4. Just as observations can be correlated and means can be correlated, proportions can also be correlated if proportions are computed from paired data rather than an average difference computed.

For example, the pairing could consist of people who work in a certain department for which invoice mistakes have been occurring during a 3-month period with too high of a frequency. So all of the employees are given a training program and the number of mistakes are recorded again after a second 3-month period. It is of interest to determine if the proportion of mistakes after the training program is less than the proportion before the training program. These are matched proportions because the same people are involved. (Note that testing for equality of the proportions is an alternative to determining if the average number of mistakes, for the department, after the training program is less than the average before the program.) A popular application of the test in genetics is the *transmission disequilibrium test*.

As in a test of two independent proportions, the counts or proportions could be represented in a 2×2 table. For the invoice application, the proportions would be the proportion of workers whose work was deemed satisfactory both before the program and after the program; unsatisfactory both before and after the program; satisfactory before but unsatisfactory afterward, and the reverse. If the last two are designated as b and c, respectively, the null hypothesis is that $b = c$ and one way to test this hypothesis is by using a chi-square test given by $\chi^2 = (b - c)^2 / (b + c)$, which obviously measures the departure of b from c relative to the sum of the two proportions. This is *McNemar's test* (1947) using the approximation defined by the χ^2 statistic.

When PASS is used for McNemar's test, the input includes $(b - c)$ and $(b + c)$. For example, if .3 is entered for $(b - c)$ and .4 for $(b + c)$, this implies that $b = .35$ and $c = .05$. With power $= .80$, and $\alpha = .05$ for a two-sided test, the required sample size is given as 36, which is the number of pairs in the sample, and the power is given as .81308. This is the exact solution, which is the default. If the approximate solution instead is requested (i.e., using the chi-square statistic), then $n = 32$. Thus, there is a noticeable difference when the two sample sizes are small, as we might expect. The PASS help file suggests using the approximate solution initially, while stating that the approximate solution is typically about 10% less than the exact solution, as was the case with this example. The reason for this suggestion is that the algorithm for the exact solution has numerical problems when $n > 2000$. Of course, if the approximate solution is far less than 2000, then so will be the exact solution, so in this case one could have safely started with the exact approach, but not knowing that the user could have started with the approximation and then switched over to the exact approach.

PASS also has a routine for determining sample size for testing two correlated proportions in a case–control design, with this being similar to the McNemar procedure.

Literature articles in which sample size determination for testing two correlated proportions is discussed include Schork and Williams (1980). Sample sizes for designing studies with correlated binary data has also been discussed by Brooks, Cottenden, and Fader (2003). See also Nam (2011) and Royston (1993).

4.2.5   Equivalence Tests for Two Proportions

Blackwelder (1982) proposed a method for "proving" the null hypothesis, as is implied by the title of the paper. [See also Blackwelder (1998).] More specifically, the general idea was to specify a difference, D, between two population proportions that was small enough that the proportions could be declared "practically" equivalent.

The *title* of Blackwelder (1982) is a misnomer, however, because as was indicated in Section 1.1, it is never possible to literally prove any hypothesis, null or alternative, using statistical methods, whenever a sample is taken from a population. The only way to obtain "proof" is to sample the entire population, which would be impractical and cost prohibitive, and thus essentially infeasible. This should be kept in mind in reading the literature on equivalence, as equivalence testing is simply a form of hypothesis testing and does not offer the user any special powers not possessed by standard hypothesis testing.

An applet is given at http://www.ucalgary.ca/~patten/blackwelder .html for calculating sample sizes for equivalence testing for stated values of D and the two proportions. The formula, assuming a one-sided test, is also given there and it is

$$n = \left[\frac{z_\alpha + z_\beta}{p_1 - p_2 - D} \right]^2 [p_1(1 - p_1) + p_2(1 - p_2)] \qquad (4.12)$$

To illustrate, let $p_1 = .5$, $p_2 = .6$, $D = .09$, $\alpha = .05$, and Power $= .80$. If we think of p_1 as being the proportion for a standard treatment and p_2 the expected proportion for a new treatment, if the difference turns out to be less than .09, then the two treatments will be declared equivalent. Using Eq. (4.11) we obtain $n = 83.9$, so $n = 84$ would be used for each sample. When the applet that is at http://www.ucalgary.ca/~patten/blackwelder.html is used, however, $n = 83$ is obtained. The solution of $n = 84$ is what is obtained using nQuery Advisor, however. This solution can also be obtained using Power and Precision, but doing so is awkward since there is no option for solving for the sample size for power of .80, as there is with other procedures. So some trial and error would have to be used to obtain the sample size that gives the desired power. Thus, it is much easier to use nQuery Advisor for this type of sample determination problem since the solution can be obtained very easily. For this example, values of D smaller than .09 would require a larger sample size (e.g., 134 for $D = .05$), while values of D larger than .09 would lead to a smaller sample size (68 for $D = .11$). (These results are obtained using the applet and differ by one unit from the results obtained using nQuery Advisor.) The direction of the change in sample size can be seen from Eq. (4.12).

4.2.6 Noninferiority Tests for Two Proportions

Equivalence tests and noninferiority tests for a single proportion were covered in Section 4.1.3. Noninferiority tests for two proportions are often needed, such as when a new drug that is safer and/or less expensive than the standard drug is introduced and a test is to be performed that will hopefully show that the new drug is not inferior to the standard drug in terms of effectiveness. Chan (2002) considered the use of noninferiority tests for two proportions using an exact method. See also Kawasaki, Zhang, and Miyaoka (2010), who proposed new test statistics for noninferiority testing for the difference of two independent binomial proportions.

4.2.7 Need for Pilot Study?

There is only one parameter in the binomial distribution and that is the one that is being tested, unlike normality-based tests since a normal distribution has two parameters. Thus, since there is no additional parameter to be estimated, there might seem to be no need for a pilot study, such as an internal pilot study. That isn't true, however, and Friede and Kieser (2004) discussed how information from an internal pilot study could lead to a recalculation of the sample size.

4.2.8 Linear Trend in Proportions

There are various ways in which a parameter can change, with one possibility being a linear trend. This can be tested using the Cochran–Armitage (Armitage, 1955) test, which is available in PASS, with the user having the option of using or not using a continuity correction. See also Nam (1987). For the case of two proportions, the computing formulas are the same as those given by Casagrande et al. (1978a). To illustrate, assume that there are three proportions, .25, .30, and .40, $\alpha = .05$, power $= .80$, and a one-sided test is used to detect an increasing trend. If the continuity correction is used, the sample size is 126 for each of the three groups, so the total is 378. The use of the continuity correction is recommended if the values of the covariate (such as dose values) are equally spaced. If there is unequal spacing, the PASS user can enter the spacing. If we use 1 2 4 as the spacing and the continuity correction is not used, in accordance with the recommendation of Nam (1987), the output shows a sample size of 116 for each group, for a total of 348.

4.2.9 Bayesian Method for Estimating the Difference of Two Binomial Proportions

The problem of determining sample size for estimating the difference of two binomial proportions using Bayesian methods was considered by Pham-Gia and Turkkan (2003). They briefly reviewed other published Bayesian approaches for one and two proportions and proposed a method such that either the expected length or maximum length of the highest posterior density (HPD) credible interval of the difference of the two population proportions is less than some predetermined quantity. In reviewing sample size determination methods for binomial data, Joseph et al. (1995) stated that sample sizes based on HPD intervals from the exact posterior distribution are generally smaller than sample sizes determined from the use of non-HPD intervals and/or normal approximations. In presenting Bayesian sample size methods for estimating the difference between two binomial proportions, Joseph, du Berger, and Bélisle (1997) made some important points, including the fact that Bayesian approaches generally lead to smaller sample sizes than frequentist approaches. This advantage is largely offset by the fact that, as these authors pointed out for the sample size criteria they gave in their Section 2, these are not closed-form solutions, so numerical methods must be employed to obtain the solutions. Undoubtedly, this partly explains why Bayesian methods of sample size determination are not generally available in sample size determination software.

4.3 MULTIPLE PROPORTIONS

There are various ways in which tests of the equality of more than two proportions can be performed. A common approach is to use a chi-square test and the sample size can be determined using software such as PASS and nQuery Advisor. The "effect size" must be specified with each and this is defined as the variance of the proportions divided by the product of the average proportion times one minus the average. That is, the effect size for k proportions is given by (from nQuery Advisor)

$$\text{Effect Size} = \sum_{i=1}^{k} (p_i - \bar{p})^2 / (k\bar{p}(1 - \bar{p}))$$

with $\bar{p} = (\sum_{i=1}^{k} p_i)/k$.

The following example illustrates the input and shows the corresponding output.

■ EXAMPLE 4.3

Assume that a sample is to be drawn from each of three populations and a proportion computed. It is believed that the three population proportions may be approximately .40, .50, and .60, respectively, and if the proportions do differ to this extent, an experimenter wants to be able to detect these differences with power of .90, using a significance level of .05.

For nQuery Advisor, the user must compute the variance, which is part of the input, and the software then computes the effect size. The variance can easily be seen to be $.02/3 = 0.00667$ so that the effect size, as defined by this software, is $0.00667/[(.5)*(.5)] = 0.02667$, with .5 denoting the average proportion. Entering the significance level, power, number of groups (3), and average proportion (.50) leads to a sample size of $n = 159$.

The same solution is obtained using PASS. Following Cohen (1988, p. 221), PASS defines the effect size as the square root of the value of the chi-square statistic computed using the assumed proportions. That is, the chi-square statistic is

$$\sum_{i=1}^{m} \frac{(O_{ik} - E_{ik})^2}{E_{ik}}$$

with O_{ik} denoting the proportion in the ith row and kth column of a 2×3 table, and E_{ik} denoting the corresponding expected proportion. For this example all of the E_{ik} are 0.5 and the value of the chi-square statistic is $4(0.01)/0.50 = 0.08$. Therefore, the effect size that PASS uses is $\sqrt{0.08} = 0.282843$. When this value is entered for the effect size, PASS gives $n = 159$ as the solution, in agreement with the solution given by nQuery Advisor, for example. ■

There is often a need to test the equality of multiple proportions, such as when comparing the work efficiency of several workers in a department. Ryan (2011, p. 592) gave an example, drawn from the author's consulting experience, involving the comparison of 20 (human) harvesters, with a desire to identify any who stand out in a positive way and whose performance traits should perhaps be studied by other workers, as well as those workers who are significantly below average and thus might need to be retrained or reassigned. This is best performed with a graphical test, whereas the chi-square test is obviously not a graphical test. Ryan (2011) showed that one of the human harvesters was significantly better than the average performance of all of them, and one harvester was significantly worse than the average performance.

An ANOM plot (but not for the data just mentioned), produced by MINITAB, showing one point above the upper decision line (UDL) is shown in Figure 4.3.

Another example of ANOM applied to proportions data was given by Homa (2007), in which she compared the referral rates of 17 providers, with spine patients who scored low on a mental health test being referred to Behavioral Medicine Services. This is not a sample size determination problem, though, since these are observational data and the sample size for each provider is the number of patient visits, which of course can't be set or predetermined. Nevertheless, it is of interest to look at the sample sizes, which of course varied among providers relative to the objective of the study, which was "to demonstrate through a case study how an analysis of means chart can be used to compare groups and to advocate the usefulness of this method in improvement work" (Homa, 2007). The ANOM analysis showed that three providers had a significantly higher rate than the overall average (using a .05 upper decision line), and three providers had a significantly lower rate (with a .05 lower decision line). Actually, multiple

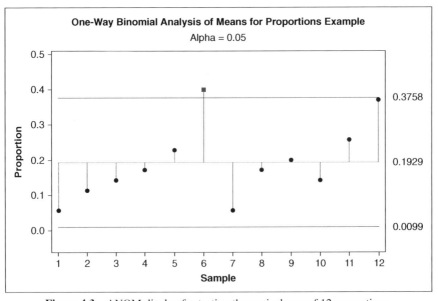

Figure 4.3 ANOM display for testing the equivalence of 12 proportions.

ANOM charts were constructed, being defined on each of several patient characteristics. The analysis led to some questions that would have to be addressed with further study.

There is almost certainly no software available for determining sample size for ANOM, and there is very little in the literature on the subject. Consequently, it is necessary to (attempt to) derive the sample size expression and we can proceed as follows. We first need to determine what magnitude of a difference we wish to detect. Since the relative strength of ANOM for proportions is in detecting an extreme proportion, the sample size might be determined for detecting a single proportion that might be a specified multiple of $\bar{p}$, such as 1.5 or 0.5, with $\bar{p}$ denoting, as before, the average of all of the plotted proportions and the other $(k - 1)$ proportions assumed to be representable by $\bar{p}$.

We immediately encounter somewhat of a potential mismatch, however, because the value of α is for testing *all* of the plotted proportions against the midline represented by $\bar{p}$, whereas we might be inclined to define β relative to testing a single large or small proportion, ignoring the other proportions.

As indicated earlier in this section, an alternative to using ANOM for testing the equality of proportions is to use a chi-square test, for which sample size determination software *is* available and was illustrated. A chi-square test is not as sensitive as ANOM for detecting a few extreme deviations, however, so if we are interested in extreme proportions in either direction, as in the human harvesters example, ANOM would be a better choice. Another problem is that it may be more difficult to specify a *logical* "effect" size for which it is desirable to detect, since a chi-square test produces a single number, as opposed to the ANOM display which shows each proportion plotted relative to the decision lines and the center line. Cohen (1988) recommended specifying an effect of .10, with the effect defined simply as χ^2/N, as discussed previously, with N denoting the sum of the counts in the $k \times 2$ table, with k denoting the number of proportions that are plotted. This effect size definition does not have any obvious intuitive meaning, however, so there are various reasons why ANOM for proportions should be used and why software should be available for determining sample size for such a procedure.

4.4 MULTINOMIAL PROBABILITIES AND DISTRIBUTIONS

The multinomial probability distribution is an extension of the binomial distribution. Although there has been some research on sample size determination for multinomial probabilities, notably by Adcock (1987, 1992, 1993) who considered Bayesian approaches and by Guenther (1977a) who considered sample size and power for hypotheses concerning multinomial probabilities with chi-square tests, sample size determination for estimating multinomial probabilities won't be pursued here. Instead, references are given for interested readers. Additional references include Bromaghin (1993) and Lee, Song, Kang, and Ahn (2002). See Nisen and Schwertman (2008) for sample size determination for chi-square tests used to test the equality of multinomial distributions.

4.5   ONE RATE

We will first consider a Poisson distribution, given by

$$f^*(x) = \frac{\exp(-\lambda)\lambda^x}{x!}$$

with λ denoting the Poisson parameter (rate) and of course X is the random variable with realization denoted by x. Although $\sum_{i=1}^{n} X_i$ has a Poisson distribution with parameter $n\lambda$, $\sum_{i=1}^{n} X_i/n$ does not. Therefore, one approach would be to use $\sum_{i=1}^{n} X_i$ as the test statistic, and Lenth's applet does use this test statistic. Assume that we wish to perform a one-sided test, with $\alpha = .05$, and want the power to be .90 for detecting an increase in λ from 1 to 1.5. Let λ_0 denote the hypothesized value of 1 and $\lambda_1 = 1.5$ denote the value that is to be detected.

We want to determine n such that $P(\sum_{i=1}^{n} X_i > c \mid \lambda = n\lambda_1) = .90$, with c determined such that $P(\sum_{i=1}^{n} X_i > c \mid \lambda = n\lambda_0) = .05$ (i.e., c is the critical value of the test). Since there is no expression for c that is a function of n, there is no equation to be solved for n. Furthermore, since the random variable is discrete, we generally cannot hit $\alpha = .05$ exactly, so we will use $\alpha < .05$. Since there is no equation to solve for n, as stated, it is necessary to use software and not all sample size determination software has this capability.

PASS does have the capability (under "means" in its main menu) but it does not perform an exact test since it determines sample size following Guenther (1977b), which utilizes the relationship between the chi-square and Poisson distributions [e.g., see Ulm (1990)]. Specifically, PASS determines the sample size by using the interval

$$\frac{\chi^2_{2d,1-\beta}}{2\lambda_1} \leq n \leq \frac{\chi^2_{2d,\alpha}}{2\lambda_0} \qquad d = 1, 2, 3, \ldots$$

with λ_0 denoting the hypothesized value of λ and λ_1 denoting the value of λ that is to be detected, with the first subscript on χ^2 denoting the degrees of freedom and the second subscript denoting the percentile of the chi-square distribution with $2d$ degrees of freedom. The value of n is found by increasing the value of d until the left interval endpoint is less than the right endpoint and the interval contains at least one integer. To illustrate, with the current example having $\lambda_0 = 1$ and $\lambda_1 = 1.5$, for a one-sided test with $\alpha = .05$ and power $= .90$, PASS gives

$n = 44$. This solution can be seen by observing that at $d = 56$ so that $2d = 112$, $\chi^2_{112,.90} = 131.558$ and $\chi^2_{112,.05} | = 88.5704$, so that the left endpoint is 43.8527 and the right endpoint is 44.2852, so that the interval barely contains $n = 44$. (It can be shown that the inequality is not satisfied at $2d = 110$, thus verifying that the solution is that obtained when $2d = 112$, so that $n = 44$.)

It should also be noted that a two-sided test is not a menu option in PASS, but the sample size for a two-sided test can be determined by specifying $\alpha/2$, as pointed out by the PASS help system.

Lenth's applet also has sample size capability for Poisson rates, as does Release 16 of MINITAB (but not in prior releases). Using Lenth's applet also results in $n = 44$ as the solution. The value of c is 55 as it can be shown that $P(\sum_{i=1}^{n} X_i > 55 | \lambda = (44)(1)) = .0456$, and $P(\sum_{i=1}^{n} X_i > 55 | \lambda = (44)(1.5)) = .9046$. Lenth gives the critical value as $c = 54$, however, whereas 55 is the largest value that would result in the null hypothesis not being rejected.

A normal approximation approach could be used, analogous to what is done with proportions, but that approximation will not work well when $\lambda < 5$, as it was in this example. An exact test is thus the preferred approach, with either PASS or Lenth's applet being good options as neither nQuery Advisor nor Power and Precision has the capability of either the exact approach or a normal approximation approach, nor does G*Power, Stata, or SiZ.

By comparison, the MINITAB solution for the preceding example is $n = 42$. For that solution, MINITAB gives the actual power of .9037 but there is no value of c that will produce .9037 for $\lambda = 42(1.5) = 63$. Thus, MINITAB could not have used an exact test and thus it is very likely the solution is obtained using a normal approximation approach, as the user does not have an option for the choice of test. It will often be desirable to first use a square root transformation for Poisson data before applying a normal approximation. Mathews (2010) gives the sample expression when that is done. Using that expression produces $n = 42.39$ so that $n = 43$ would be used. Thus, it is very probable that MINITAB used a normal approximation without a square root transformation.

Regarding other approaches, van Belle (2008, p. 420) gave a rule of thumb for the sample size that is the application of Eq. (3.7) to the Poisson case and also assuming the use of the square root transformation of Poisson data since $\sqrt{X}$ is approximately $N(\sqrt{\lambda}, 0.25)$. Substitution of these quantities into Eq. (3.7) produces $n = 4/(\sqrt{\lambda_0} - \sqrt{\lambda_1})^2$. Note that this could be used only for a power of .80 and a significance level for a two-sided test of .05. For detecting an increase in λ from 9 to 16, this formula gives $n = 16$, but this applies to the transformed variable $\sqrt{X}$, not to X. Therefore, it cannot be compared against the results obtained using sample size determination software for the Poisson parameter, as such calculations would be for the Poisson distribution, for which the mean and the variance are assumed to be equal. [It can be shown, however, that the sample size approximation is poor for a change in a normal mean from $\sqrt{9} = 3$ to $\sqrt{16} = 4$ when the variance is assumed to be 0.25, as Eq. (3.2) or the use of software produces $n = 2$. Recall that Eq. (3.7) has been criticized as being inaccurate, however, as discussed in Section 3.6. Thus, it is probably best not to use approximations based on that formula. Furthermore, of course, two approximations are being used in applying the van Belle rule of thumb, as an adequate approximation to normality is also being assumed. With today's computing power it is both unnecessary and undesirable to rely heavily on approximations.]

4.5.1 Pilot Study Needed?

As with the binomial distribution, the Poisson distribution has only one parameter, so there is no nuisance parameter to be estimated. Therefore, assuming that there is a good handle on what the null hypothesis should be, a pilot study might be considered to determine if the rate specified in the alternative hypothesis is reasonable, although what rate the user wants to detect might already have been determined with some certainty. Thus, there will not necessarily be a strong motivation for a pilot study when testing a Poisson rate, except in clinical trials work when there are three phases. Friede and Schmidli (2010) presented formulas for adjusting the sample size for Poisson-distributed data and for Poisson-distributed data with overdispersion (excess variability). In a thesis on sample size determination with an auditing application, Pedersen (2010) used a zero-inflated Poisson model (a model used to overcome problems posed by an excessive number of zeros with Poisson data) and considered sample sizes for both frequentist and Bayesian approaches.

4.6 TWO RATES

When a company has two (or more) plants, and one plant seems to be having trouble making a particular product, it would be desirable to compare the rate of nonconformities for the plants and do this repeatedly at specified intervals and to do this until the null hypothesis of equal rates cannot be rejected.

Specifically, assume that the rate at the better of two plants is 2 for some time period and the objective is to determine the (common) sample size so that a rate of 4 at the other plant is to be detected with probability (power) of .90. This might be addressed as a one-sample problem, using 2 as the desired value since that is the value for the first plant and the company personnel would then determine what would constitute an unacceptable rate for the second plant relative to that baseline value. This would permit the use of software such as MINITAB or Lenth's applet, as illustrated in Section 4.4. Unfortunately, there is apparently very little commercial software that can be used to determine sample size for testing the equality of two Poisson rates.

MINITAB does have a two-sample Poisson rate procedure in Release 16, which uses an unspecified iterative algorithm for determining the sample size. For example, if we specify a null hypothesis in which two Poisson rates are equal, then the "baseline rate" used by MINITAB, which is the ratio of the two Poisson rates under the null hypothesis, is 1.0. If the first Poisson rate is 0.8 and the second Poisson rate is 0.6 under the alternative hypothesis, so that the comparison rate is $0.8/0.6 = 1.33$, with $\alpha = .05$ and power $= .90$, the output gives a sample size of $n = 180$ for each of the two samples for a one-sided test.

This agrees with the formula for the sample size of the unconstrained maximum likelihood test given by Gu, Ng, Tang, and Schucany (2008), which is

$$n = \left[\frac{\left(c/\rho + c^2\right)\left(z_\alpha + z_\beta\right)^2}{(1-c)^2} \right]$$

with $\rho = 1$ when the null hypothesis is that the sampling rates are equal and the two fixed sampling frames are also equal, and c is the ratio of the two Poisson rates under the null hypothesis divided by the ratio of the first rate to the second rate under the alternative hypothesis, provided that the ratio exceeds the ratio under the null hypothesis. Thus, for this example,

$$n = \left[\frac{(0.75 + 0.75)^2(1.645 + 1.28155)^2}{(1 - .75)^2} \right]$$
$$= 179.859$$

so that $n = 180$ would be used.

PASS also has the capability for a two-sample Poisson test, with its test being one of the four types of tests covered by Gu et al. (2008). The user has five options for the test statistic, with the unconstrained maximum likelihood test in which the two Poisson means are estimated separately being the default. Unlike MINITAB's routine, the two-sample Poisson routine in PASS requires that the ratio of the two means be specified in both the null and alternative hypotheses. The use of PASS for the unconstrained maximum likelihood test also gives $n_1 = n_2 = 300$, in agreement with MINITAB. (The same sample size is obtained if use of the constrained maximum likelihood test is assumed, for which the two Poisson means are estimated jointly.)

Gu et al. (2008), however, performed simulations and found that the asymptotic test derived from the variance-stabilizing transformation proposed by Huffman (1984) was the most reliable asymptotic test, being conservative but having high power. This is the last of the five options available in PASS.

Gu et al. (2008) gave the sample size formulas for all of the methods that they covered, with the formula for their preferred test, based on the variance-stabilizing transformation, being

$$n = \left[\frac{z_\alpha \sqrt{c/\rho + c} + z_\beta \sqrt{1 + c/\rho}}{2 \left(1 - \sqrt{c}\right)} \right]^2 - \frac{3}{8}$$

with $\rho = R/d$ and R is the ratio under the null hypothesis of the first Poisson mean (i.e., rate) divided by the second Poisson mean, $c = R/R'$, with R' denoting the ratio of the Poisson means under the alternative hypothesis, and $d = t_1/t_0$, with t_1 and t_0 denoting the fixed sampling frames (i.e., time intervals) for the two Poisson processes.

Continuing with the example given earlier in this section, for this test PASS gives the sample size as 319 for each sample. Except for this result, the sample sizes are almost identical (300, 300, 302, and 296, respectively) for the first four options in PASS.

Using hand computation, we obtain

$$n = \left[\frac{z_\alpha \sqrt{c/\rho + c} + z_\beta \sqrt{1 + c/\rho}}{2 \left(1 - \sqrt{c}\right)} \right]^2 - \frac{3}{8}$$

$$= \left[\frac{1.645\sqrt{0.75 + 0.75} + 1.28155\sqrt{1 + .75}}{2 \left(1 - \sqrt{.75}\right)} \right]^2 - \frac{3}{8}$$

$$= 191.338$$

so $n = 192$ would be used. Notice that this sample size is almost 7% greater than the sample size obtained for the unconstrained maximum likelihood test.

Nelson (1991) gave a normal approximation approach and provided a computer program (written in BASIC) for performing the computations, but a normal approximation approach won't work when the Poisson rates are small, as will be the case in many applications.

A method for determining sample size and power in comparing two Poisson rates has been given by Thode (1997) and by Hand, Stamey, and Young (2011). See also Stamey and Katsis (2007) for the case of rates that are underreported. Gu et al. (2008) examined the proposed methods for testing two Poisson rates when the null hypothesis for the ratio of the rates does not equal 1. They provided sample size formulas for each approach and gave their recommendations. Shiue and Bain (1982) considered the determination of the experiment length needed to achieve a specified power for an approximate test when the two intervals are equal and when they are unequal. Ng and Tang (2005) considered methods for testing the equality of Poisson means when the intervals are unequal and gave sample size formulas for that case.

Although not well known, the distribution of the difference of two Poisson random variables is due to Skellam (1946), and is referred to as the Skellam distribution. Menon, Massaro, Lewis, Pencina, Wang, and Lavin (2011) used this exact distribution in a proposed procedure. They gave an example to illustrate their methodology, which is as follows. Suppose there is interest in the relapse rate per year of an infectious disease for two treatments. The rate for the standard treatment is expected to be 6.25, and 5.15 for the new treatment. Assume that the target power for detecting this difference is .90 and a one-sided test with $\alpha =$ .05 is to be performed. They gave $n = 87$ as the sample size to be used for each group. (Their method is in the `skellam` package that is in R.) By comparison, when MINITAB is used, the solution is $n = 81$, so the exact procedure requires a slightly larger sample size.

4.7 BAYESIAN SAMPLE SIZE DETERMINATION METHODS FOR RATES

Bayesian sample size determination methods for both one and two Poisson rates were given by Stamey, Young, and Bratcher (2006), who gave two actual quality control examples and compared the results to sample sizes determined using frequentist methods.

4.8 SOFTWARE

Unlike the case with sample means, there is some disagreement among software that handles sample size determination for proportions, as was indicated in Section 4.1.2. As another example, for the case of a hypothesized proportion of .50, an upper-tailed test with no continuity correction, and an assumed true proportion of .60, with power of .80, Lenth's applet gives a sample size of 153, as does MINITAB, Stata, and Power and Precision, but PASS gives 146. There is disagreement because the latter uses a combination of a normal approximation approach and an exact approach, whereas the others use a normal approximation approach throughout.

There are, of course, applets that can be used for determining sample size with one or two proportions, in addition to Lenth's applet, although not all of these can be recommended. One of these other applets is at http://statpages.org/ proppowr.html but it is not clear what alternative hypothesis is being assumed.

There is very little available software for determining sample size for testing the equality of two Poisson rates. Lenth's applet can be used for one rate, but not for the test of the equality of two rates. PASS and MINITAB can be used for this purpose, however, as was illustrated, but sample size for two rates cannot be determined using either nQuery Advisor, Power and Precision, G*Power, or Stata.

4.9 SUMMARY

This chapter contained considerable discussion of the options that a user has in determining sample size for either one or two proportions. Certain software do not provide options, however, and the user needs to be cognizant of the method that is being used to determine sample size. Software for rates is not as plentiful as software for proportions, and this is especially true for two rates.

APPENDIX

(a) Derivation of Eq. (4.2)—No Continuity Correction

As with any sample size formula derivation, the first step is to obtain the expression for β since the formula will be a function of β. The test statistic is

$$Z = \frac{\hat{p} - p_0}{\sqrt{\dfrac{p_0(1 - p_0)}{n}}} \tag{A.1}$$

which is approximately $N(0,1)$ when n is large only if $p = p_0$, with the latter denoting the hypothesized value of p. The term "power" has meaning only if $p \neq p_0$ and as pointed out in Chapter 1, null hypotheses are almost always false anyway. We will let p_1 denote the actual value of p.

The sample size expression in Eq. (4.2) does not depend on the direction of the inequality, but for the derivation we will assume that it is an upper-tailed test so that the critical value of Z is z_α. The null hypothesis is erroneously not rejected if

$$\frac{\hat{p} - p_0}{\sqrt{\dfrac{p_0(1 - p_0)}{n}}} < z_\alpha \tag{A.2}$$

Since the left side of Expresssion (A.2) is not approximately $N(0,1)$ when $p = p_1$, it is necessary to modify that expression to create an expression that is approximately $N(0,1)$. Since $E(\hat{p}) = p_1$, the expected value of the left side of expression

(A.2) is $(p_1 - p_0)/\sqrt{p_0(1 - p_0)/n}$. Since $\hat{p}$ is the only random variable on the left side, the variance of the expression *might seem to be*

$$\text{Var}\left(\frac{\hat{p} - p_0}{\sqrt{\dfrac{p_0(1 - p_0)}{n}}}\right) = \frac{p_1(1 - p_1)/n}{p_0(1 - p_0)/n}$$

Therefore, the appropriate standardization would be

$$\frac{\dfrac{\hat{p} - p_0}{\sqrt{\dfrac{p_0(1 - p_0)}{n}}} - \dfrac{p_1 - p_0}{\sqrt{\dfrac{p_0(1 - p_0)}{n}}}}{\sqrt{\dfrac{p_1(1 - p_1)/n}{p_0(1 - p_0)/n}}} < \frac{z_\alpha - \dfrac{p_1 - p_0}{\sqrt{\dfrac{p_0(1 - p_0)}{n}}}}{\sqrt{\dfrac{p_1(1 - p_1)/n}{p_0(1 - p_0)/n}}}$$

$$< \frac{z_\alpha\sqrt{\dfrac{p_0(1 - p_0)}{n}} - (p_1 - p_0)}{\sqrt{\dfrac{p_1(1 - p_1)}{n}}} = C\text{(say)}$$

Thus, $\beta = \Phi\,(C)$, so that $C = \Phi^{-1}(\beta)$. Therefore,

$$z_\alpha\sqrt{\frac{p_0(1 - p_0)}{p_1(1 - p_1)}} - \frac{p_1 - p_0}{\sqrt{\dfrac{p_1(1 - p_1)}{n}}} = \Phi^{-1}(\beta) = z_\beta = -z_\beta$$

so

$$-\frac{p_1 - p_0}{\sqrt{\dfrac{p_1(1 - p_1)}{n}}} = -z_\beta - z_\alpha\sqrt{\frac{p_0(1 - p_0)}{p_1(1 - p_1)}}$$

Solving this last equation for n produces

$$n = \left[\frac{z_\alpha\sqrt{p_0(1 - p_0)} + z_\beta\sqrt{p_1(1 - p_1)}}{p_1 - p_0}\right]^2 \qquad \text{(A.3)}$$

For a two-sided test, z_α would be replaced by $z_{\alpha/2}$.

The sample size expression given by Eq. (A.3) is what is given by Fleiss et al. (2003) and used by the software nQuery as well as Russ Lenth's software. These book authors, Lenth, and the developers of the single proportion routine in nQuery would undoubtedly agree with the derivation given here. However, under the classical Neyman–Pearson theory of hypothesis testing, parameters that appear in test statistics, and hence in sample size formulas that are derived from those test statistics, are set equal to their values under the null hypothesis. When this is done here, Eq. (A.3) becomes

$$n = \left[\frac{(z_\alpha + z_\beta)\sqrt{p_0(1 - p_0)}}{p' - p_0} \right]^2 \tag{A.4}$$

which is the expression given by Chow et al. (2008, p. 86). Thus, there is disagreement about the formula for n, although the sample sizes should not differ very much between the two formulas unless p' differs more than slightly from p_0. Fleiss et al. (2003) derived their sample size expression from the expression for power at p'. Since this is based on the assumption that p' is the true proportion, this results in p' being in more than just the denominator in the expression for n.

(b) Derivation of Eq. (4.6)—No Continuity Correction

We can proceed analogously to the derivation of Eq. (4.1). That is, we start with the test statistic

$$Z = \frac{\hat{p}_1 - \hat{p}_2 - 0}{\sqrt{\dfrac{2\bar{p}(1 - \bar{p})}{n}}} \tag{A.5}$$

with 0 representing the value of $p_1 - p_2$ under the null hypothesis, n is the assumed common sample size for samples from the two populations, and $\bar{p} = (\hat{p}_1 + \hat{p}_2)/2$ for a common sample size.

As in the derivation of the sample size expression for a single proportion, we will assume an upper-tailed test so that the null hypothesis of $p_1 = p_2$ should be rejected in favor of the alternative hypothesis, $p_1 > p_2$. Under the alternative hypothesis, the expected value and the variance of the Z-statistic in Eq. (A.3) are approximately

$$\frac{p_1 - p_2}{\sqrt{\dfrac{2\bar{p}^*(1 - \bar{p}^*)}{n}}} \quad \text{and} \quad \sqrt{\frac{[p_1(1 - p_1) + p_2(1 - p_2)]/n}{2\bar{p}^*(1 - \bar{p}^*)/n}}$$

respectively, with $\bar{p}^* = (p_1 + p_2)/2$. The results are approximate because the denominator in Eq. (A.3), which contains the random variable $\bar{p}$, is treated as a constant. Then,

$$\frac{z_\alpha - \dfrac{p_1 - p_2}{\sqrt{\dfrac{2\bar{p}^*(1 - \bar{p}^*)}{n}}}}{\sqrt{\dfrac{[p_1(1 - p_1) + p_2(1 - p_2)]/n}{2\bar{p}^*(1 - \bar{p}^*)/n}}} = \Phi^{-1}(\beta)$$

so

$$\frac{\sqrt{\dfrac{2\bar{p}^*(1 - \bar{p}^*)}{n}}\,z_\alpha - (p_1 - p_2)}{\sqrt{\dfrac{p_1(1 - p_1) + p_2(1 - p_2)}{n}}} = \Phi^{-1}(\beta) = z_\beta = -z_\beta$$

Thus,

$$z_\alpha \left[\frac{\sqrt{2\bar{p}^*(1 - \bar{p}^*)}}{\sqrt{p_1(1 - p_1) + p_2(1 - p_2)}} \right] = -z_\beta + \sqrt{n} \left[\frac{(p_1 - p_2)}{\sqrt{p_1(1 - p_1) + p_2(1 - p_2)}} \right]$$

and solving this equation for n produces Eq. (4.6), after substituting $(p_1 + p_2)/2$ for $\bar{p}^*$ That is,

$$n = \left(\frac{z_\alpha \sqrt{2\bar{p}^*(1 - \bar{p}^*)} + z_\beta \sqrt{p_1(1 - p_1) + p_2(1 - p_2)}}{(p_1 - p_2)} \right)^2$$

before $(p_1 + p_2)/2$ is substituted for $\bar{p}^*$, with that substitution then producing Eq. (4.6).

(c) Explanation of Eq. (4.9)—Using Continuity Correction for Two Proportions

In using the continuity correction for the two-proportion case, we proceed analogously to the one-sample case. Specifically, if the alternative hypothesis is $p_1 - p_2 > 0$, then we should think of p_1 "starting" (loosely speaking, in terms of continuity correction) at $p_1 - 1/2n$. Similarly, we should think of p_2 as "ending" at $p_2 + 1/2n$. The numerator of the statistic should then be $p_1 - 1/2n - (p_2 + 1/2n) = p_1 - p_2 - 1/n$. If the alternative hypothesis had been $p_1 - p_2 < 0$, the numerator would have been $p_1 - p_2 + 1/n$. Let $p_1 - p_2 = a$ for the case $p_1 - p_2 > 0$ and $-a$ for the case $p_1 - p_2 < 0$. We then have $a - 1/n$ and $-a + 1/n$, so that the negative of the latter is the former. The sample size will, of course, be the same for the two cases, so we want to use $|-a+1/n|$ in computing the required sample size. As explained by Fleiss et al. (2003, p. 72), the sample size formula gives the impression that only one continuity correction is being employed because the second continuity correction effectively cancels out the round-off error. [See also the explanation of this given by Levin and Chen (1999, p. 64).]

REFERENCES

Adcock, C. J. (1987). A Bayesian approach to calculating sample sizes for multinomial sampling. *The Statistician*, **36**, 155–159.

Adcock, C. J. (1992). Bayesian approaches to the determination of sample sizes for binomial and multinomial sampling—some comments on the paper by Pham-Gia and Turkkan. *The Statistician*, **41**, 399–401.

Adcock, C. J. (1993). A improved Bayesian approach for calculating sample sizes for multinomial sampling. *The Statistician*, **42**(2), 91–95.

Afshartous, D. (2008). Sample size determination for binomial proportion confidence intervals: An alternative perspective motivated by a legal case. *The American Statistician*, **62**, 27–31.

Agresti, A. and B. A. Coull (1998). Approximate is better than "exact" for interval estimation of binomial proportions. *The American Statistician*, **52**(2), 119–126.

Armitage, P. (1955). Tests for linear trends in proportions and frequencies. *Biometrics*, **11**(3), 375–386.

Berkson, J. (1978). In dispraise of the exact test. *Journal of Statistical Planning and Inference*, **2**, 27–42.

Blackwelder, W. (1982). Proving the null hypothesis in clinical trials. *Controlled Clinical Trials*, **3**, 345–353.

Blackwelder, W.C. (1998). Equivalence Trials. In *Encyclopedia of Biostatistics, Volume 2*, 1367–1372. New York: Wiley.

Brittain, E. and J. J. Schlesselman (1982). Optimal allocation for the comparison of proportions. *Biometrics*, **38**, 1003–1009.

Bromaghin, J. F. (1993). Sample size determination for interval estimation of multinomial probabilities. *The American Statistician*, **47**(3), 203– 206.

Brooks, R. J., A. M. Cottenden, and M. J. Fader (2003). Sample sizes for designed studies with correlated binary data. *Journal of the Royal Statistical Society, Series D*, **52**, 539–551.

Campbell, M. J., S. A. Julious, and D. G. Altman (1995). Estimating sample sizes for binary, ordered categorical, and continuous outcomes in two group comparisons. *British Medical Journal*, **311**, 1145–1148.

Casagrande, J. T., M. C. Pike, and P. G. Smith (1978a). An improved approximate formula for calculating sample sizes for comparing two binomial distributions. *Biometrics*, **34**, 483–486.

Casagrande, J. T., M. C. Pike, and P. G. Smith (1978b). The power function of the "exact" test for comparing two binomial proportions. *Applied Statistics*, **78**, 176–180.

Cesana, B. M., G. Reina, and E. Marubini (2001). Sample size for testing a proportion in clinical trials: A "two-step" procedure combining power and confidence interval expected width. *The American Statistician*, **55**, 265–270.

Chan, I. S. F. (2002). Power and sample size determination for noninferiority trials using an exact method. *Journal of Biopharmaceutical Statistics*, **12**, 457–469.

Chernick, M. R. and C. Y. Liu (2002). The saw-toothed behavior of power versus sample and software solutions: Single binomial proportion using exact methods. *The American Statistician*, **56**(2), 149–155.

Chow, S.-C, J. Shao, and H. Wang (2008). *Sample Size Calculations in Clinical Research*, 2nd edition. Boca Raton, FL: Chapman & Hall/CRC.

Clopper, C. J. and E. S. Pearson (1934). The use of confidence or fiducial limits illustrated in the case of the binomial. *Biometrika*, **26**, 404–413.

Cohen, J. (1988). *Statistical Power Analysis for the Behavioral Sciences*. Philadelphia: Lawrence Erlbaum Associates.

Conover, W. J. (1980). *Practical Nonparametric Statistics*, 2nd edition. New York: Wiley.

D'Agostino, R. B., W. Chase, and A. Belanger (1988). The appropriateness of some common procedures for testing equality of two independent binomial proportions. *The American Statistician*, **42**(3), 198–202.

Farrington, C. P. and G. Manning (1990). Test statistics and sample size formulae for comparative binomial trials with null hypothesis of non-zero risk difference or non-unity relative risk. *Statistics in Medicine*, **9**, 1447–1454.

Fleiss, J. L., A. Tytun, and H. K. Ury (1980). A simple approximation for calculating sample sizes for comparing independent proportions. *Biometrics*, **36**, 343–346.

Fleiss, J. L., B. Levin, and M. C. Paik (2003). *Statistical Methods for Rates and Proportions*, 3rd edition. Hoboken, NJ: Wiley.

Friede, T. and M. Kieser (2004). Sample size recalculation for binary data in internal pilot study designs. *Pharmaceutical Statistics*, **3**(4), 269–279.

Friede, T. and H. Schmidli (2010). Blinded sample size reestimation with count data: Methods and applications in multiple sclerosis. *Statistics in Medicine*, **29**, 1145–1156.

Gould, A. L. (1983). Sample sizes required for binomial trials when the true response rates are estimated. *Journal of Statistical Planning and Inference*, **8**, 51–58.

Gordon, I. and R. Watson (1996). The myth of continuity-corrected sample size formulae. *Biometrics*, **52**, 71–76.

Gu, K., H. K. T. Ng, M. L. Tang, and W. Schucany (2008). Testing the ratio of two Poisson rates. *Biometrical Journal*, **50**(2), 283–298.

Guenther, W. C. (1977a). Power and sample size for approximate chi-square tests. *The American Statistician*, **31**, 83–85.

Guenther, W. C. (1977b). *Sampling Inspection in Statistical Quality Control*. Griffin's Statistical Monographs, No. 37. London: Griffin.

Hand, A. L., J. D. Stamey, and D. M. Young (2011). Bayesian sample-size determination for two independent Poisson rates. *Computer Methods and Programs in Biomedicine*, **104**(2), 271–277.

Homa, K. (2007). Analysis of Means used to compare providers' referral patterns. *Quality Management in Health Care*, **16**(3), 256–264.

Huffman, M. (1984). An improved approximate two-sample Poisson test. *Applied Statistics*, **33**(2), 224–226.

Joseph, L., D. B. Wolfson, and R. du Berger (1995). Some comments on Bayesian sample size determination. *The Statistician*, **44**(2), 167–171.

Joseph, L., R. Du Berger, and P. Bélisle (1997). Bayesian and mixed Bayesian/likelihood criteria for sample size determination. *Statistics in Medicine*, **16**(2), 769–781.

Kawasaki, Y., F. Zhang, and E. Miyaoka (2010). Comparisons of test statistics for noninferiority test for the difference between two independent binomial proportions. *American Journal of Biostatistics*, **1**(1), 23–30.

Khuri, A. I. (1978). A conservative sample size for the comparison of several proportions. *Communications in Statistics—Theory and Methods*, **7**(13), 1283–1293.

Lee, M.-K., H.-H. Song, S.-H. Kang, and C. W. Ahn (2002). The determination of sample sizes in the comparison of two multinomial proportions from ordered categories. *Biometrical Journal*, **44**, 395–409.

Levin, B. and X. Chen (1999). Is the one-half continuity correction used once or twice to derive a well-known approximate sample size formula to compare two independent binomial distributions? *The American Statistician*, **53**, 62–66.

Levy, P. S. and S. Lemeshow (1991). *Sampling of Populations: Methods and Applications*. New York: Wiley.

Mathews, P. (2010). *Sample Size Calculations: Practical Methods for Engineers and Scientists*. Fairport Harbor, OH: Mathews Malnar and Bailey, Inc.

McNemar, Q. (1947). Note on the sampling error of the difference of two correlated proportions or percentages. *Psychometrika*, **12**(2), 153–157.

Menon, S., J. Massaro, J. Lewis, M. Pencina, Y.-C. Wang, and P. Lavin (2011). Sample size calculation for Poisson endpoint using the exact distribution of difference between two Poisson random variables. *Statistics in Biopharmaceutical Research*, **3**(3), 497–504.

M'Lan, C. E., L. Joseph, and D. B. Wolfson (2008). Bayesian sample size determination for binomial proportions. *Bayesian Analysis*, **3**(2), 269–296.

Nam, J.-M. (1987). A simple approximation for calculating sample sizes for detecting linear trends in proportions. *Biometrics*, **43**, 701–705.

Nam, J.-M. (2011). Power and sample size requirements for non-inferiority in studies comparing two matched proportions where the events are correlated. *Computational Statistics and Data Analysis*, **55**, 2880–2887.

Nelson, L. S. (1991). Power in comparing Poisson means: II. Two-sample test. *Journal of Quality Technology*, **23**(2), 163–166.

Newcombe, R. G. (1998). Two-sided confidence intervals for the single proportion: Comparison of seven methods. *Statistics in Medicine*, **17**, 857–872.

Ng, H. K. T. and M. L. Tang (2005). Testing the equality of two Poisson means using the rate ratio. *Statistics in Medicine*, **24**, 955–965.

Nisen, J. A. and N. C. Schwertman (2008). A simple method of computing the sample size for chi-square test for the equality of multinomial distributions. *Computational Statistics and Data Analysis*, **52**(11), 4903–4908.

Pedersen, K. (2010). Sample size determination in auditing accounts receivable using a zero-inflated Poisson model. M.S. thesis, Worcester Polytechnic Institute.

Pham-Gia, T. and N. Turkkan (1992). Sample size determination in Bayesian analysis. *The Statistician*, **41**, 389–397.

Pham-Gia, T. and N. Turkkan (2003). Determination of exact sample sizes in the Bayesian estimation of the difference of two proportions. *The Statistician*, **52**, 131–150.

Royston, P. (1993). Exact conditional and unconditional sample size for pair-matched studies with binary outcome: A practical guide. *Statistics in Medicine*, **12**, 699–712.

Ryan, T. P. (2007). *Modern Engineering Statistics*. Hoboken, NJ: Wiley.

Ryan, T. P. (2011). *Statistical Methods for Quality Improvement*, 3rd edition. Hoboken, NJ: Wiley.

Samuels, M. L. and T. C. Lu (1992). Sample size requirements for the back-of-the-envelope binomial confidence interval. *The American Statistician*, **46**(3), 228–231.

Schader, M. and F. Schmid (1989). Two rules of thumb for the approximation of the binomial distribution by the normal distribution. *The American Statistician*, **43**, 23–24.

Schork, M. and G. Williams (1980). Number of observations required for the comparison of two correlated proportions. *Communications in Statistics—Simulation and Computation*, **B9**(4), 349–357.

Shiue, W.-K. and L. J. Bain (1982). Experiment size and power comparisons for two-sample Poisson tests. *Applied Statistics*, **31**,130–134.

Skellam, J. G. (1946). The frequency distribution of the difference between two Poisson variates belonging to different populations. *Journal of the Royal Statistical Society, Series A*, **109**, 296.

Stamey, J. and A. Katsis (2007). Sample size determination for comparing two Poisson rates with underreported counts. *Communications in Statistics—Simulation and Computation*, **36**(3), 483–492.

Stamey, J., D. M. Young, and T. L. Bratcher (2006). Bayesian sample-size determination for one and two Poisson rate parameters with applications to quality control. *Journal of Applied Statistics*, **33**(6), 583–594.

Suissa, S. and J. J. Shuster (1985). Exact unconditional sample sizes for the 2 × 2 binomial trial. *Journal of the Royal Statistical Society, Series A*, **148**, 317–327.

Thode, H. C. Jr. (1997). Power and sample size requirements for tests of differences between two Poisson rates. *The Statistician*, **46**(2), 227–230.

Tobi, H.; P. B. van den Berg, and L. T. de Jong-van den Berg (2005). Small proportions: What to report for confidence intervals? *Pharmacoepidemiology Drug Safety*, **14**(4), 239–247. Erratum: **15**(3), 211.

Ulm, K. (1990). A simple method to calculate the confidence interval of a standardized mortality ratio. *American Journal of Epidemiology*, **131**(2), 373–375.

Upton, G. J. G. (1982). A comparison of alternative tests for the 2 × 2 comparative trial. *Journal of the Royal Statistical Society, Ser A*, **145**, 86–105.

Ury, H. K. and J. L. Fleiss (1980). On approximate sample sizes for comparing two independent proportions with the use of Yates' correction. *Biometrics* **36**, 347–351.

van Belle, G. (2008). *Statistical Rules of Thumb*, 2nd edition. Hoboken, NJ: Wiley.

Vollset, S. E. (1993). Confidence intervals for a binomial proportion. *Statistics in Medicine*, **12**(9), 873–890 (author's reply: **13**, 809–824).

Walter, S. D. (1977). Determination of significant relative risks and optimal sampling procedures in prospective and retrospective comparative studies of various sizes. *American Journal of Epidemiology*, **105**, 387–397.

Williams, M. S., E. D. Ebel, and B. A. Wagner (2007). Monte Carlo approaches for determining power and sample size in low-prevalence applications. *Preventive Veterinary Medicine*, **82**, 151–158.

EXERCISES

4.1. Derive the sample size of 296 that was given, just after Eq. (4.6), in an example in Section 4.2.

4.2. The website for the American Academy of Periodontology states that 30 percent of adults over the age of 50 have periodontal disease. Literature handed out by a dentist (true story) stated that 3 out of 4 adults over the age of 35 have periodontal disease. The state dental board doesn't believe the literature but decides to perform a hypothesis test, using .30 as the null hypothesis and wanting the power to be (at least) .80 for an assumed true proportion of .75. Would a large or small sample be needed to detect .75 as the true value when the hypothesized value is .30 and a one-sided test is performed? Do the necessary hand computation or use software and determine the necessary sample size, using $\alpha = .05$.

4.3. Explain why it isn't necessary to select a value for $\sigma_{\hat{p}}$ for a one-sample test of a proportion.

4.4. Determine the sample size necessary for detecting a true proportion of .40 in a one-sided test with the null hypothesis being that the proportion is .50. Use $\alpha = .05$.

4.5. Assuming a one-sided test with $\alpha = .05$, determine the sample size necessary to detect an increase in the Poisson parameter from 5 to 6 with a power of .80.

4.6. Show by using the letters for Eq. (4.8) in Eq. (4.5) that the former is equal to the square of the latter.

CHAPTER 5

Regression Methods and Correlation

We run into some problems when we try to apply sample size determination methods to regression models, as will be seen in this chapter. The types of problems encountered vary with the type of model used and the number of regression variables in the model.

There are many important applications of regression over a wide variety of fields, however, so it is highly desirable to try to overcome these problems. For example, many colleges and universities have used regression prediction equations to predict a prospective student's college grade point average (GPA) if the student were admitted, and to make an admittance decision based partly on that result. Several researchers have investigated the minimum sample size for regression models developed for this purpose and this is discussed in Section 5.1.2.1.

5.1 LINEAR REGRESSION

The general form for a multiple regression model is typically written

$$Y = \beta_0 + \beta_1 X_1 + \beta_2 X_2 + \cdots + \beta_m X_m + \epsilon \tag{5.1}$$

with Y the dependent variable, $X_1, X_2, \ldots, X_m$ the independent variables (also called the predictors or regressors), and ϵ the error term, with the error terms assumed to be independent and to have a normal distribution with a mean of zero and a common variance of σ_ϵ^2.

The simplest approach to determining sample size is to adopt the Draper and Smith (1998) rule-of-thumb and use at least 10 observations for each predictor in a linear regression model. This recommendation had also been made by Halinksi and Feldt (1970) and Miller and Kunce (1973). That isn't possible in many types of

Sample Size Determination and Power, First Edition. Thomas P. Ryan.
© 2013 John Wiley & Sons, Inc. Published 2013 by John Wiley & Sons, Inc.

applications, however, especially in chemometric applications where the number of predictors will often exceed the number of observations. So determination of sample size for regression problems will often be necessary, with the sample size that is obtained perhaps compared with the sample size using the Draper and Smith (1998) rule-of-thumb.

5.1.1 Simple Linear Regression

The simple linear regression model is

$$Y = \beta_0 + \beta_1 X + \epsilon$$

That is, there is just a single independent variable, X.

Work on determining sample size to estimate β_1 when both X and Y are random (the usual case in practice but not in textbooks) dates at least from Thigpen (1987).

Unfortunately, if we take an analytical approach to sample size determination, we can run into problems, depending on how we proceed, even when there is only a single predictor. Adcock (1997) explained that it is necessary not only to specify the nonzero value of β_1 that constitutes the alternative hypothesis in simple linear regression, but also to supply estimates of σ_ϵ^2 and the variance of the predictor values. Of course, the latter can be estimated reasonably well if the predictor values are to be fixed, but it may be very difficult to estimate if the values are not fixed. For random X, the same approach might be used as was discussed in Section 2.1; that is, use the range of likely values divided by 6 in place of s_x.

We can avoid those problems, however, if we do not focus on testing β_1 but instead specify the value of r^2 (the square of the Pearson correlation between X and Y) that would be considered acceptable and that we want to detect. This would be for a test of $\rho = 0$ as the null hypothesis, with ρ designating the population correlation between X and Y. That is, the test would be outside the realm of regression but would apply to the regression model. This is perfectly reasonable because if a simple linear regression model is written in "correlation form," the slope coefficient is the correlation between X and Y. That is, the model would be written as $Y - \bar{Y} = \beta^*(X - \bar{X}) + \epsilon$, with β^* then being the correlation coefficient.

Another problem, not addressed by Adcock (1997), is that it is not sufficient just to reject H_0: $\beta_1 = 0$, as the model could still have poor predictive value. We can also avoid this problem by focusing on r^2 and using sample size determination software that has this option.

Despite this, undoubtedly many users will want to focus on β_1 when it has an easy and important physical interpretation. Therefore, we will address how to proceed when that is the focal point. As explained by Ryan (2009a, p. 20), if we adapt the work of Wetz (1964) to the test of H_0: $\beta_1 = 0$, we would conclude that the model is useful only if the value of the t-statistic for testing the hypothesis is at least twice the critical value. We can actually use this rule-of-thumb to circumvent the problem of having to specify values of σ_ϵ^2 and the variance (or the standard deviation) of the predictor values, although in doing so we do run into some other problems.

This is illustrated in the following example.

■ **EXAMPLE 5.1**

Consider the use of Lenth's applet, which requires that the user enter values for s_x, the standard deviation of the X-values, s_e, the standard deviation of the residuals (the observed values minus the values from the fitted model), and the "detectable beta," which is defined as "the clinically meaningful value of the regression coefficient that you want to be able to detect." The input requirements for PASS are essentially the same, except that the user must enter the standard deviation of the residuals rather than the error standard deviation, which is essentially just a semantic difference. (There are many other options for sample size determination software for simple linear regression, including the user-written command `sampsi_reg` for Stata.)

When a t-test is used to test H_0: $\beta_1 = 0$, the t-statistic is

$$ t = \frac{\hat{\beta}_1}{s_e / \sqrt{S_{xx}}} $$

with $S_{xx} = \sum_{i=1}^n (x_i - \bar{x})^2$. Since $\sqrt{n-1}\, s_x = \sqrt{S_{xx}}$, it follows that we may write the t-statistic as

$$ t = \frac{\hat{\beta}_1}{s_e / (\sqrt{n-1}\, s_x)} = \left(\frac{s_x}{s_e}\right) \hat{\beta}_1 \sqrt{n-1} $$

If we apply the adaptation of the Wetz (1964) rule-of-thumb, we would want to have $t = (s_x/s_e)\hat{\beta}_1\sqrt{n-1} \geq 2t_{\alpha/2,n-2}$ for a two-sided test. Since the right side will slightly exceed 4 for most sample sizes, we might enter $s_x = s_e = \hat{\beta}_1 = 1$ into an applet or software. This would be a reasonable starting point because both power and the value of the t-statistic depend only on the ratio, s_x/s_e, not on the individual values. Furthermore, these are the default values that the user of Lenth's applet encounters. The objective would be to see if the sample size that is produced is at least 18, since the left side of the last inequality would then be at least $\sqrt{17} = 4.12$, and thus be at least slightly greater than 4, as desired. Lenth's applet produces $n = 11$ if power is to be at least .80, with power being .8385 for that sample size.

Similarly, when PASS is used, entering "1" for "Standard Deviation of Residuals" and for "Standard Deviation of Xs," with slope of 0 specified for B0 (the null hypothesis) and 1 for Bl (the alternative hypothesis), power $= .80$ and $\alpha = .05$ for a two-tailed test, the software gives $n = 11$ and power $= .8385$, in agreement with Lenth's applet.

If a sample of that size were taken resulting in $\hat{\beta}_1 = 1$ and $s_x = s_e$, the value of the t-statistic would be $\sqrt{10} = 3.16$, which is far short of $2t_{\alpha/2,n-2} = 2t_{.025,9} = 2(2.262) = 4.524$. Thus, although the power is .8385 for detecting a value of β_1 that is 3.16 times the standard error of $\hat{\beta}_1$, the Wetz (1964) criterion is not met because 3.16 is less than 4.524. Consequently, it would be a good idea to increase the sample size and ignore a target value of .80 for the power, as that is just an arbitrary value anyway. It is necessary to use $n \geq 19$ in order for the Wetz criterion to be met; using $n = 19$ produces a power of .9839. This satisfies the Draper–Smith rule-of-thumb (as did $n = 11$) and may also satisfy the Wetz criterion, depending on the sample values.

This ad hoc procedure seems to be a reasonable way to overcome the problems posed by the input requirements for determining sample size when an applet or software is used, especially since quantities such as s_e depend on how well the model explains the dependent variable, and a value for s_x will generally be hard to determine if the values of the regressor are not preselected. (Regressor values are random in most applications.) Furthermore, the focal point should be determining the sample size that will enable the user to determine if the model is useful, not being able to detect a (perhaps) arbitrary value of β_1 for an arbitrary power value of .80. Therefore, even if there is a theoretical basis for an experimenter to believe that β_1 should be equal to a certain value in a particular application, it would still be desirable to use the ad hoc approach given in this section and compare the sample sizes that are obtained using each approach, using the result from the ad hoc approach as a benchmark. Of course, the ad hoc approach does rely on inputted values that almost certainly won't be the true values, but that will always be the case whenever sample sizes are determined in any type of application.

We can contrast the results for this example with the result obtained using the Soper applet for linear regression (http://www.danielsoper.com/statcalc/calc01.aspx). With that applet, the user enters the number of predictors, value of α, minimum acceptable power, and effect size, and the applet returns the sample size. For example, using $\alpha = .05$ with simple linear regression, a minimum acceptable power of .80, and an effect size of 2.33, the applet gives a sample size of 7.

It is easier to relate to an R^2 value in regression than to relate to an effect size, which is more appropriate for experimental design applications and doesn't have an obvious interpretation in regression problems. The relationship between the two is given by $R^2 = f^2/(f^2 + 1)$, with f^2 the usual notation for effect size.

Thus, $f^2 = R^2/(1 - R^2)$, which doesn't have a meaningful physical interpretation since it is the proportion of the variation in the dependent variable that is explained by the model divided by the proportion that is not explained by the model.

It was determined for this example that $n = 19$ should be used. Since $t_{.025,17} = 2.10982$, $2t_{.025,17} = 4.21963$. We can use the latter to solve for R^2 since the relationship between the value of the t-statistic and the value of R^2 in simple linear regression is given by $R^2 = t^2/(n - 2 + t^2)$. [See, for example, Ryan (2009a, p. 20).] Performing the computation produces $R^2 = .5516$, which leads to $f^2 = 1.04737$.

Since $n = 19$ produces power $= .9839$ using Lenth's applet and the same for PASS, we would hope that entering $\alpha = .05$, power $= .9839$, and effect size $= 1.04737$ in Soper's applet would produce a sample size of 19, which indeed is what happens.

What is the practical value of all of this? It is useful to consider certain rules-of-thumb such as those given by Draper and Smith (1981) and Wetz (1964), but of course we won't know if the latter is satisfied until we take a sample, whose desirable size we are trying to determine! If the regressor values will be selected, then s_x can be computed, or at least estimated, and a detectable value for β_1 should not be difficult to determine. With Lenth's applet and PASS, however, it is also necessary to specify a value for s_e, in addition to the desired power, although in PASS a value for r_{xy}, the correlation between X and Y, can be used in lieu of s_e. The latter would be a good choice if the user has a good idea of what the correlation might be, and should certainly be easier to specify than s_e, which doesn't have the intuitive appeal of a correlation coefficient.

Soper's applet is easier to use for linear regression as the detectable effect size can be determined without difficulty if the applet user has a minimum acceptable R^2 value in mind, as it is then just a matter of solving for the effect size from the value of the smallest acceptable R^2 value. Then it is just a matter of specifying the minimum acceptable power and seeing if the sample size that results is acceptable when other criteria (e.g., sampling cost) are considered. Note that this does not incorporate the Wetz (1964) criterion, but specifying a minimum acceptable R^2 value essentially serves as a replacement for that criterion since, as indicated previously, R^2 is a function of t^2. Given the selected sample size, a user might then take a sample of that size and see if the Wetz criterion is met. If so, then the regression equation should be at least reasonably useful.

Soper's applet uses an iterative procedure to arrive at the sample size, with the procedure explained at http://www.danielsoper.com/statcalc/calc01.aspx.

It is important to note that no method of determining sample size will ensure that the resultant regression equation will be useful because that depends on the relationship between X and Y exhibited by the data. ∎

5.1.2 Multiple Linear Regression

The multiple linear regression case is far more difficult than simple linear regression and practically intractable because the values of multiple linear regression parameters generally don't have any meaning when the predictor values are random (Ryan, 2009a, p. 168). If the parameter values don't have any meaning, then a confidence interval on a parameter value similarly would not have any meaning, and it then logically follows that determining sample size so as to be able to detect regression parameters with specific parameter values also seems highly questionable. This is apparently not well understood, however, as Maxwell (2000) and Kelley and Maxwell (2003) discussed determining sample size in such a way as to give a confidence interval for each β_i that is sufficiently narrow. [*Note*: Other authors of regression books have not taken such a strong position regarding the interpretation of regression parameters and coefficients, but Cook and Weisberg (1999) stated: "In some problems, this simple description of a regression coefficient cannot be used, particularly if changing one term while holding others fixed doesn't make sense.... In a study of the effects of economic policies on quality of life, for example, changing one term like the prime interest rate may necessarily cause a change in other possible terms like the unemployment rate. In situations like these, interpretation of coefficients can be difficult."]

Recognizing the complexities involved, Adcock (1997) stated: "What to do in the multiple-regression case remains a topic for further study."

More recently, Dattalo (2008, p. 29) gave effect sizes of small, medium, and large for R^2, following the general idea of Cohen (1988) of designating effects of 0.02, 0.15, and 0.35 as small, medium, and large, respectively. Since $R^2 = f^2/(f^2 + 1)$, with f^2 denoting the effect size, the corresponding values of R^2 are .02, .13, and .26, for small, medium, and large, respectively. Obviously, f^2 and R^2 will be equal, to two decimal places, when f^2 is close to zero. Lenth (2001) appropriately criticized the use of the small, medium, and large designations, which clearly doesn't make any sense for regression models, and the same can be said for other applications. Indeed, Cohen (1988), who used effect size throughout his book, admitted (p. 413) that there wasn't a strong need for it in regression in stating "... the need to think in terms of f^2 is reduced, and with it, the need to rely on conventional operational definitions of 'small,' 'medium,' and 'large' values for f^2. We nevertheless offer such conventions for the frame of reference that they provide, and for use in power surveys and other methodological investigations." My advice is to simply forget about f^2 altogether.

An acceptable value of R^2 depends on the particular application and, as a rough rule-of-thumb, R^2 generally varies inversely with sample size and also increases as regressors are added to a model, but for most applications, $R^2 \geq .90$ is generally considered desirable, although much smaller values of R^2 are viewed as important in some applications. Thus, the threshold values of R^2 that result from the arbitrary designation of effect sizes given by Cohen (1988) will not lead to acceptable R^2 values for most applications.

In contrast to the values given by Dattalo (2008), we could proceed as follows. Since $R^2 = SSR/SST$, with SSR the sum of squares due to regression and SST the total sum of squares, the F-statistic for testing the significance of a regression model can be written

$$F = \frac{\dfrac{R^2}{k}}{\dfrac{1 - R^2}{n - k - 1}} \tag{5.2}$$

for a multiple linear regression model with k regressors. The reader is asked to verify this result in Exercise 4.1, which can easily be done using the fact that F is (more customarily) defined as

$$F = \frac{\dfrac{SSR}{k}}{\dfrac{SSE}{n - k - 1}}$$

Since the Wetz (1964) criterion was defined in terms of the F-statistic for the regression model, with the criterion being that the computed F-value should be at least four times the critical value, we could use that to obtain a benchmark for a "good" R^2 value by solving Eq. (4.2) for R^2 as a function of F, and then applying the Wetz criterion.

Solving for R^2 produces

$$R^2 = \frac{kF}{n - k - 1 + kF} \tag{5.3}$$

The Wetz (1964) criterion could then be applied to produce

$$R^2_{\text{desired}} = \frac{k4F_{.05,k,n-k-1}}{n - k - 1 + k4F_{.05,k,n-k-1}} \geq a \tag{5.4}$$

with a a number such as .7 or .8. Of course, this lower bound on desirable R^2 values depends on the sample size through the $F_{.05,k,n-k-1}$ tabular value, but this might be used to solve for n for fixed k and for a benchmark R^2 value. Alternatively, following the original discussion, Eq. (5.4) might be used to identify desirable R^2 values for given values of n and k. For example, with $k = 3$ and $n = 30$ (just meeting the 10:1 rule-of-thumb), we obtain $R^2_{\text{desired}} \geq .58$. This is a reasonable lower bound because a lower value than this would not be acceptable in the vast majority of applications involving three regressors.

Alternatively, we could solve for n for fixed k and a lower bound on R^2, such as, say, .80. If we set R^2_{desired} in Eq. (5.4) at .80 and use $k = 3$, we obtain

$n = 4.0 + 3F_{.05,3,n-4}$. We obtain $n = 14.8$ from inspection of an F-table, which would round to $n = 15$. This does not come close to satisfying the 10:1 rule-of-thumb, although that guideline will not be met in many applications.

We can see from Eq. (5.4) that R^2 will be large, using the Wetz (1964) criterion, whenever the Wetz criterion is met and $n - k - 1$ is small, approaching 1 as $n - k - 1$ approaches 0. (Of course, there is an exact fit whenever the sample size equals the number of model parameters, which is the same as saying that $n - k - 1 = 0$.) Making that quantity small, however, would be an artificial way of trying to produce a desirable R^2 value. This relates to the discussion in Draper and Smith (1981) regarding how R^2 can be inflated when the number of observations is not much larger than the number of distinct sets of regressor values.

We can't make a direct comparison of the results obtained using the Wetz (1964) criterion and the results obtained using Soper's applet because the former does not involve power. Nevertheless, it is of interest to see some results using Soper's applet for $k = 3$. Using the latter, if we want to detect $R^2 \geq .80$ (so that the minimum detectable effect is 4.0) and set power nominally at .80 with $\alpha = .05$, the applet gives $n = 8$. With such a sample size, the error variance would be estimated with only four degrees of freedom. Furthermore, the $n:k$ ratio is poor. Power would have to be set at .9998 or higher in order to obtain $n = 15$, which was the value obtained based on the Wetz (1964) criterion.

Soper's applet gives a small value of n when a large value of R^2 is used (to solve for f^2) because the objective is to *detect* a large effect when the null hypothesis is that the effect size is zero. Wetz's criterion, on the other hand, is not used for sample size determination, but could be used for that purpose in a roundabout way, as was done earlier in this section. Since power is not involved in Wetz's criterion, we might suspect that the sample sizes obtained indirectly through the use of that criterion may correspond to the results obtained using Soper's applet if the power selected for the latter is virtually 1.0, as was the case in the example just given.

Soper's applet uses the noncentral F-distribution, whereas Wetz's criterion uses the central F-distribution, thus making a direct analytical comparison somewhat difficult. A question could be raised as to whether or not such a comparison is even appropriate since the Wetz criterion was not intended to be used to solve for sample size, although it could be used to do so indirectly.

Nevertheless, the following computations may be illuminating. If we let $a = .7$ in Eq. (5.4) and solve for n, we obtain $n \leq k + 1 + (12k/7)F_{.05,k,n-k-1}$. Of course, this is not a simple expression for n because the third term on the right side of the inequality is a function of n, so we can't obtain a closed-form expression. It is simple to solve for n by using an F-table, however, and it is more convenient to write the inequality as $n - k - 1 \leq (12k/7)F_{.05,k,n-k-1}$, since the left side is the denominator degrees of freedom for the F-statistic. By multiplying the entries in each column of the table by $(12k/7)$, we can then look

Table 5.1 Sample Sizes for Models with $k = 1$–6 Predictors Under Certain Sample Size Guidelines

	Wetz		Power = .8		
k	$(R^2 > .70, \text{Power} = .8)$	$(R^2 > .70)$	"Large" Effect $(0.35, R^2 = .26)$	"Medium" Effect $(0.15, R^2 = .13)$	"Small" Effect $(0.02, R^2 = .02)$
1	6	11	25	55	387
2	9	16	31	68	476
3	10	19	36	77	539
4	12	24	40	85	590
5	13	28	43	92	635
6	14	32	46	98	674

for the largest value of $n - k - 1$ that is less than the corresponding value of $(12k/7)F_{.05,k,n-k-1}$. For example, when $k = 2$, $n - k - 1 = 13$ is slightly less than $(24k/7)F_{.05,2,13} = 13.063$. Therefore, $n = 16$ is used.

Alternatively, we might let $a = .8$, reasoning that R^2 should be at least .8 for sample sizes typically used if the model has at least two or three predictors and the correlations between them are not large. This would result in smaller sample sizes selected than are obtained when $a = 0.7$, however, because the multiplier of $F_{.05,k,n-k-1}$ is then k instead of $12k/7$.

Consider Table 5.1, which gives the required sample sizes obtained through indirect use of the Wetz criterion (in column 2). The other columns give the sample sizes obtained by using the Power and Precision software, with the R^2 values entered, not the effect sizes, as there is no option to enter the latter. There are some differences, especially for the "small" effect, when those R^2 values are converted to effect sizes with four decimal places and those values are entered in Soper's applet. The differences are small, usually 1, except at the small effect, where the differences are about 2% of the Power and Precision values. (Similarly, differences exist if four decimal place R^2 values are inputted in Power and Precision corresponding to each of the three exact effect sizes.)

Since power is not part of the Wetz (1964) criterion, we might guess that the power associated with each of the Wetz sample sizes would be virtually 1. It can be shown using Soper's applet that the power values do range from .99 for $k = 1$ to .99999+ for $k = 6$, with the "+" indicating that the power is greater than .99999 but the Soper applet allows only five decimal places.

The values in the last three columns, using Cohen's three effect sizes, are shown simply for comparison, as the R^2 values are too low to be of practical value and the sample size values in the last column are absolutely nonsensical, as regression datasets are generally much smaller than that.

Although we might view the sample sizes obtained from indirect use of the Wetz criterion as being somewhat smaller than desirable, there are many well-known regression datasets with approximately these combinations of k and n. For example, the famous stack loss dataset of Brownlee (1960) has $k = 3$ and $n = 21$ and the Gorman and Toman (1966) dataset had $k = 6$ and $n = 31$, differing only slightly from the corresponding Wetz (k, n) combinations. Both of these datasets have been analyzed extensively in the literature, and are used for illustration in Ryan (2009a).

Of course, we should bear in mind that Wetz (1964) did not propose sample size guidelines; I am simply obtaining guidelines by indirect use of the Wetz criterion. The sample sizes given are simply those that would result in R^2 being slightly in excess of .70 if the Wetz criterion is met when a set of regression data is analyzed.

One point that is sometimes made (http://www.listserv.uga.edu/cgi-bin/wa?A2=ind0107&L=spssx-l&P=29839) is that the requisite sample size depends not just on the number of predictors but also on the correlations between them. The logic behind such thinking is undoubtedly that the amount of information provided by the predictors is lessened when there is at least moderate correlations between them, necessitating a larger sample than would be required if the predictor correlations were small. Predictor correlations are not incorporated into the Power and Precision software nor into Soper's applet. They are also not built into PASS or nQuery, and the latter cannot be used to determine sample size for multiple regression with a general number of predictors. If suitable software were available, these correlations would have to be specified a priori, which would generally be very difficult or impossible without the availability of prior data. Nevertheless, sample size determination methods that incorporate correlations between the predictors have been proposed by Hsieh, Bloch, and Larsen (1998).

When PASS is used for determining sample size in multiple linear regression, the user specifies the number of predictors that will be included in the regression model without being tested and the R^2 value that should result from the inclusion of those predictors. (Zero is one of the options for the number of such predictors; correlations between predictors is not an input option.) Then the user specifies the number of predictors that are to be tested and the increase in R^2 that one wishes to detect. If the incremental R^2 is large, the necessary sample size will be small since the null hypothesis is that the incremental R^2 is zero. For example, if no predictors are to be automatically included and four predictors are to be tested, with desired power $= .90$ $\alpha = .05$, with $R^2 = .70$ anticipated for those four predictors, PASS gives $n = 13$. This is too small a sample size for a model with four predictors, however, but a small value of n should be expected because of the large difference between 0 and .70. If we substitute in Eq. (5.3), we obtain $R^2 = .66$. Even though this is close to the .70 used in the PASS sample size determination, there is no reason why they should be the same since a value for power is being specified for PASS but power is not involved in Eq. (5.3), nor in its development.

If the predictor values are fixed, as when an experimental design is used, the correlations between the predictor values would then be either zero or very small numbers, so software that did not incorporate predictor intercorrelations as input would not be a problem. Notice that even with predictor intercorrelations, which opens up the possibility that all of the predictors would be used if variable selection methods were applied to the dataset, the PASS input requirement for multiple linear regression is much simpler than is the case for simple linear regression.

Other software for determining sample size relative to R^2 includes a program described by Mendoza and Stafford (2001).

Krishnamoorthy and Xia (2008) considered the case of sample size determination for testing a nonzero null hypothesis value of R^2.

If there is interest simply in determining sample size so that R^2 can be estimated with a suitably small error of estimation, this was addressed by Algina and Olejnik (2000).

5.1.2.1 Application: Predicting College Freshman Grade Point Average

An important sample size question in the use of regression models is: "How large should the sample size be for developing a regression model to predict what a prospective student's college freshman grade point average would be if the student were admitted?" Many colleges and universities use such regression models and base their admittance decisions partly on the predictions obtained using such models. Of course, the worth of such models depends on whether or not all, or at least almost all, of the important variables are in the model. That is an issue of variable selection and will not be discussed here.

Similar to other sample size determination problems, the parameters of the selected regression model must be estimated, and the larger the sample size, the smaller the variance of those estimators and the smaller will be the variance of the predictions. Sawyer (1983) concluded that total group predictions based on 70 or more students works as well as predictions obtained using larger samples, whereas separate prediction equations for males and females should be satisfactory if based on as few as 50 students.

5.2 LOGISTIC REGRESSION

The logistic regression model is usually written

$$\pi\left(X_1, X_2, \ldots X_k\right) = \frac{\exp\left(\beta_0 + \beta_1 X_1 + \cdots + \beta_k X_k\right)}{1 + \exp\left(\beta_0 + \beta_1 X_1 + \cdots + \beta_k X_k\right)} \tag{5.5}$$

for the general case of k regressors, $X_1, X_2, \ldots, X_k$, with $\pi(X_1, X_2, \ldots, X_k) = P(Y = 1|X_1 = x_1, X_2 = x_2, \ldots, X_k = x_k)$, with the dependent variable, Y, being binary. Alternatively, since $1 - \pi = 1/[1 + \exp(\beta_0 + \beta_1 X_1 + \cdots + \beta_k X_k]$, $\pi/(1 - \pi) = \exp(\beta_0 + \beta_1 X_1 + \cdots + \beta_k X_k)$, so

$$\log[\pi/(1 - \pi)] = \beta_0 + \beta_1 X_1 + \cdots + \beta_k X_k$$

thus writing the right-hand side in the form of a linear model.

Hosmer and Lemeshow (2000, p. 339) stated: "There has been surprisingly little work on sample size for logistic regression. The available methods to address sample size selection have been implemented in just a few specialty software packages." Not much has changed since they made that statement.

Throughout this book there has been discussion of the use of pilot studies to obtain parameter estimates that can be used as software input to determine sample sizes, with internal pilot studies having some advantages over external pilot studies. Flack and Eudey (1993) illustrated the use of an external pilot study, a dental study involving 19 people. They cautioned, however, that the parameter estimates in logistic regression are, at least when maximum likelihood is used, large-sample approximations, but only a small sample (of 19) was used in this study to obtain the parameter estimates. Consequently, they suggested that a sensitivity analysis be performed by varying the parameter estimates and observing the resultant changes in the associated sample size values. Muller and Pasour (1997) examined the bias that results when only significant tests from a prior study result in power being calculated for the main study.

One point that cannot be overemphasized is that a continuous response variable should *not* be dichotomized, as doing so discards information and this results in a loss of power for a fixed sample size, or the need for a larger sample size for a fixed power. See, for example, Taylor, West, and Aiken (2006).

As discussed by Ryan (2009a, Chapter 9), there are more complexities inherent in multiple logistic regression than in multiple linear regression, and this also applies to sample size determination. As in linear regression, we will first consider the case of simple logistic regression.

5.2.1 Simple Logistic Regression

If we wanted to develop an approach to sample size determination analogous to what was done in Section 5.1.1 for simple linear regression, we would need a measure of model adequacy. Software utilizes the Wald test, which is analogous to the *t*-test in linear regression. Although the Wald test has received some criticism in the literature, we will use it here since it is used frequently in practice.

In linear regression, ordinary least squares is usually the method of estimation, so sample size determination software tacitly assumes the use of that method. In logistic regression, maximum likelihood is generally used, but will often not be the best estimation method (see the discussion in Ryan, 2009b). In particular, the maximum likelihood solution will not exist when complete separation exists. An example of this is when there is one continuous covariate and all of the values of the covariate at $Y = 1$ are greater than all of the values of the covariate at $Y = 0$. Near separation exists when there is only slight overlap of the two sets of values and when that happens the maximum likelihood estimates will tend to blow up, as will the standard errors of their estimators. Because of this problem and other problems with maximum likelihood estimators in logistic regression, various alternative approaches have been proposed but they will not all be discussed in this chapter.

Nevertheless, we will initially assume the use of maximum likelihood and will start with the sample size determination methods that have been proposed. Whittemore (1981) was probably the first to propose a method for determining sample size in logistic regression and provided tables of required sample sizes. Those tables for power values of .90, .95, and .99, but not .80. Graphs were also given to aid in sample size selection. The recommended approach was for small response probabilities only, however (say, $\pi < .1$), and when that is the case, the data will generally be sparse (i.e, there will be only a small percentage of $Y = 1$ values), necessitating the use of some method other than maximum likelihood.

Whittemore (1981) did assume the use of maximum likelihood, however, and showed that the proposed method is quite sensitive to the distribution of the corresponding covariates. Very large sample sizes can result from application of the method, with an example discussing possible sample sizes of 15,425 and 17,584. Even though this is an era in which larger amounts of data are being handled, those would be extremely large datasets.

Another sample size determination method was proposed by Self, Mauritsen, and Ohara (1992), but their method can be used only with discrete predictors, not continuous predictors. [Their method was extended to the class of generalized linear models by Shieh (2000).] See also Bull (1993), who considered the special case of a three-level predictor, including a three-level ordinal predictor, and Alam, Rao, and Cheng (2010), who proposed a variation of the Whittemore (1981) method and also critiqued the Hsieh et al. (1998) methods, pointing out that they are very sensitive to the choice of β_0. Therefore, they suggested that a pilot study be performed so that a reasonable value for β_0 might be selected.

Dattalo (2008, p. 32), for example, pointed out that sample size determination in simple logistic regression can be determined for a normally distributed covariate by using the sample size formula for a two-sample t-test, as previously stated by Hsieh et al. (1998) and Vaeth and Skovlund (2004). This follows from the fact that for a normally distributed covariate, the log odds value β_1 is zero if and only if the group means for the two response categories, assuming equal variances, are the same. Since Y has two values, 0 and 1, there are thus "two groups" of values, as in a two-sample t-test. The general idea with this approach is to avoid the considerable complexities inherent in sample size computations for logistic regression, as indicated here in Section 5.2 and also mentioned by Vaeth and Skovlund (2004). They stated that their method is exact when applied to linear regression, and approximate when applied to logistic regression and Cox regression because it relies on asymptotic theory. Of course, we should generally be concerned about the latter, especially when the use of software leads to a sample size that is not very large. Simulations were performed that showed the adequacy of their method, although there were some problems with small samples and highly skewed predictor distributions.

Similarly, sample size could be determined by focusing on the odds ratio, which is defined as $(\pi/(1 - \pi))$, with $\pi = P(Y = 1 | X = x)$, as indicated previously, and $1 - \pi = P(Y = 0 | X = x)$. That is, the odds ratio implicitly incorporates the two groups, as in the two-sample t-test. The applet of Demidenko (2007) solves for sample size in simple logistic regression for a binary covariate (only) with user-inputted values of the proportion of $X = 1$ values and $P(Y = 1 | X = 0)$, as illustrated in the following example.

■ **EXAMPLE 5.2**

Using the applet of E. Demidenko (http://www.dartmouth.edu/~eugened /power-samplesize.php), if we specify power $= .80$, $\alpha = .05$, 50% of the X-values are "1", and $P(Y = 1 | X = 0) = .50$, which would correspond to a binary covariate having no predictive ability at all, and specify a "detectable" odds ratio of 3, the applet gives a sample size of $n = 121$. Of course, an odds ratio of 3 would imply $\pi = .75$ and $1 - \pi = .25$, which would be a reasonable odds ratio. Of course, a specified odds ratio larger than 3 would require a smaller sample size, with $n = 84$ for an odds ratio of 4, and a larger sample size needed for a smaller odds ratio. For example, $n = 278$ is required for an odds ratio of 2.

Although the applet does not provide a graph of sample size plotted against detectable odds ratio as an option, such a graph can be produced by using a reasonable number of data points. Doing so produces the graph in Figure 5.1.

The computed sample sizes are based on the assumed use of the Wald test, which corresponds to the t-test in linear regression, as stated previously. Despite that correspondence, the Wald test has received some criticism [see, e.g., Hosmer and Lemeshow (2000, p. 17)]. The applet also assumes the use of maximum likelihood, which, as stated previously, would be a poor choice of estimation method for certain data configurations, as well as small sample sizes. Nevertheless, the applet results can be used as at least a rough general guideline, and Demidenko (2008) defends the use of the Wald test.   ■

5.2.1.1 *Normally Distributed Covariate*
The software Power and Precision can also be used to obtain sample sizes for logistic regression models, as can other software including SiZ and PASS. [Broadly, the `powercal` command in Stata can be used to compute sample size and power for generalized linear models, a class that includes logistic regression models. See Newson (2004) for details.]

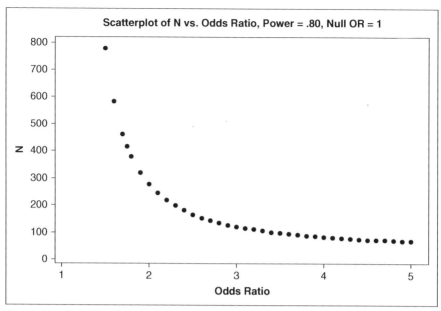

Figure 5.1 Relationship between sample size and detectable odds ratio; power $= .80$; null hypothesis: equal proportion of $x = 0$ and $x = 1$; $P(Y = 1|X = 0) = .5$.

For the assumption that X has a normal distribution, PASS uses the following expression, given by Hsieh et al. (1998):

$$n = \frac{\left(z_{\alpha/2} + z_\beta\right)^2}{\pi^*(1 - \pi^*) B^2} \tag{5.6}$$

with $z_{\alpha/2}$ and z_β as previously defined, $\pi^* = P(Y = 1)$ at the mean of X, μ_x, and $B = \sigma_x \beta_1$, with β_1 determined from $P(Y = 1)$ at $\mu_x + \sigma_x$.

For example, assume that $H_0: \beta_1 = 0$ is tested using a two-sided test with $\alpha = .05$, $\sigma = 5$, and power is to be .90. To obtain B expressed as a multiple of the standard deviation of X, we could proceed as follows. For example, if we wish to detect $P(Y = 1) = .65$ at $\mu_x + \sigma_x$, this assumption implies an assumption of a specific value of β_1, which in turn leads to the corresponding value of B. This can be explained as follows. It is well known [see, e.g., Ryan (2009a, p. 314)] that $P(Y = 1) = .5$ occurs at $X = -\beta_0/\beta_1$. [This can be verified by substitution in Eq. (5.5).] Let that value of $X = \mu_x$ so that $X = \mu_x + \sigma_x = -\beta_0/\beta_1 + 5$. Then from Eq. (5.5) we have

$$\pi(X) = \frac{\exp(\beta_0 + \beta_1 X)}{1 + \exp(\beta_0 + \beta_1 X)}$$

so that

$$.65 = \frac{\exp\left[\beta_0 + \beta_1\left(-\beta_0/\beta_1 + 5\right)\right]}{1 + \exp\left[\beta_0 + \beta_1\left(-\beta_0/\beta_1 + 5\right)\right]}$$

and thus

$$.65 = \frac{\exp\left(5\beta_1\right)}{1 + \exp\left(5\beta_1\right)}$$

Solving this equation for β_1, we obtain $\beta_1 = [\log(.65/.35)]/5 = 0.123808$. Since, as indicated, $B = \sigma_x \beta_1$ in Eq. (5.6), $B = 5(0.123808) = 0.619038$. Then, using Eq. (5.6), we obtain

$$\begin{aligned}
n &= \frac{\left(z_{\alpha/2} + z_\beta\right)^2}{\pi^*(1 - \pi^*)\,B^2} \\
&= \frac{(1.95996 + 1.28155)^2}{(0.5)(0.5)(0.619038)^2} \\
&= 109.678
\end{aligned}$$

so that $n = 110$ would be used. This is the sample size given by SiZ, whereas PASS gives $n = 109$.

Some discrepancies between software can be expected because of the use of different sample size formulas. For example, nQuery uses a different formula [given as Eq. (4) in Hsieh et al. (1998)], so when nQuery is used, the sample size is given as $n = 138$, which obviously differs considerably from the sample sizes given by SiZ and PASS. The formula used by nQuery is

$$n = \frac{\left[z_{\alpha/2} + z_\beta \exp\left(-\beta^2/4\right)\right]^2}{\pi_1 \beta^2}\left[1 + 2\pi_1\Delta\right]$$

with

$$\Delta = \frac{\left[1 + \left(1 + \beta^2\right)\exp\left(-5\beta^2/4\right)\right]}{1 + \exp\left(-\beta^2/4\right)}$$

Here β^2 is the square of the log odds value, $\beta = \log[\pi_2(1 - \pi_1)/(\pi_1(1 - \pi_2))]$, with π_1 and π_2 denoting the value of π at $X = \mu_x$ and $X = \mu_x + \sigma_x$, respectively.

Hsieh et al. (1998) suggested that this formula not be used when the odds ratio $\pi_2(1 - \pi_1)/\pi_1(1 - \pi_2)$ is at least 3, since it will then overestimate the required sample size. Here it is 1.86 and the fact that the sample size for this example was much larger than the sample sizes obtained using PASS and SiZ was noted. This raises the question of whether the formula should be used at all.

Note that B is not part of the input with either PASS or Power and Precision, for example, as with Power and Precision the user would enter $P(Y = 1)$ at a value for X other than μ_x, in addition to entering $P(Y = 1)$ at μ_x, which we will later designate as $P_1(\mu_x)$. With PASS, the user would enter the value for $P(Y = 1)$ at μ_x and at $\mu_x + \sigma_x$, or enter the first of these two and the odds ratio.

Regarding these software input requirements, the following statement by Novikov, Fund, and Freeman (2010) is worth noting, with P_1 used in place of π and $E(X) = \mu_x$: "As, in our experience, the investigator is unlikely to recognize the difference between P_1 and $P1(E(X))$ and will generally supply the more natural P_1, we explore the impact that this will have on the sample sizes calculated by these methods." The sidebar explanation that is provided in PASS indicates that when both probabilities are entered, the first one is the probability at μ_x and the second one corresponds to $\mu_x + \sigma_x$. This is the same input requirement for SiZ and similarly the user of nQuery has the same two input options, with this clearly indicated by both software packages. What is being inputted into Power and Precision is also clearly indicated but, as with the other software, this does place a burden on the user with the user perhaps not being clear on what is required, as suggested by Novikov et al. (2010), or simply overlooking the explanations. In referring to nQuery, PASS, and Power and Precision, Novikov et al. (2010) also stated: "The above-mentioned packages use different algorithms for the calculation, and in certain circumstances the resulting estimates can be quite different, especially when the hypothesized effect is large."

The example that they gave to illustrate that is as follows. With $\alpha = .05$ for a two-sided test, power $= .80$, $P_1(\mu_x) = 0.5$ and the user wants to detect an odds ratio as large as 3.49, PASS gives the solution as $n = 20$, whereas the solution from Power and Precision is $n = 44$, as can be verified by a user who has both software packages, although the user would have to first compute $P(Y = 1|X = \mu_x + \sigma_x)$ for input in Power and Precision, which is .778. Obviously, there is a huge difference in the two sample sizes!

Accordingly, Novikov et al. (2010) proposed a method that utilized the sample size formula for a two-sample t-test with unequal variances and unequal sample sizes given by Schouten (1999) and given previously in Section 3.7. (As indicated previously, the two-sample idea comes from the fact that there are two groups of observations for Y: 0 and 1.) The method proposed by Novikov et al. (2010) is somewhat involved, however, and requires three preliminary steps before Schouten's formula is used, one of which involves solving an equation numerically. They provided a SAS program for all of the necessary computations.

Novikov et al. (2010) performed simulation studies to examine the accuracy of their proposed method and compared it to the methods of Hsieh et al. (1998) and Demidenko (2007). They also examined the effect of the user specifying

$P1(E(X))$ instead of P_1, which is the overall probability that $Y = 1$. Power was determined using the Wald test. Novikov et al. (2010) found that all three methods performed well for detecting small effects but that their proposed method is superior for detecting large effects. They also found that the method given by Hsieh (1989), which is an extension of the formula given by Whittemore (1981) and is used by the software nQuery, is based on the sampling distribution of the log of the odds ratio and overestimates the sample size, especially for a large response probability. As Novikov et al. (2010) stated, this result is not surprising since the method given by Whittemore (1981) was intended to be used for a small response probability, as stated previously. (Overestimation was evident in Example 5.2.)

5.2.1.2 Binary Covariate

Hsieh et al. (1998) gave the following sample size formula for a single binary covariate. In their notation it is

$$n = \frac{\left\{ z_{\alpha/2} \left[P(1 - P/B) \right]^{1/2} + z_\beta \left[P1(1 - P1) + P2(1 - P2)(1 - B)/B \right]^{1/2} \right\}^2}{(P1 - P2)^2(1 - B)}$$

(5.7)

Here B denotes the proportion of the sample with $X = 1$; $P1$ and $P2$ are the event rates at $X = 0$ and $X = 1$, respectively; and the overall event rate, P, is given by $P = (1 - B)P1 + BP2$.

Hosmer and Lemeshow (2000, p. 339) stated that, for a single binary covariate, sample size determination is equivalent to determining the sample size for testing the equality of two proportions, and stated that the sample size formula for the latter can be used. That requires some clarification, however, because the $\bar{p}$ that is embedded in Eq. (5.6) is just a simple average of two proportions under the assumption of equal sample sizes, whereas the P in Eq. (5.7) is a weighted average since the proportion of responses at $X = 0$ and $X = 1$ probably won't be the same. Hosmer and Lemeshow (2000) gave an example using Eq. (5.6) and compared the sample size obtained using that formula with the sample size obtained using the Whittemore (1981) approach, with the latter being much larger than the sample size obtained using Eq. (5.6).

When software is used, the user must specify whether the covariate has a normal distribution or is binary. For example, in PASS the user selects "logistic regression" and then indicates whether the covariate is normally distributed or binary. In Power and Precision, the user first selects "Logistic" and then chooses the option for either "Logistic regression, one continuous predictor" (normality is not mentioned but that is apparently assumed) or "Logistic regression, one categorical predictor (two levels)." Not all software provides these options, however, as the simple logistic regression routines in nQuery and SiZ have the capability only for a normal covariate.

5.2.2 Multiple Logistic Regression

The simplified approach discussed by Hsieh et al. (1998) and Vaeth and Skovlund (2004) for simple logistic regression can, according to these authors, be applied to multiple logistic regression by using variance inflation factors (VIFs). As explained by Hsieh et al. (1998), Whittemore (1981) showed that for a set of normally distributed covariates, $Var(\hat{\beta}_i)$ can be approximated by inflating the variance when only the corresponding predictor is used in the model. The inflation is accomplished by dividing that variance by $(1 - R_i^2)$, with R_i^2 denoting the square of the correlation between X_i and the other covariates in the model. [This is the VIF that is used in linear regression; see Ryan (2009a, p. 170).]

The necessary sample size is inflated in the same way. That is, the sample size necessary for testing $\beta_i = 0$ is inflated by dividing it by $(1 - R_i^2)$. Hsieh et al. (1998) reported that this inflation factor also "seems to work well for binary covariates."

Hosmer and Lemeshow (2000, p. 346) were critical of this ad hoc approach, however, stating: "We think that the sample size suggested by equation (8.49) may be unnecessarily large but could be the starting point for a more in depth sample size analysis using pilot data [to] do some model fitting." They distinguish between the sample size needed to detect a particular nonzero value of a model parameter with a desired power and the number of observations needed to fit a selected model.

There can be problems interpreting coefficients in logistic regression models due to multicollinearity, just as happens with linear regression models when multicollinearity is present, so determining sample size from hypothesis tests of regression parameters is not necessarily a good idea. It would be better to use the increase in R^2 when the covariate that is being tested is added as a criterion in testing a covariate and its parameter, but such an approach would have its own problems because there are multiple R^2 statistics that have been proposed for logistic regression and no one statistic stands out as being clearly superior to the other ones. See Menard (2000) and Sharma (2006). This would hinder any attempt to focus attention on determining sample size so as to try to ensure that the logistic regression model will be of value in terms of explaining the variability in the response variable. Therefore, developing a sample size determination approach that parallels the development for linear regression using the Wetz criterion (as in Sections 5.1 and 5.1.2) would be even more challenging than for linear regression and will not be attempted here. (Since such an approach has apparently not been given in the literature, it is also not available in software since software methods generally follow methods given in the literature, and generally lag the publication of those methods by several years.)

The concern that Hosmer and Lemeshow (2000) expressed over the sample size inflation factor given by Hsieh et al. (1998) is indirectly supported by the results of Peduzzi, Concato, Kemper, Holford, and Feinstein (1996), who found that at least 10 events per covariate are needed to avoid problems of bias in the regression coefficients in both directions and similarly both underestimation and overestimation of variances of the estimators. For general models in which the number of parameters is greater than the number of covariates, they concluded that there should be at least 10 events *per parameter*.

Peduzzi et al. (1996) are indirectly stating that the necessary increase in the sample size should be (at least roughly) a linear function of the number of covariates or the number of parameters, if the two differ.

An online sample size rule-of-thumb that was motivated by the results of Peduzzi et al. (1996) is $n = 10k/p$ (see http://www.medcalc.org/manual/ logistic_regression.php), with $k =$ the number of covariates and $p =$ the smaller of the anticipated proportion of events and nonevents in the population. Long (1997, p. 54) stated in referring to maximum likelihood (ML): "It is risky to use ML with samples smaller than 100." So a person who felt that way would probably want to round $10k/p$ up to 100, if necessary, although $10k/p$ might exceed 100 if the model has more than a few covariates or the dataset is sparse (i.e., unbalanced), so that p is small.

This would be a simple rule-of-thumb for practitioners to follow, whereas the Hsieh et al. (1998) adjustment depends on an adjustment factor that may be unknown, and will be only monotonically related to an increase in the number of covariates. More specifically, when a variable selection algorithm is applied to linear regression or logistic regression, a point of diminishing returns is reached (as measured, say, by R^2) in terms of addition of covariates. This is often, but not always, due to multicollinearity if the data are observational. If a designed experiment is used, however, R_i^2 may be increasing very little, if at all, when covariates are added. Then the Hsieh et al. (1998) adjustment factor would fail badly, according to the results of Peduzzi et al. (1996). The Hsieh et al. (1998) adjustment factor is also flawed in another way as it is inappropriate to use a Pearson correlation coefficient or multiple correlation coefficient to measure the correlation between continuous covariates and binary covariates, a mixture that occurs quite frequently with logistic regression data.

This is useful information because software capability for multiple logistic regression is limited. PASS and nQuery use the Hsieh et al. (1998) inflation factor as the user specifies the value of R_i^2 and there is no restriction on the number of covariates. The user of SiZ specifies $\sqrt{R_i^2}$. Power and Precision will handle only two continuous predictors and the user specifies the correlation between them.

So what should a user do? The problem with trying to use the results of Peduzzi et al. (1996) is that the user needs to know approximately what percentage of events and nonevents to expect for the covariates of interest. Software could then be used to arrive at a sample size, with the user facing a dilemma if the percentage multiplied times the sample size from the software output is not at least 10 times the number of covariates or 10 times the number of parameters in the tentative model, whichever is appropriate. If that condition is not met, it might be safer to use a sample size that is large enough that the expected number of events meets the ≥ 10 rule-of-thumb.

Logistic regression is a generalized linear model. Self and Mauritsen (1988) considered sample size determination for such models, with logistic regression models considered as a special case. Lindsey (1997) gave a simple general formula for exact calculations of sample size for any member of the linear exponential family. This includes generalized linear models with a known or fixed dispersion parameter. Kodell, Lensing, Landes, Kumar, and Hauer-Jensen (2010) considered a specific application involving radiation measures and considered sample size deteremination when a logistic model is used as well as other generalized linear models.

5.2.2.1 Measurement Error

For the case of two continuous covariates, with one being an exposure variable that is subject to measurement error, an applet is given at `http://biostat.hitchcock.org/MeasurementError/Analytics/PowerCalculations forLogisticRegression.asp` and is based on the work of Tosteson, Buzas, Demidenko, and Karagas (2003), which allows the incorporation of covariate measurement error, with the user specifying (estimating) the correlation between the observed measurement and the true measurement, as well as the correlation between the exposure variable and the other covariate.

This applet will not compute sample size, however, but will give the power for a selected sample size as one point on a graph that shows the power for various values of the odds ratio for a one standard deviation increase in the exposure variable. The graph actually has two lines/curves—one for measurement error and the other for no measurement error, as shown in Figure 5.2. Of course, such graphs are always useful because the inputted values will almost certainly not be the true values.

5.2.3 Polytomous Logistic Regression

The response variable in logistic regression can have more than two categories. When this is the case, it is called *polytomous logistic regression*. This is used much less frequently than binary logistic regression. Readers are referred to Section 8.1 of Hosmer and Lemeshow (2000) for information on polytomous logistic regression. Software for sample size determination does not generally include capability for polytomous logistic regression. Another problem is that polytomous logistic regression can be undermined by near separation just as in binary logistic regression, and the maximum likelihood estimators will not exist when there is compete separation. (How the latter can occur in polytomous logistic regression should be apparent from the discussion in Section 5.2.1, as it is just a matter of extending that discussion to more than two levels.)

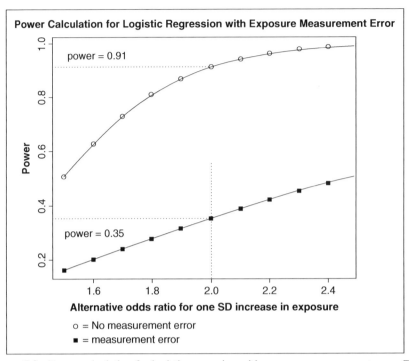

Figure 5.2   Power calculation for logistic regression with exposure measurement error. Correlation between true and observed exposure $= 0.5$. Odds ratio for covariate $= 1.5$. Prevalence with no exposure $= 0.5$. Correlation between exposure and covariate $= 0$. Sample size $= 100$. Significance level $= 0.05$.

5.2.4   Ordinal Logistic Regression

In both binary and polytomous logistic regression, the levels of the dependent variable are nominal. This is appropriate if the response variable is, say, gender or race, but not if, for example, ranks of people are involved, such as executive titles or army ranks.

Assume that the response variable has k ordered categories and there is a treatment group and a control group of subjects for each category. The formula for sample size, as given by Whitehead (1993) [see also Walters (2004) and Simon (2008)], is

$$n = \frac{6 \left(Z_{\alpha/2} + Z_{\beta}\right)^2}{\log(OR)^2 \left[1 - \sum_{i=1}^{k} \bar{\pi}_i^3\right]}$$

with OR denoting the odds ratio given in Section 5.2.1 and $\bar{\pi}_i$ being the average of the proportion of patients in the treatment and control groups for the ith category.

Sample size determination for ordinal logistic regression models has also been addressed by Vaughan and Guzy (2002), who presented an algorithm for exploring subsets of data from previous studies to enable a study to be designed with a desired power. Its use with SAS Software was illustrated.

See Section 8.2 of Hosmer and Lemeshow (2000) for information on ordinal logistic regression models, as they cover three different types of such models.

5.2.5 Exact Logistic Regression

One potential problem with all of the sample size methods for logistc regression that have been given in the literature is that they all assume the use of maximum likelihood (ML) as the method of estimation. As shown by King and Ryan (2002), the use of ML can result in very poor parameter estimates under certain conditions. There are a few alternatives to maximum likelihood in logistic regression, one of which is *exact logistic regression* (Cox, 1970, pp. 44–48). See also Mehta and Patel (1995). Quoting from the SAS Software documentation at `http://support.sas.com/rnd/app/da/new/daexactlogistic.html`: "Exact logistic regression has become an important analytical technique, especially in the pharmaceutical industry, since the usual asymptotic methods for analyzing small, skewed, or sparse data sets are unreliable." Ammann (2004) showed in a medical application of ML logistic regression, which had a small sample, that the exact p-value for testing for the inclusion of one of the predictors was .046, whereas the ML p-value was .231, thus giving totally different pictures regarding the worth of that predictor. Ammann (2004) stated that it would not have been possible to increase the number of patients without considerable effort. Thus, an estimation method that is not encumbered by small-sample bias should have been used. Such bias is well known (see, e.g., Firth, 1993), as the ML estimators are only asymptotically unbiased. So there could be major problems when there are small samples, as in the example cited by Ammann (2004).

Another alternative is a method due to Firth (1993), which might be the best overall method to use, although that has not yet been determined. Firth's method is penalized maximum likelihood, which reduces the amount of bias in the maximum likelihood estimator by adding a small amount of bias into the score function.

In addition to SAS Software, exact logistic regression is available in other software, including LogXact, Egret, and Stata. Sample size determination for exact logistic regression is apparently not available with any software, however.

5.3 COX REGRESSION

Cox regression, also known as proportional hazards regression, is used very extensively in survival analysis. Ryan and Woodall (2005) indicated that Cox (1972) was the second most frequently cited statistics paper and it now has well over 20,000 citations.

The Cox model can be written

$$h_Y(t) = h_0(t)\exp(\beta_1 X_1 + \beta_2 X_2 + \cdots + \beta_k X_k) \qquad (5.8)$$

where $X_1, X_2, \ldots, X_k$ denote a set of predictor variables, $h_Y(t)$ denotes the hazard function of Y at time t, $h_0(t)$ is an arbitrary baseline hazard function computed, at time t, by possibly using zero as the value of each predictor variable, and the β_i are parameters to be estimated. [The hazard function is the probability of failure (i.e., death in survival analysis) at time t divided by the probability of survival until time t.]

The parameters are estimated using Cox regression and their interpretation is similar to the interpretation of the parameters in a multiple logistic regression model.

As in logistic regression, there are different, equivalent forms of the Cox regression model, with a linear model representation resulting from dividing both sides of Eq. (5.8) by $h_0(t)$ and then taking the log of each side of the equation, so as to give

$$\log(h_Y(t)/h_0(t)) = \beta_1 X_1 + \beta_2 X_2 + \cdots + \beta_k X_k \qquad (5.9)$$

Of course, this is very similar to what is done in logistic regression to produce a linear model. Another similarity is that maximum likelihood is used to estimate the parameters, with iterations performed until the log(likelihood) appears to have converged. Unfortunately, the use of maximum likelihood in Cox regression can sometimes cause the same type of problems that can exist with logistic regression. Specifically, the parameter estimates can either blow up or fail to exist. This was demonstrated in Ryan (2009b). Thus, there will be conditions under which an alternative to Cox regression should be used, and one such alternative is the method due to Firth (1993), which was mentioned in Section 5.2.5 and which was developed for the class of generalized linear models. That class includes Cox regression.

The practitioner who is trying to determine sample size is faced with a dilemma as it usually won't be apparent until the data have been collected that maximum likelihood is a poor choice for that set of data, but the sample size has been determined under the assumption that maximum likelihood will be used and sample size formulas have not been presented in the literature for alternative estimation methods such as those of Firth (1993).

As indicated in Section 4.2.1, the method given by Vaeth and Skovlund (2004) can be used in Cox regression (when Cox regression can be appropriately used, that is). This is not the method that is used in the software discussed in this book and therefore won't be illustrated here.

Sample size determination for Cox regression is available in Stata and PASS. For Stata, this is based on the method of Hsieh and Lavori (2000), which reduces to the method of Schoenfeld (1983) for a binary covariate. This is discussed and illustrated in Section 9.2. The procedure in PASS assumes use of the model given in Eq. (5.8) and also uses the formula given by Hsieh and Lavori (2000), which is the same type of inflation formula given by Hsieh et al. (1998) for logistic regression. That is, the sample size for testing the null hypothesis that $\beta_1 = 0$ is determined in part by the correlation that X_1 has with the other covariates, with the formula given by

$$n = \frac{(Z_{\alpha/2} + Z_\beta)^2}{(1 - R^2)\sigma^2 B^2}$$

with B being the value of β_1 that an experimenter wishes to detect.

Whether or not the inflation factor is appropriate can perhaps be questioned, just as Hosmer and Lemeshow (2000) questioned the similar formula of Hsieh et al. (1998).

■ **EXAMPLE 5.3**

Assume that we wish to determine the sample size for testing a parameter in a Cox regression model, with $\alpha = .05$ for a two-sided test and the desired power is .90. With the null hypothesis being that the parameter value is zero, we want to detect a value of 0.5 when the standard deviation of the corresponding covariate is 1.5, there are no censored observations, and the value of R^2 when the covariate is regressed against the other covariates in the model (using linear regression) is 0.30. The output from PASS shows that the required sample size is 27 and the power is .903. If the computation had been performed by hand, the result would have been

$$\begin{aligned} n &= \frac{(Z_{\alpha/2} + Z_\beta)^2}{(1 - R^2)\sigma^2 B^2} \\ &= \frac{(1.96 + 1.28155)^2}{(1 - .3)(2.25)(0.5)^2} \\ &= 26.686 \end{aligned}$$

so that $n = 27$ would be used, in agreement with the PASS output.   ■

5.4 POISSON REGRESSION

Poisson regression is used when regression is applied to count data and the dependent variable is distributed as approximately a Poisson distribution. As with logistic regression, the estimation procedure is iterative. The parameter estimates are usually obtained as maximum likelihood estimates, using iteratively reweighted least squares. Although exact Poisson regression is an alternative to maximum likelihood, and will often be preferable for small samples, there is apparently no software that will determine sample size for exact Poisson regression. Some software does have capability for using exact Poisson regression, however, such as Stata.

The model for Poisson regression is

$$\log(\text{Rate}) = \beta_0 + \beta_1 X_1 + \beta_2 X_2 + \cdots + \beta_k X_k$$

so

$$\text{Rate} = \exp(\beta_0 + \beta_1 X_1 + \beta_2 X_2 + \cdots + \beta_k X_k) \qquad (5.10)$$

and the model for the count variable is then n times the right-hand side, with n as usual denoting the sample size, which could be determined using software unless the user is already set on a sample size. That is,

$$\text{Count} = Y = n\left[\exp(\beta_0 + \beta_1 X_1 + \beta_2 X_2 + \cdots + \beta_k X_k)\right]$$
$$= \exp[\ln(n) + \beta_0 + \beta_1 X_1 + \beta_2 X_2 + \cdots + \beta_k X_k]$$

Signorini (1991) proposed a method for determining sample size and that method is incorporated into G*Power and PASS, with these being the only major sample size determination software with capability for Poisson regression. Specifically, power or sample size is determined for the model in Eq. (5.10) for the null hypothesis $\beta_1 = 0$ versus the alternative hypothesis $\beta_1 = B1$ (using the notation in PASS).

When X_1 is the only regression variable in the model, the minimum sample size, n, is determined from (Signorini, 1991)

$$n \geq \phi \frac{\left[z_{\alpha/2}\sqrt{\text{Var}(\hat{\beta}_1|\beta_1 = 0)} + z_\beta\sqrt{\text{Var}(\hat{\beta}_1|\beta_1 = B1)}\right]^2}{\mu_T \exp(\beta_{10})B1^2} \qquad (5.11)$$

where ϕ denotes a measure of overdispersion, μ_T is the mean exposure time, β_{10} denotes the value of β_1 under the null hypothesis, z is the standard normal deviate, and this is for a two-sided test. For a one-sided test, $z_{\alpha/2}$ would be replaced by z_α.

To illustrate, the null and alternative hypotheses are generally expressed in terms of $\exp(\beta_1)$ rather than β_1 itself. Thus, $\exp(\beta_1) = 1$ under the null hypothesis that $\beta_1 = 0$, and we will assume that we want to detect, with a one-sided test, a reduction to $\exp(B1) = 0.7$, which implies that $B1 = -0.356675$. $\text{Var}(\hat{\beta}_1) = e^{-\beta_1^2/2}$ is the asymptotic variance under the assumption that X has a standard normal distribution, with the variance form for other distributions of X given in Table 1 of Signorini (1991). Thus, for this distributional assumption, $\text{Var}(\hat{\beta}_1|\beta_1 = 0) = e^0 = 1$ and $\text{Var}(\hat{\beta}_1|\beta_1 = -0.356675) = \exp[(-0.5)(-0.356675)^2] = 0.938372$.

Thus, for $\alpha = .05$ and power $= .95$ and assuming no overdispersion (so that $\phi = 1$), the necessary minimum sample size is

$$
n = \phi \frac{\left[z_\alpha \sqrt{\text{Var}(\hat{\beta}_1 | \beta_1 = 0)} + z_\beta \sqrt{\text{Var}(\hat{\beta}_1 | \beta_1 = B1)} \right]^2}{\mu_T \exp(\beta_{10}) B1^2}
$$

$$
= \frac{\left[1.645 \sqrt{1} + 1.645 \sqrt{(0.938372)} \right]^2}{(1)(1)(-0.356675)^2}
$$

$$
= 82.44 \tag{5.12}
$$

Thus, the sample size would be rounded up to $n = 83$, in agreement with the solution given by PASS. Table 2 of Signorini (1991) gives $n = 82$, presumably because there was rounding to the nearest integer, but as has been stated previously, the rounding must be up to ensure that the power is at least equal to the desired power. For those readers who wish to consult Signorini (1991), it is worth noting that the same thing happens when the alternative hypothesis is $\exp(B1) = 0.5$, for example, as use of Eq. (5.12) leads to $n = 20.05$, so that Table 2 of Signorini (1991) gives $n = 20$, whereas PASS properly gives $n = 21$. Such one-unit differences are really inconsequential, however, because an asymptotic variance expression is being used, which would not apply to such small samples. So both solutions are thus potentially incorrect. It should also be noted that Signorini (1991) did not discuss one-sided and two-sided tests, but simply gave Eq. (5.11), which obviously applies to two-sided tests, whereas the entries in Table 2 of Signorini (1991) are obviously for one-sided tests. Thus, there is the potential for confusion.

When there are other regression variables in the model, PASS, for example, follows the lead of Hsieh et al. (1998) for multiple logistic regression and Hsieh and Lavori (2000) for Cox regression with multiple covariates and inflates the sample size for Poisson regression with a single covariate by $1/(1 - R^2)$, with R^2 denoting the square of the correlation between the covariate that corresponds to the parameter that is being tested and the other covariates in the model.

Thus, using the example given earlier in this section, if there were other covariates in the model and $R^2 = .90$, the sample size would be $10(82.44) = 824.4$, so $n = 825$ would be used, which is the solution given by PASS. The latter uses the formula

$$
n = \phi \frac{\left[z_{\alpha/2} \sqrt{\text{Var}(\hat{\beta}_1 | \beta_1 = 0)} + z_\beta \sqrt{\text{Var}(\hat{\beta}_1 | \beta_1 = B1)} \right]^2}{\mu_T \exp(\beta_0) B1^2 (1 - R^2)}
$$

for a two-sided test, with R^2 denoting the square of the multiple correlation coefficient when the variable of interest is regressed on the other regression variables in the model. It can be observed that this is the formula due to Signorini (1991) given earlier in this section, divided by $(1 - R^2)$.

Thus, the sample size is larger when there are other regression variables in the model since $(1 - R^2) < 1$. Although there has apparently not been any published research to confirm this, this inflation factor may be suspect for use in Poisson regression with multiple covariates, just as it is for logistic regression, as discussed in Section 5.2.2.

Just as was done for logistic regression, Shieh (2001) offered an improvement over the approach given by Signorini (1991) for Poisson regression. Specifically, Shieh's (2001) method incorporated the limiting value of the maximum likelihood estimates of nuisance parameters under the composite null hypothesis. Since it is based on maximum likelihood estimates, the method may not work very well when maximum likelihood is not the best method of estimation, but as indicated previously, this isn't going to be known until the data have been collected.

5.5 NONLINEAR REGRESSION

Determining sample size for nonlinear regression would be a very formidable task because there are so many possible nonlinear regression models. Therefore, it is not surprising that sample size capability for nonlinear regression is not available in any of the leading software (e.g., it is not available in PASS), nor has it apparently been discussed in the literature.

5.6 OTHER TYPES OF REGRESSION MODELS

There are other types of regression models (probit regression, random coefficient regression, etc.) but there is no widely available sample size determination software for such models, nor has there apparently been any research on sample size determination for such models.

5.7 CORRELATION

Correlation is related to linear regression in the following way. If X is a *random* variable, we may properly speak of the *correlation* between X and Y. [Note that the term "correlation" is frequently used (improperly) when the values of X to be used in a regression model are preselected rather than occurring as realizations of a random variable, but the practice is longstanding and not likely to change.]

Correlation refers to the extent that the two random variables are related, with the strength of the relationship measured by the (sample) correlation coefficient, r_{xy}. There are many types of correlation coefficients, whose use depends on whether the variables are continuous, binary, ordinal, and so on. Some of these are mentioned briefly in Chapter 11, with references that discuss sample size determination.

The most commonly used correlation coefficient, which is for measuring the strength of the linear relationship between two continuous random variables that have a joint bivariate distribution (a seldom checked requirement), is the Pearson sample correlation coefficient. It is computed as

$$r_{xy} = \frac{S_{xy}}{\sqrt{S_{xx}S_{yy}}} \tag{5.13}$$

with $S_{xx} = \sum(X - \bar{X})^2$, $S_{xy} = \sum(X - \bar{X})(Y - \bar{Y})$, and $S_{yy} = \sum(Y - \bar{Y})^2$. Formally, the population correlation coefficient, ρ_{xy}, is defined as the covariance between X and Y divided by the standard deviation of X times the standard deviation of Y. When those parameters are estimated by the sample statistics, the result reduces to Eq. (5.13).

The possible values of r_{xy} range from -1 to $+1$. The former represents perfect negative correlation, as would happen if all the points fell on a line with a negative slope, and the latter represents perfect positive correlation. In regression there is nothing really "negative" about negative correlation, though, as a strong negative correlation is just as valuable as a strong positive correlation as far as estimation and prediction are concerned, although usually the Xs in a regression model are positively correlated with Y. A zero correlation between X and Y would signify that it would not be meaningful to construct a linear regression equation using that regressor, and the same could be said if the correlation is small.

Although a user could solve for the sample size for a hypothesis test of H_0: $\rho = 0$ against a logical alternative, we would certainly expect there to be a nonzero correlation between Y and any particular X that is being considered for a simple linear regression model. Thus, this would be a somewhat meaningless exercise. (Recall the statement made in Section 1.1 that null hypotheses are almost always false; this would be an example of that.)

What would not be meaningless, however, would be to proceed along the lines of what was discussed in Section 5.1.1 regarding Soper's applet.

Since R^2 discussed in that section equals r_{xy}^2, the discussion there directly applies to correlation. That is, one could decide upon a minimally acceptable value of r_{xy} to allow the user to claim a meaningful (linear) correlation between X and Y, then convert that to R^2 and then to the corresponding effect size and use Soper's applet. To illustrate, assume that 0.7 is chosen as the dividing line between an acceptable and unacceptable correlation. Thus, $R^2 = .49$ and the effect size, f^2, is 0.96. With Soper's applet we obtain $n = 11$ if the power is specified as .80 and $\alpha = .05$; we obtain $n = 14$ if the power is .90.

When the user-written command `sampsi_rho` for Stata is used, a sample size of $n = 11.22$ results when 0.7 is specified as the value of the correlation coefficient under the alternative hypothesis and power of .80 and a one-sided test are specified. When the power is increased to .90, Stata gives 14.38 as the sample size. (The actual powers are .832 and .914, respectively.) These are also, oddly, the values of n, to the nearest integer, that result when Power and Precision is used and a *two*-sided test is specified. When a one-sided test is specified, the sample sizes that the software gives are 9 and 11, respectively, for powers of .80 of .90, respectively. PASS, which uses theoretical results given by Guenther (1977), gives 13 and 17, respectively, for these two power values when a two-sided test is used and 11 and 14 for a one-sided test, with nQuery giving 14 and 17 for the two-sided test and 11 and 14 for the one-sided test. The corresponding results given by G*Power are 14 and 17 and 11 and 13, respectively, thus not agreeing with either nQuery or PASS. The disagreement is small, although the percentage disagreement is not small. Lenth's applet agrees with PASS without giving the user the option of choosing between a one-sided and two-sided test. It is not clear why the results given by Power and Precision for a two-sided test are off more than slightly.

Among other applets, the one at `http://www.quantitativeskills.com/sisa/statistics/corrhlp.htm` can be used for both two-sided tests and one-sided tests and, without specific additional input, gives necessary sample sizes for all combinations of $\alpha = .10, .05, .01$, and $.001$, and power values of .6, .7, .8, and .9. The results agree with the aforementioned results given by PASS.

When there is more than one independent variable that is of interest relative to a dependent variable, determining sample size to detect a certain minimum (nonzero) value of a multiple correlation coefficient may be of interest. Gatsonis and Sampson (1989) addressed this issue and presented tables for sample size determination.

5.7.1 Confidence Intervals

Of course, a confidence interval for ρ of a desired width could also be constructed, and would be a more practical approach because testing a null hypothesis of zero doesn't accomplish very much. To illustrate, assume as in the preceding example that $\hat{\rho} = .7$ and we want a 95% two-sided confidence interval to be of width 0.1. In order to accomplish this, the sample size must be 404, according to PASS. Since that is a very large sample, a width of .20 might have to be used. This requires a sample size of 105, which might still be larger than practical in certain applications.

Interestingly, nQuery provides a hypothesis test for ρ that can be either one-sided or two-sided, but sample size can be determined for only a one-sided confidence bound. Because of asymmetry of the distribution of r_{xy}, the required sample size will depend on whether an upper limit or lower limit is desired. For example, if $\hat{\rho} = .7$ and an upper limit of .8 is specified, nQuery gives $n = 54$, but $n = 93$ results if a lower limit of .6 is specified. These results are in agreement with the results given by PASS, which has the capability for one-sided confidence bounds in addition to two-sided intervals.

Although G*Power has the capability for testing several different types of correlation coefficients, no confidence intervals of any type are provided. Similarly, although MINITAB has the capability for sample size determination for some types of confidence intervals, this does not include a confidence interval for ρ. Power and Precision does not have the capability to compute sample sizes for confidence interval widths directly, but a user can enter a number for the population correlation and the limits are displayed. Thus, the user could use some directed trial and error to arrive at a sample size for a confidence interval of a desired width as a by-product of the hypothesis tests. Unfortunately, when a one-sided hypothesis test is specified, the output gives the limits for a two-sided confidence interval, so the hypothesis test and confidence interval results are not connected.

5.7.2 Intraclass Correlation

There are different types of intraclass correlation coefficients, with intraclass correlation originally for paired measurements, such as measurements made on the same subject. This is the way that intraclass correlation is incorporated into PASS, with sample size determined relative to the hypothesis test that the intraclass correlation is equal to a specified value.

For example, if the null hypothesis of no intraclass correlation is tested against the alternative hypothesis that the intraclass correlation is 0.6, the number of subjects must be input into PASS, which will give the number of observations to use per subject. (In a random effects linear model, with treatments the random factor, this is the number of treatments rather than the number of people.) When $\alpha = .05$, power $= .90$, and 5 is entered for the number of subjects, PASS gives $n = 7$ observations per subject. This is a one-sided test, as a two-sided test is not an option, unlike the options that are available for testing a Pearson correlation coefficient, which include a two-sided test and an upper and lower one-sided test. See Bonett (2002) for sample size determination for estimation of intraclass correlation coefficients.

5.7.3 Two Correlations

It is sometimes of interest to test whether two correlation coefficients are equal, such as determining if two different methods of school instruction correlate equally with student test performance. This is completely analogous to testing whether the slopes of two simple linear regression models are equal because if both X and Y are put in correlation form, the (single) regression coefficient in the equation is the linear (Pearson) correlation between X and Y. So testing for the equality of two correlation coefficients would indirectly test the equality of the slopes of the two simple linear regression models.

Segmented regression refers to the fitting of two or more linear regression models to a set of data, with the different models fit for nonoverlapping ranges of the data. For example, a simple linear regression model might be fit for $12 \leq X \leq 18$ and a different simple linear regression model fit for $19 \leq X \leq 30$. This decision might be based on subject-matter knowledge. If the assumption of the need for two models is not well founded, however, a test of the equality of the two correlation coefficients might be performed, with a decision made to fit two models only if the sample correlations differ by at least a specified amount. The task is then to determine the sample size for each group, after specifying the desired power and significance level.

Power and Precision and PASS are two software packages that can be used for solving for sample size. Of course, the two correlation coefficients should be reasonably close to one; otherwise, neither simple linear regression model would provide a good fit to the data.

So let's specify one correlation at .80 and the other at .90, with this difference of .10 being the minimum difference that we want to detect. Using either Power and Precision or PASS, the sample size for each group is found to be 154, so the total number of observations will be 308. Such a large number may not be obtainable, however. If so and if power of .80 is acceptable, 116 observations would be required for each group, for a total of 232. Of course, larger sample sizes would be required if the difference between the two correlations was less than .10. Depending on the type of application, the required sample sizes might not be attainable, even for a power of .80 and a difference of .10.

The applet mentioned in Section 5.7 gives results that agree with the results given by PASS and Power and Precision for this example and provides sample sizes for one- and two-sided tests of the null and alternative hypotheses for all combinations of $\alpha = .10, .05, .01, .001$ and power $= .6, .7, .8,$ and $.9$.

5.8 SOFTWARE

Overall, software for sample size determination for regression models is somewhat of a problem. First, software is not available for all types of regression models and there are some problems with existing software, both in terms of different software producing different solutions, as noted in Section 5.2.1.1 for logistic regression because different algorithms are being used, and in terms of what the user must input. It is best not to focus on individual regression coefficients in multiple linear regression and multiple logistic regression, but rather determine sample size by using a measure of model worth, such as R^2. Although this is straightforward in linear regression because there is one commonly used form of R^2, there are multiple forms of R^2 that have been proposed for logistic regression.

Another problem with software is the absence of capability for determining sample size when a necessary alternative to maximum likelihood should be used, such as the method proposed by Firth (1993).

5.9 SUMMARY

Sample size determination for regression models is difficult (and almost inadvisable when the focus is on individual regression coefficients) because of the problems involved in trying to interpret regression coefficients. A new method that involves the Wetz criterion was presented for linear regression but there is no way to avoid guesswork unless there is prior information available. Another problem is that the common use of maximum likelihood as the method of estimation can create problems in logistic regression (binary and polytomous), as well as in Cox regression. These problems can overshadow problems caused by using a sample size that is too small or too large when these methods are employed. Furthermore, even in simple linear regression there are quantities that must be specified which will generally be unknown and may be difficult to estimate, such as the variance of the predictor when it is a random variable, as discussed in Section 5.1.1. Problems were noted with a proposed method of determining sample size for multiple logistic regression, and although a simple rule-of-thumb might be preferable, analogous to the 10:1 rule-of-thumb for multiple linear regression, it would be difficult to construct a simple rule motivated by the results of Peduzzi et al. (1996) because it may be difficult to estimate how many events there should be for combinations of planned or anticipated values of the predictor variables. Of course, there is also parameter estimation error in virtually all practical applications of sample size determination and Taylor and Muller (1996) have looked at the bias this creates for linear models.

REFERENCES

Adcock, C. J. (1997). Sample size determination: A review. *The Statistician*, **46**(2), 261–283.

Alam, M. K., M. B. Rao, and F.-C. Cheng (2010). Sample size determination in logistic regression. *Sankya*, **72B**, Part 1, 58–75.

Algina, J. and S. Olejnik (2000). Determining sample size for accurate estimation of the squared multiple correlation coefficient. *Multivariate Behavioral Research*, **35**(1), 119–136.

Ammann, R.A. (2004). Correspondence. Bone Marrow Transplantation, **34**, 277–278. (Available at `http://www.cytel.com/Papers/2004.08_Letter_nature.pdf`.)

Bonett, D. G. (2002). Sample size requirements for estimating intraclass correlations with desired precision. *Statistics in Medicine*, **21**(9), 1331–1335.

Brownlee, K. A. (1960). *Statistical Theory and Methodology in Science and Engineering*. New York: Wiley.

Bull, S. B. (1993). Sample size and power determination for a binary outcome and an ordinal response when logistic regression is planned. *American Journal of Epidemiology*, **137**, 676–684.

Cohen, J. (1988). *Statistical Power Analysis for the Behavioral Sciences*. 2nd edition. New York: Routledge Academic.

Cook, R. D. and S. Weisberg (1999). *Applied Regression Including Computing and Graphics.* New York: Wiley.

Cox, D. R. (1970). *The Analysis of Binary Data.* London: Chapman and Hall.

Cox, D. R. (1972). Regression models and life tables. *Journal of the Royal Statistical Society, Series B,* **34**, 187–220.

Dattalo, P. (2008). *Determining Sample Size: Balancing Power, Precision, and Practicality.* New York: Oxford University Press.

Demidenko, E. (2007). Sample size determination for logistic regression revisited. *Statistics in Medicine,* **26**(18), 3385–3397.

Demidenko, E. (2008). Sample size and optimal design for logistic regression with binary infection. *Statistics in Medicine,* **27**, 36–46.

Draper, N. R. and H. Smith (1981). *Applied Regression Analysis,* 2nd edition. New York: Wiley. (The current edition is the 3rd edition, 1998.)

Firth, D. (1993). Bias reduction of maximum likelihood estimates. *Biometrika,* **80**, 27–38.

Flack, V. F. and T. L. Eudey (1993). Sample size determinations using logistic regression with pilot data. *Statistics in Medicine,* **12**, 1079–1084.

Gatsonis, C. and A. R. Sampson (1989). Multiple correlation: Exact power and sample size calculations. *Psychological Bulletin,* **106**(3), 516–524.

Gorman, J. W. and R. J. Toman (1966). Selection of variables for fitting equations to data. *Technometrics,* **8**, 27–51.

Guenther, W. C. (1977). Desk calculation of probabilities for the distribution of the sample correlation coefficient. *The American Statistician,* **31**(1), 45–48.

Halinksi, R. S. and L. S. Feldt (1970). The selection of variables in multiple regression analyses. *Journal of Educational Measurement,* **7**(3), 151–158.

Hosmer, D. W. Jr. and S. Lemeshow (2000). *Applied Logistic Regression,* 2nd edition. New York: Wiley.

Hsieh, F. Y. (1989). Sample size tables for logistic regression. *Statistics in Medicine,* **8**, 795–802.

Hsieh, F. Y. and P. W. Lavori (2000). Sample-size calculations for the Cox proportional hazards regression model with nonbinary covariates. *Controlled Clinical Trials,* **21**, 552–560.

Hsieh, F. Y., D.A. Bloch, and M. D. Larsen (1998). A simple method of sample size calculation for linear and logistic regression. *Statistics in Medicine,* **17**, 1623–1634.

Kelley, K. and S. E. Maxwell (2003). Sample size for multiple regression: Obtaining regression coefficients that are accurate, not simply significant. *Psychological Methods,* **8**, 305–321. (Available at http://citeseerx.ist.psu.edu/viewdoc/download?doi=10.1.1.163.5835&rep=rep1&type.pdf.)

Krishnamoorthy, K. and Y. Xia (2008). Sample size calculation for estimating or testing a nonzero squared multiple correlation coefficient. *Multivariate Behavioral Research,* **43**(3), 382–410.

King, E. N. and Ryan, T. P. (2002). A preliminary investigation of maximum likelihood logistic regression versus exact logistic regression. *The American Statistician,* **56**, 163–170.

Kodell, R. L., S. Y. Lensing, R. D. Landes, K. S. Kumar, and M. Hauer-Jensen (2010). Determination of sample sizes for demonstrating efficacy of radiation countermeasures. *Biometrics,* **66**, 239–248.

Kraemer, H. C. and S. Thiemann (1987). *How Many Subjects? Statistical Power Analysis in Research.* Newbury Park, CA: Sage Publications.

Lenth, R. V. (2001). Some practical guidelines for effective sample size determination. *The American Statistician*, **55**, 187–193.

Lindsey, J. K. (1997). Exact sample size calculations for exponential family models. *The Statistician*, **46**(2), 231–237.

Long, J. S. (1997). *Regression Models for Categorical and Limited Dependent Variables*. Thousand Oaks, CA: Sage Publications.

Maxwell, S. E. (2000). Sample size and multiple regression analsyis. *Psychological Methods*, **5**, 434–458.

Mehta, C. R. and N. R. Patel (1995). Exact logistic regression: Theory and examples. *Statistics in Medicine*, **14**, 2143–2160.

Menard, S. (2000). Coefficients of determination for multiple logistic regression analysis. *The American Statistician*, **54**, 17–24.

Mendoza, J. L. and K. L. Stafford (2001). Confidence intervals, power calculation, and sample size estimation for the squared multiple correlation coefficient under the fixed and random regression models: A computer program and useful standard tables. *Educational and Psychological Measurement*, **61**(4), 650–667.

Miller, D. E. and J. T. Kunce (1973). Prediction and statistical overkill revisited. *Measurement and Evaluation in Guidance*, **6**(3), 157–163.

Müller, K. E. and V. B. Pasour (1997). Bias in linear model power and sample size due to estimating variance. *Communications in Statistics—Theory and Methods*, **26**(4), 839–852.

Newson, R. (2004). Generalized power calculations for generalized linear models and more. *The Stata Journal*, **4**(4), 379–401.

Novikov, I., N. Fund, and L. S. Freedman (2010). A modified approach to estimating sample size for simple logistic regression with one continuous covariate. *Statistics in Medicine*, **29**(1), 97–107.

Peduzzi, P., J. Concato, E. Kemper, T. R. Holford, and A. R. Feinstein (1996). A simulation study of the number of events per variable in logistic regression analysis. *Journal of Clinical Epidemiology*, **49**(12), 1373–1379.

Ryan, T. P. (2009a). *Modern Regression Methods*, 2nd edition. Hoboken, NJ: Wiley.

Ryan, T. P. (2009b). Maximum Likelihood. Course developed for The Institute for Statistics Education.

Ryan, T. P. and W. H. Woodall (2005). The most-cited statistical papers. *Journal of Applied Statistics*, **32**(5), 1–14.

Sawyer, R. (1983). Determining minimum sample sizes for multiple regression grade prediction equations for colleges. *American Statistical Association Proceedings of the Social Statistics Section*, pp. 379–384. (Also as Research Report No. 83, American College Testing Program, February 1984.)

Schoenfeld, D. A. (1983). Sample size formula for the proportional-hazards regression model. *Biometrics*, **39**, 499–503.

Schouten, H. J. A. (1999). Sample size formula with a continuous outcome for unequal group sizes and unequal variances. *Statistics in Medicine*, **18**, 87–91.

Self, S. G. and R. H. Mauritsen (1988). Power/sample size calculations for generalized linear models. *Biometrics*, **44**, 79–86.

Self, S. G., R. H. Mauritsen, and J. Ohara (1992). Power calculations for likelihood ratio tests. *Biometrics*, **48**, 31–39.

Sharma, D. R. (2006). Logistic regression, measures of explained variation, and the base rate problem. Ph.D. dissertation. Department of Statistics, Florida State University. (Available at http://etd.lib.fsu.edu/theses/available/etd-06292006-153249/unrestricted/dissertation_drs.pdf.)

Shieh, G. (2000). On power and sample size calculations for likelihood ratio tests in generalized linear models. *Biometrics*, **56**, 1192–1196.

Shieh, G. (2001). Sample size calculations for logistic and Poisson regression models. *Biometrika*, **88**(4), 1193–1199.

Signorini, D. F. (1991). Sample size for Poisson regression. *Biometrika*, **78**(2), 446–450.

Simon, S. (2008). Sample size for an ordinal outcome. (Electronic resource: www.pmean.com/04/ordinalLogistic.html.)

Taylor, D. J. and K. E. Müller (1996). Bias in linear model power and sample size calculation due to estimating noncentrality. *Communications in Statistics—Theory and Methods*, **25**(7), 1595–1610.

Taylor, A. B., S. G. West, and L. S. Aiken (2006). Loss of power in logistic, ordinal logistic, and probit regression when an outcome variable is coarsely categorized. *Educational and Psychological Measurement*, **66**(2), 228–239.

Thigpen, C. C. (1987). A sample size problem in simple linear regression. *The American Statistician*, **41**, 214–215.

Tosteson, T. D., J. S. Buzas, E. Demidenko, and M. Karagas (2003). Power and sample size calculations for generalized regression models with covariate measurement error. *Statistics in Medicine*, **22**(7), 1069–1082.

Vaeth, M. and E. Skovlund (2004). A simple approach to power and sample size calculations in logistic regression and Cox regression models. *Statistics in Medicine*, **23**(11), 1781–1792.

Vaughn, C. and S. Guzy (2002). Redesigning experiments with polychotomous logistic regression: A power computation application. Paper 26-27. SUGI27.

Walters, S. J. (2004). Sample size and power estimation for studies with health related quality of life outcomes: A comparison of four methods using the SF-36. *Health and Quality of Life Outcomes*, **2**, 26. (Open access; available at www.hqlo.com/content/2/1/26 and www.hqlo.com/content/pdf/1477-7525-2-26.pdf.)

Wetz, J. M. (1964). Criteria for judging adequacy of estimation by an approximating response function. Ph.D. thesis. Department of Statistics, University of Wisconsin.

Whitehead, J. (1993). Sample size calculations for ordered categorical data. *Statistics in Medicine*, **12**, 2257–2271. (Erratum: April 30, 1994; **13**(8), 871.)

Whittemore, A. S. (1981). Sample size for logistic regression with small response probability. *Journal of the American Statistical Association*, **76**, 27–32.

EXERCISES

5.1. Verify Eq. (5.2).

5.2. Use the Demidenko applet at http://www.dartmouth.edu/~eugened/power-samplesize.php to determine the required sample size for a one-variable logistic regression problem with a binary covariate, such that 40% of the covariate values are equal to 1 and when the covariate value is 0,

60% of the response values are equal to 1, and the detectable odds ratio is 2.5. Use a significance level of .05 and power of .90.

5.3. A scientist comes to you and asks you to determine the sample size that she should obtain when linear regression is to be used. There is to be just a single predictor so this will be simple linear regression. The predictor, however, is a random variable. The scientist tells you that she wants to have a good regression model with $R^2 \geq .75$. She realizes that a very small sample size is not a good idea but there is a sampling cost involved, which is not small. She has heard of the Wetz criterion and believes the criterion should be met. Assume the use of $\alpha = .05$.

5.4. An experimenter makes the following statement: "Because of the difficulty in determining sample size in simple linear regression, especially since my predictor will be random and samples in my field are costly, I am simply going to use the Draper and Smith rule-of-thumb and use a sample size of 10. Then I will enter the sample quantities from my experiment into PASS, including the sample size of 10 that I used, and see what power my experiment had, as given by PASS." Critique that statement.

5.5. How would you advise a researcher to determine sample size for multiple binary logistic regression?

5.6. The regression methods discussed in the chapter all rely on maximum likelihood as the method of estimation (ordinary least squares is equivalent to maximum likelihood under the assumption of normality), even though maximum likelihood could be a poor choice, depending on the data (King and Ryan, 2002). Of course, when the sample size is being determined, there are no data, unless there are data available from a pilot study or similar study. Therefore, what is the first step that you would recommend for a user once the data have been collected?

CHAPTER 6

Experimental Designs

Designed experiments are often costly and consequently there has long been interest in determining adequate sample sizes, with such interest dating at least from Harris, Horvitz, and Mood (1948).

In examining sample size determination for experimental designs, we need to consider replicated and unreplicated designs separately. Included in the latter category are fractional factorial designs, which are generally not replicated. In this chapter we will question whether they should be replicated, and what would be gained by using replication. We will also consider whether certain types of blocking designs, such as Latin square designs, should be replicated.

Another thing to keep in mind is that a large number of experimental runs, which may result if the experimenter wants to detect a somewhat small effect, could, depending on the application, generally not be performed in a short period of time. This could create a time effect if the results did vary over time. An experimenter might not anticipate this, however, with the consequence that a time effect may not be designed into an experiment so that time can be separated from the error term. If not, the error term may be considerably inflated and the power of hypothesis tests reduced. This should be kept in mind in determining the sample size for experiments that cannot be performed quickly.

Since sample sizes will be determined so that effects of specified magnitudes can be detected with high probability, we will almost totally restrict attention to fixed factors until Section 6.13, since effect sizes are not used with random factors (variance components are used instead). Sample size determination for designs with random factors is discussed briefly in Section 6.13.

We should also keep in mind that experimentation should ideally be sequential so that more than a single experimental design should be used. For example, a two-level screening design might be used in the first stage to identify the important factors, followed by a design with more levels that would be used to try to identify

Sample Size Determination and Power, First Edition. Thomas P. Ryan.
© 2013 John Wiley & Sons, Inc. Published 2013 by John Wiley & Sons, Inc.

optimum levels of the important factors as well as to identify interaction terms that might be needed in the model.

Daniel (1976) recommended that 33 to 50% of the resources be spent on the first experiment, and Box, Hunter, and Hunter (1978) recommended that at most 25% of the resources be used for the first experiment. (The latter did not discuss this topic in the 2nd edition, 2005, of their book.) This means that sample size (i.e., design size) must be determined for each design that is part of the sequence. It is especially important that this be planned carefully so that the budget is not exceeded. (Recall the discussion in Section 2.7 on the cost of sampling.) For some experimentation objectives it may not be readily apparent that sequential experimentation should be performed, whereas for other objectives, such as determining optimum operating conditions, the use of at least two experimental designs is routine and common practice. This is the case in response surface experimentation, which is discussed in Section 6.6. In general, once the linear effect of important factors is identified, it is desirable to see if any of those factors additionally have any nonlinear effects, such as quadratic effects.

6.1   ONE FACTOR—TWO FIXED LEVELS

Consider the simplest case of one factor with two fixed (i.e., predetermined) levels, with the data independent between the two levels. The data could be analyzed using either a pooled-t test in Eq. (1.1) or by using analysis of variance, with the results being equivalent.

Assuming that the number of observations to be made at each of the two levels is the same and the variances at each level are equal and known (admittedly a strong assumption), the formula for the sample size at each level, $n/2$, assuming a two-sided test, is given by

$$\frac{n}{2} = \frac{(z_{\alpha/2} + z_\beta)^2 (2\sigma^2)}{\Delta^2} \qquad (6.1)$$

(See the chapter Appendix for the derivation.) Here, as in previous chapters, Z_α is the standard normal variate for the selected value of α, Z_β is the standard normal variate for $1 - \text{power} = \beta$, and Δ is the difference between the two means. If $\alpha = .05$, $\beta = .20$ (corresponding to a desired power of .80), and we express Δ generally as $k\sigma$, then

$$\frac{n}{2} = \frac{(1.96 + 0.84)^2 (2\sigma^2)}{(k\sigma)^2} = \frac{15.68}{k^2} \qquad (6.2)$$

Thus, $n/2$ is a decreasing function of k as a greater sample size is needed to detect a small difference than to detect a large difference.

Especially when human subjects are involved, the experimenter will at times have a fixed number of subjects available to participate in a study. In that case, it is useful to solve for Z_β and ultimately determine power as a function of $n/2$ and either Δ or $k\sigma$. Doing so produces

$$Z_\beta = \frac{\Delta\sqrt{\frac{n}{2}} - Z_{\alpha/2}\sigma\sqrt{2}}{\sigma\sqrt{2}}$$

If we let $\Delta = k\sigma$, this simplifies to

$$Z_\beta = \frac{k\sqrt{n}}{2} - Z_{\alpha/2}$$

Then $\beta = 1 - \Phi(k\sqrt{n}/2 - Z_{\alpha/2})$, with $\Phi(\cdot)$ denoting the normal cumulative distribution function. Thus,

$$\text{Power} = 1 - \beta = \Phi\left(\frac{k\sqrt{n}}{2} - Z_{\alpha/2}\right) \tag{6.3}$$

To illustrate, for the current example and using $k = 1$,

$$\text{Power} = 1 - \beta = \Phi\left(\frac{\sqrt{31.36}}{2} - 1.96\right) = \Phi(.84) = .80,$$

as was specified.

When data are not independent between the two levels, such as when a paired-t test is used, the two samples are collapsed into one set of differences ("before" minus "after," say), and sample size determination then proceeds the same as when there is only one sample (i.e., as in Section 3.3).

Although the computations are relatively simple when there are two levels, software can be used, if desired. For example, when MINITAB is used, the power and sample size routine for comparing two means assumes that a t-test is being used, even though the user must specify σ. Of course, if we knew σ, then we wouldn't use t! We can't replace Z by t in Eq. (6.1) and obtain an expression that could be used to solve for the sample size because a t-variate depends on the degrees of freedom for the t-statistic in the hypothesis test, which in turn depends on the sample size. Thus, an iterative approach must be used for determining sample size whenever a t-statistic is used in hypothesis testing. MINITAB does not provide the capability for determining sample size when σ is either assumed to be known or estimated without using data from the two samples that are to be taken in a two-sample procedure. That is, there is not a two-sample Z procedure whereas the user does have the option of determining sample size for either a one-sample t or a one-sample Z.

The Power Pack applet developed by Russell Lenth (http://homepage. stat.uiowa.edu/~rlenth/Power/) is one of many other available software that could be used. It works the same way as does MINITAB for this test. That is, σ for each population must be specified, but the computation is performed using the t-distribution. Thus, if the pooled-t test is selected, the user must specify either equal or unequal sigmas; then the computation of power for specified sample sizes or for "true difference of the means," whichever is selected, is based on the use of the t-distribution.

For example, if $\sigma_1 = \sigma_2 = 1$, a two-tailed test is to be performed, the minimum true difference between the means that one wishes to detect is also 1 (i.e., $k\sigma = 1$ in the notation of this section), equal sample sizes for the two groups are specified, and a desired power of .80 is used, then the applet produces $n_1 = n_2 = 17$, with a power of .807. (Of course, the applet does not give fractional sample sizes, so the power will almost certainly not be equal to the specified value.)

We can verify this sample size by proceeding analogously to the example used at the start of this section. That is, if we proceed as in Eq. (6.3) but use t instead of z, we have

$$\text{Power} = 1 - \beta = \Phi^* \left(\frac{k\sqrt{n}}{2} - t_{\alpha/2,((n_1+n_2)/2)} \right)$$

If we use $n_1 = n_2 = 17$ and $n = 34$, with Φ^* denoting the cdf of a t-distribution with 32 degrees of feedom, we obtain Power $= .807$, which is the value given by the applet.

6.1.1   Unequal Sample Sizes

We might expect that it would be logical to have $n_1 = n_2$. This would indeed be reasonable if $\sigma_1 = \sigma_2$, but not if they differed more than slightly. The logic is as follows. If one population had considerable variability, we would expect to need a large sample size in order to have an estimator of the population mean (i.e., the sample mean), with acceptable variability, whereas a smaller sample size would suffice for a population with less variability.

To illustrate this point, consider the following simple example. Let one (very small) population consist of the numbers 12, 23, 29, 32, and 34, and let the other population consist of the numbers 13, 15, 18, 19, and 20. For the first population, no sample of size three would have a sample mean that is close to the population mean of 26 (the closest would be 28, the average of the middle three numbers), whereas the average of the middle three numbers of the second population differs from the population mean by only 0.3. Because the population standard deviations differ considerably (9.91 versus 3.26), the sample sizes should also differ.

Lenth's applet can be used to determine either equal or unequal sample sizes for the two-sample t-test. The user has three options: (1) equal sample sizes, (2) choose n_1 and n_2 independently, and (3) optimal allocation, which sets $n_1/n_2 = \sigma_1/\sigma_2$, with this allocation minimizing the standard error of the difference of the sample means. To illustrate, continuing with the example in which the two population standard deviations are 9.91 and 3.26, respectively, if a difference in means of 4 is to be detected with power of .80, using a two-sided test with $\alpha = .05$, the applet gives $n_1 = 66$ and $n_2 = 21$, with power $= .7997$, if we try to come as close to .80 as possible, and $n_1 = 66$ and $n_2 = 22$ with power $= .8043$ if we require that the power be at least .80.

Such software options are clearly desirable because there will be many applications in which it will not be plausible to assume $\sigma_1 = \sigma_2$. Although a pooled-t test then cannot be used, an approximate t-test (often called the Welch t-test) can be used. If both sample sizes are large, then a z-test could be used as each standard deviation would then be a good estimator of the corresponding population standard deviation.

The Power and Precision software, for example, does not allow for unequal sample sizes, nor does MINITAB, and problems ensue when one attempts to use either nQuery Advisor or PASS. The former has a Satterthwaite t-test procedure for unequal variances but the routine can be used only to solve for power, not sample sizes. If $n_1 = 66$ and $n_2 = 22$ are entered in addition to the other input, the power is given as .80, in general agreement with the Lenth applet solution. The solution given by PASS is also in general agreement, as selecting the procedure "Tests for Two Means (Two-Sample T-Test) [Differences]" and using an allocation ratio of 0.329 ($= 3.26/9.91$) results in 66 and 22 for the two sample sizes, respectively, with the power given as 0.80453.

See Luh and Guo (2010) for sample size determination with unequal variances.

6.2 ONE FACTOR—MORE THAN TWO FIXED LEVELS

When a factor has more than two levels, analysis of variance (ANOVA) is used to analyze the data. We will assume that the design is a completely randomized design (CRD). That is, the levels are assigned at random to the experimental units and the design is run with random order. For example, if there were six experimental units for each of three levels, the 18 experimental runs would be made in a random order.

The sample size hand computation is naturally more involved when there are more than two levels, but it can be done without too much difficulty, if hand computation is desired to gain understanding.

With more than two levels, one obvious question is: What "effect" is used in determining sample size? That is, should it be the largest pairwise effect, or should it be the F-statistic for testing the equality of the means, or something else? The user of Lenth's applet, for example, can determine sample size based on either the F-test or on multiple comparisons such as Tukey's Honestly Significant Difference [see, e.g., http://en.wikipedia.org/wiki/Tukey's_test or Gravetter and Wallnau (2009)] or the set of t-tests. It might also be of interest to solve for n based on the smallest difference of the effects of two levels of interest. This is discussed, for example, in Sahai and Ageel (2000, p. 63).

When an F-statistic is the criterion, power is computed using the value of the *noncentrality parameter*. Unfortunately, it is not possible to give a simple definition of a noncentrality parameter, and this is due in large part to the fact that noncentrality parameters for various tests in experimental design are defined differently by different writers. For example, in one-way ANOVA with k means, the noncentrality parameter is often given as $\sum_{i=1}^{k}[n_i(\tau_i - \bar{\tau})^2/\sigma^2]$, where n_i denotes the number of observations in level i, k is the number of means, $\tau_i = \mu_i - \mu$, with μ_i the mean for the ith level and μ the overall mean (i.e., the expected value of each individual observation under the null hypothesis that the treatment means are all equal, and $\bar{\tau} = \sum_{i=1}^{k} n_i \tau_i / \sum_{i=1}^{k} n_i$) Of course, σ^2 is the variance of the individual observations under the null hypothesis. Note that the expression simplifies to $n \sum_{i=1}^{k}(\tau_i^2/\sigma^2)$ when there are an equal number of observations for each level. Some authors (e.g., Sahai and Ageel, 2000, p. 57) have given $\sum_{i=1}^{k}[n_i(\tau_i - \bar{\tau})^2/2\sigma^2]$ as the form of the noncentrality parameter, and other authors have used the square root of this expression. [See., for example, the discussion of this in Giesbrecht and Gumpertz (2004, p. 61).] These different, conflicting expressions do impede understanding somewhat.

One very general and simple explanation of a noncentrality parameter given by Minitab, Inc. at http://www.minitab.com/en-US/support/answers/answer.aspx?log=0&id=733&langType=1033 is that noncentrality parameters "reflect the extent to which the null hypothesis is false." More specifically, it is a standardized measure of the difference between the hypothesized value of a parameter and the actual (assumed) value. We can see this if we think about the noncentrality parameter for a t-test, although it isn't necessary to use the noncentrality parameter for that test to compute power and to solve for a sample size, as was shown in Section 3.11. Nevertheless, in the present context it is helpful to do so. If the null hypothesis for such a test is H_0: $\mu = 72$, the noncentrality parameter is $(\mu - 72)/(\sigma/\sqrt{n})$, with μ denoting the true mean. Thus, the noncentrality parameter is the difference between the true mean and the hypothesized mean divided by the standard deviation of the point estimator of μ, which is $\bar{x}$, with its standard deviation being $\sigma/\sqrt{n}$.

For simplicity of exposition, we will now assume that the n_i are equal, so that the (first) noncentrality parameter expression simplifies to $n \sum_{i=1}^{k} \tau_i^2/\sigma^2$. If we think about that explanation relative to the noncentrality parameter, under the null hypothesis the $\tau_i = 0$, which is equivalent to saying that the k means are all equal to the overall mean, μ. Although mathematically unnecessary, it is somewhat useful to think of the noncentrality parameter as $n \sum_{i=1}^{k}(\tau_i - 0)^2/\sigma^2$. This is useful because the hypothesized value won't necessarily be zero in all types of sample size determination problems. This view of the form of a noncentrality parameter is intuitive because it is the difference between the true state of nature and the hypothesized state, divided by a standardization factor, σ^2, and multiplied by the number of observations sampled from each of the k populations. Of course we are continuing to assume fixed factors, whereas as will be seen in Section 6.13, expressions for noncentrality parameters with random factors are not so simple and intuitive.

Although noncentrality parameters were not discussed in previous chapters, the presentation, such as in Chapter 3, could have been along these lines. Equations (3.2), (3.4), and (3.6) show the sample size expression in each equation being a function of the squared difference of the actual parameter value and the hypothesized value, just as is being discussed here. For a pooled-t test, the noncentrality parameter is $\delta/\sqrt{2\sigma^2/n}$ or the square of this quantity, if preferred, with δ denoting the difference in the population means.

For practitioners who have an interest in seeing how the power is determined rather than just relying on sample size and power software, there are a few options. One option would be to work directly with the noncentral F-distribution, which is available in the R programming language, MATLAB, and Mathematica, as well as in Power and Precision.

■ **EXAMPLE 6.1**

To illustrate, let's assume that there are three fixed levels so that the null hypothesis is that the three population means are equal. In order to compute power for a specific example, we need to specify the true state of nature. That is, what is the effect of each level of the factor? The estimate of each effect is given by $\hat{\tau}_i = \hat{\mu}_i - \hat{\mu}$, with $\hat{\mu}$ the average of all the observations and $\hat{\mu}_i$ the average of the observations for the ith factor level. It is conventional in Analysis of Variance (ANOVA) with a fixed factor to assume that $\sum_{i=1}^{k} \hat{\tau}_i = 0$ for k levels of the factor. This is logical because the sum of the observations from the overall mean must be zero. Let's assume that $\tau_1 = 1$, $\tau_2 = 0$, and $\tau_3 = -1$. Then, assuming an experiment with ten observations obtained at each of the three levels, $\sigma^2 = 1$, and $\alpha = .05$, the noncentrality parameter is $n \sum_{i=1}^{3} \tau_i^2/\sigma^2 = 10[(1)^2 + (-1)^2]/1 = 20$. The tail probability of a noncentral F-distribution with 2 degrees of freedom for the numerator and 12 for the denominator (i.e., the power), as given by Power and Precision, is .9733. Thus, there is a high probability that the F-test will reject the hypothesis of equal population means for these values of the τ_i. And similarly if some other combination of τ_i values had produced $n \sum_{i=1}^{3} \tau_i^2 = 10(2) = 20$. Of course, in practice it may be very difficult to even determine a value for $n \sum_{i=1}^{3} \tau_i^2$, much less values for the individual τ_i. This general type of problem occurs with *all* types of sample size determination problems, however, as certain parameter values must of course be specified in order to solve for n. ■

An obvious problem with computations of this type is that if we knew the effect of each level of a factor, we wouldn't need to conduct an experiment! The more means that are involved, the more difficult it will be to think in terms of a value for the noncentrality parameter. Accordingly, it will often be easier to compute power for specific values of contrasts, such as $\mu_1 - \mu_2$. Software can also be used when this approach is taken.

Similarly, software can be used when specific methods of multiple comparisons are used, such as Tukey and Scheffé. The general textbook recommendation, however, has been that specific comparisons or contrasts should not be made unless the overall F-test for the equality of all the means is rejected. Because of this and because of the fact that the choice of a comparison procedure can depend on whether or not the experimenter wants to be conservative and also on whether or not the comparisons to be made are determined before looking at the data, we will not give much attention to sample size determination for multiple comparisons in this chapter, with the topic treated somewhat briefly in Section 6.2.1.

To illustrate the computation of sample size for this example such that the power will be .80, if we use, say, either Lenth's applet or Power and Precision, we need to compute $\sigma_\tau^2 = \sum_{i=1}^{3} \tau_i^2/d.f.$, where here $d.f.$ (degrees of freedom) is $3 - 1 = 2$ since there are three levels. Thus, $\sigma_\tau^2 = 2/2 = 1$ for the current example. Using Lenth's applet, we find that 6 observations per level are necessary to provide power of approximately .80 (actually .8053). Of course, we know that it must be less than 10 observations per level since that produced a power of .9733.

Since power of .80 is an arbitrary choice, it is usually a good idea to do at least a small-scale sensitivity study to see how power changes with the sample size. For this example, if we use 7 observations per level instead of 6, the power increases to .877. That is a sizable jump for just a one-unit increase in the number of observations, so depending on cost and resources, at least 7 observations may be preferred. Figure 6.1 shows the power values for n_i from 6 to 10.

Of course one problem with these calculations – which is common to all of the designs covered in this chapter – is that it is necessary to specify the error variance, which of course is generally unknown.

At this point it is worth noting how the case of one factor with more than two levels was handled by Cohen (1988), who defined a measure f as $f = \sigma_m/\sigma$, with σ the (assumed equal) standard deviation of each population, and σ_m the Standard deviation of the population means" defined, using the author's notation, as

$$\sigma_m = \sqrt{\frac{\sum_{i=1}^{k}(m_i - m)^2}{k}}$$

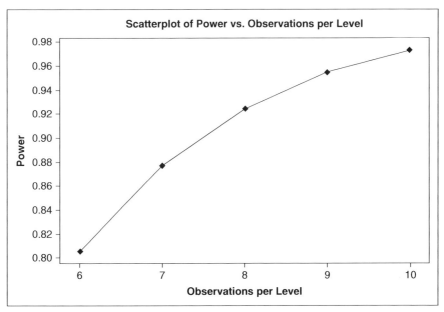

Figure 6.1   Power for various numbers of observations per level relative to Example 6.1.

for k means (levels of the factor), with m_i denoting the ith population mean and m denoting the means of the k population means, assuming equal sample sizes. This, of course, is a rather loose definition since population means are fixed and do not have a standard deviation. Thus, this should be viewed as simply a measure of spread of the population means.

Given this definition of f, Cohen (1988, pp. 284–285) considered small, medium, and large values of f to be .10, .25, and .40, respectively, which is the same set of designations that the Power and Precision software uses for Analysis of Variance with a single factor. Cohen was obviously influenced by what happens in the behavioral sciences and stated (p. 284) that "values of f as large as .50 are not common in the behavioral sciences."

Comparing this set of numbers with the three corresponding numbers (.10, .30, and .50) given in Section 2.5 shows that the three designations given by Cohen depend on the type of test that is being performed. There has been some confusion about this in the literature.

It was stated in Section 2.5 that such designations have been criticized by Lenth (2001) and others. One obvious deficiency is that practical significance is ignored with such a classification. The following illustration of this should be helpful.

Of course, σ and the population means will generally be unknown, so for illustration we will let them be estimated by their natural sample estimators for the following example of three levels of a factor and seven observations per level.

1	2	3
4.62	4.64	4.65
4.61	4.63	4.63
4.63	4.62	4.63
4.62	4.63	4.64
4.62	4.63	4.65
4.63	4.64	4.63
4.61	4.62	4.65

Let f be estimated by

$$\hat{f} = \sqrt{\frac{\sum_{i=1}^{3}(\bar{x}_i - \bar{\bar{x}})^2}{3}} \Big/ \hat{\sigma}$$

with $\hat{\sigma}$ denoting the square root of the pooled variance from an ANOVA table and $\bar{\bar{x}}$ denoting the average of the three means. Since the means are 4.62, 4.63, and 4.64, respectively, so that $\bar{\bar{x}} = 4.63$, we thus obtain $\hat{f} = \sqrt{(0.0002/3)}/0.00882 = 0.926$. Thus, the value of $\hat{f}$ is *more than double* what is considered to be a "large" value, yet the means differ by only 0.01. Thus, it is not practical to try to extend Cohen's (1988) effect sizes to general applications, and, in fairness to him, he did not try to do so. It is judicious to ignore Cohen's designations, except perhaps in behavioral science applications.

6.2.1 Multiple Comparisons and Dunnett's Test

When there are more than two levels of a fixed factor, there is often interest in performing multiple comparison tests involving subsets of the population means. For example, if a study involves three population means, the comparison of the first two means might be of particular interest, as well as the comparison of the second and third means. The question then arises as to how knowing that multiple comparisons are to be performed affects the determination of sample size. Witte, Elston, and Cardon (2000) addressed this issue, with the adjustment they gave being a (conservative) Bonferroni adjustment. Specifically, if m comparisons are to be performed, Witte et al. (2000) gave the Bonferroni adjustment as replacing z_d by $z_{d/m}$ in Eq. (3.6). They concluded: "the increase in sample size required for multiple comparisons (or tests) is not as great as might perhaps be expected. In particular, the relative sample size—allowing for the Bonferroni adjustment—is approximately linearly related to the logarithm of the number of comparisons made." Bang, Jung, and George (2005) gave a simple method for determining sample size and power for a simulation-based multiple testing procedure that they claimed is superior to a Bonferroni adjustment. Pan and Kupper (1999) determined optimal sample sizes for four multiple comparison procedures: Scheffé, Bonferroni, Tukey, and Dunnett. Schwertman (1987) presented a method for determining sample size to detect the largest pairwise difference in means for a single factor.

Although some multiple comparison tests require equal sample sizes, it is worth noting that unequal sample sizes are preferred when Dunnett's test is used. This is a test in which all of the treatments are compared against a control and these are the only comparisons that are made. Since the data for the control are thus being "Worked more" than the data for any one of the treatments, we might suspect that it would be desirable to use more observations for the control.

We can use PASS to show that this is indeed what should be done. If the minimum detectable difference is specified as 1.5σ and $\alpha = .05$, the power is .664 with equal sample sizes of 20 per group for two groups (treatments) plus the control, compared to a power of .883 when the sample sizes are 10, 20, and 30, with 30 being used for the control group. Thus, the total number of subjects is 60 in both cases, but the power figures differ greatly.

Generally, we want to have equal sample sizes for designs so that the data are balanced, but this is an exception.

6.2.2 Analysis of Means (ANOM)

Although ANOVA has been the assumed method of analysis to this point in the chapter, an alternative method that is inherently graphical is Analysis of Means (ANOM), for which the same assumptions must be met as in ANOVA. The latter and ANOM have different null hypotheses, as with ANOVA the null hypothesis is that all of the means are equal, whereas with ANOM there is a null hypothesis for each mean, with that null hypothesis being that the mean is equal to the average of all of the means. With ANOM, the alternative hypothesis is that at least one of the means differs from the others, whereas with ANOM the objective is to see whether or not one or more means differ from the average of all of the plotted means. Thus, what is being tested is different for the two procedures, so the results will not necessarily agree. In particular, when $k - 1$ sample averages are bunched tightly together but the kth sample average (i.e., the other one) differs considerably from the $k - 1$ averages, the F-value in ANOVA would likely be relatively small (thus indicating that the population means are equal), whereas the difference would probably be detected using ANOM. Conversely, if the differences between adjacent sample averages are both sizable and similar,

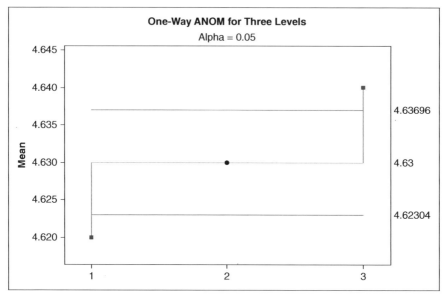

Figure 6.2 ANOM display for one factor and three levels.

the (likely) difference in the population means is more apt to be detected with ANOVA than with ANOM.

ANOM applied to the data given in Section 6.2 results in Figure 6.2.

The display shows that, with $\alpha = .05$, the first and third means differ significantly from the overall average.

There is no software available for determining sample sizes for ANOM, but some tables and power curves are available for that purpose at the back of Nelson, Wludyka, and Copeland (2005), which are also given in Nelson (1983). (See also P. R. Nelson, 1985.)

To use those tables and figures, the user must specify a value for Δ, which is defined as

$$\Delta = \max_{i,j} \frac{|\mu_i - \mu_j|}{\sigma}$$

In words, this is the largest standardized difference between two means that a user wishes to detect. For this example, $\Delta = 2.27$, and interpolating in Table B.2 of Nelson et al. (2005) shows that a sample size of 7 (which was used in this example), gives a power of approximately .90 of detecting the difference.

Nelson (1983) compared ANOM and ANOVA in terms of the sample sizes required for each to attain a certain power for a specified value of Δ and found that ANOM compared very favorably to ANOVA. For example, for power = .90, $\alpha = .05$, and $\Delta = 2$, the required sample size for ANOM is the same as for ANOVA for $3 \leq k \leq 7$, and is either the same or one less for $8 \leq k \leq 16$.

6.2.3 Unequal Sample Sizes

As when there are two levels, it may be desirable to have unequal sample sizes when there are more than two levels. Although ANOVA with assumed equal variances is the standard approach, it will not always be appropriate to assume equal variances, as stated previously. Of course, in both cases there must be a way to obtain estimates of the either equal or unequal variances. If the variances are believed to be unequal and the resultant data corroborate this belief, then heteroscedastic ANOVA (Bishop and Dudewicz, 1978) would have to be used. Cohen (1988, p. 394), however, gave examples of conditions under which it would be desirable to have unequal sample sizes (such as highly unequal population sizes) when the variances are assumed to be equal.

It should be noted, however, that this should be an issue only if populations are small, as different population sizes of, say, 10,000, 20,000, and 30,000 are of no concern if sample sizes normally encountered in practice are to obtained from each population. This is because the standard error of a mean for a finite population is

$$\hat{\sigma}_{\bar{x}} = \hat{\sigma}/\sqrt{n}\left(\sqrt{\frac{N-n}{N-1}}\right)$$

with the parenthetical expression being the *finite population correction factor*. If samples of size 10 are to be taken from each of three populations of sizes 10,000, 20,000, and 30,000, the values of the correction factor will vary only slightly for the three population sizes.

Unlike the case of two means, Lenth's applet cannot be used to solve for unequal sample sizes, nor can Power and Precision, which, as stated previously, does not have that capability for two means. Similarly, MINITAB and nQuery cannot be used to solve for unequal sample sizes based on unequal variances.

Although Cohen (1988) does illustrate how to use his tables for the unequal sample size case, these tables are based on values of f that will not be suitable for many types of application outside the behavioral sciences.

PASS does have the capability for unequal sample sizes, however, as the user enters the desired relationship between the sample sizes. To illustrate, assume that a factor has three levels, $\sigma = 10$, and the user enters 0.167, 0.334, and 0.501 for the "group allocation ratios" in the "One Way Analysis of Variance" procedure, which of course is the same as the pattern 1 2 3 using integers. The three sample sizes will then have the same ratios as the ratios of these three numbers, so if the user enters hypothesized means of 10, 20, and 20, respectively, with a desired power of .90 and $\alpha = .05$, the software gives the three sample sizes as 5, 10, and 15, respectively, which is in agreement with the specified sample size pattern. The power is .9421. The pattern 1 2 3 produces the same sample sizes for this example and it is best either to use a pattern with the first number being a 1 or to use decimal fractions that add to 1. This is because the sample sizes must obviously be integers and the algorithm searches for the smallest multiple of the first number that will meet the power requirement, with the sample sizes for the other groups determined by the specified pattern. The user should NOT enter a pattern with the first integer greater than one because that can result in sample sizes that are larger than necessary to give the specified power. For this example, if the pattern 2 4 6 had been entered, the software gives 6, 12, and 18 as the group sample sizes, with the power of .9759 far exceeding .90. Thus, the wrong answer is obtained because the first sample size is being increased in increments of 2 and thus misses the optimal sample size of 5.

If the power is well above the specified power, the user might want to experiment and specify a lower desired power, realizing that the actual power might be close to the original desired power. For example, if the specified power is lowered to .85, the sample sizes are then 4, 8, and 12, and the power is .8690. This is closer to .90 than .9421, and since of course there is a cost associated with sampling, the 4, 8, and 12 combination might actually be preferable.

Consequently, unless PASS is used, when variances are believed to be unequal and infinite populations are involved, an experimenter might take an ad hoc approach and solve for a single n that would be the appropriate sample size for testing a single mean with a postulated value of σ, which in this case would be the average of the assumed values of σ of each population. Then solve for the n_i such that the values of $\sigma_{\bar{x}_i} = \sigma_i/\sqrt{n_i}$ are approximately equal.

6.2.4   Analysis of Covariance

Analysis of Covariance, generally represented by the acronym ANCOVA or ANACOV, is an extension of ANOVA and is when there is a need to adjust for the effect of a quantitative variable (i.e., a covariate) that would likely affect the results of comparisons between the levels of a factor in ANOVA. Sample size determination for ANCOVA is not widely available in software, but it is available in PASS, which uses the approach given by Keppel (1991). Another approach was given by Borm, Fransen, and Lemmens (2007), which was restricted to the comparison of two treatments and thus was not a general approach.

The adjustment that is made is a natural one, as the adjustment is the correlation between the covariate and the response variable. To illustrate with a simple example, let's assume that a factor has three levels and the objective is to determine the sample size so as to detect means of 1, 2, and 3 for the three levels, respectively. Let's further assume that the within-level standard deviation is 1, the desired power is .90, and the significance level is .05. If the correlation between the covariate and the response variable is .50, then PASS gives $n = 5$ as the number of observations per level, with the actual power being .9244. What would be the value of n if the correlation were smaller, or even zero, or ignored? If the correlation were .30, then $n = 6$ and if the correlation is either 0 or ignored and ANOVA used instead, then $n = 8$. Again the power is .9244. These results are intuitive because the use of a covariate helps explain some of the variability in the response variable and thus reduces the amount of unexplained variability in essentially the same way that an additional variable reduces the unexplained variability in a regression analysis. The smaller the unexplained variability, then the smaller the sample size needed in ANCOVA.

6.2.5 Randomized Complete Block Designs

A randomized block design is a one-factor design with a single blocking factor. It is used when there is an extraneous factor that is likely to have an effect on the experimental values and accordingly should be separated from the error term. This design is one of the menu items for Lenth's applet. Let's assume the same scenario as in Example 6.1 in terms of σ^2, α, and σ_τ^2. Significance of the blocking factor is of interest only as an indicator of whether or not a randomized complete block design was an appropriate design to use. Using Lenth's applet, if 6 blocks are used so that the number of observations for each treatment level is 6 (one per block), the power is .7592—less than the .8053 value obtained without blocking. Why is that? Blocking reduces the degrees of freedom for the error term, which reduces power. Because of this loss of power, blocking should be used only when there is a strong belief that there is an identifiable extraneous factor that will affect experimental results, so that blocking should be done to remove that effect.

Note that even if the number of blocks is such that the treatment and error degrees of freedom for a particular completely randomized design (CRD) and some randomized complete block design (RCBD) are the same, the power values will differ because the number of observations that each level mean is computed from will differ. Remember from Section 6.2 that the noncentrality parameter for a one-factor CRD design with k levels is $\sum_{i=1}^{k}[n_i(\tau_i - \bar{\tau})^2/\sigma^2]$, so it will increase if the n_i increase and there is no other change. For example, assume a CRD with 3 levels and 7 observations per level, relative to a RCBD with 10 blocks. The error $d.f.$ is 18 in both cases and the treatment $d.f.$ is 2. The RCBD will have greater power because each mean is computed from 10 observations versus 7 observations for the CRD. The RCBD has a power of .9648 (still assuming $\sigma^2 = \sigma_\tau^2 = 1$ and $\alpha = .05$), compared to .877 for the CRD, as noted previously. Of course, the power values can always be computed "semimanually" by computing the value of the noncentrality parameter and entering that into software. The expression for the noncentrality parameter of the RCBD (e.g., see Giesbrecht and Gumpertz, 2004, p. 92) is equivalent to the expression for the noncentrality parameter of the CRD under the assumption of blocks being fixed, or under the (standard) assumption that there is no block $\times$ treatment interaction when blocks are random. Using the Power and Precision software for this example also gives a power of .9648, in agreement with the power obtained using Lenth's applet.

PASS also has (some) capability for a RCBD. Instead of specifying σ^2 and σ_τ^2, however, the user enters σ and the hypothesized means for each block, which of course is more intuitive than σ_τ^2. PASS cannot be used to solve for the number of blocks, however; it simply gives the power for the entered number of blocks.

6.2.6 Incomplete Block Designs

An incomplete block design is a design for which every level of the factor does not appear in each block. A balanced incomplete block (BIB) design has all factor levels appearing the same number of times across the blocks, and pairs of levels appearing the same number of times within the blocks. Because of these requirements regarding balance, there are restrictions on the number of blocks that can be used, which means that there are restrictions on the choice of sample size.

Most software for sample size determination are of no help with BIB designs, and this applies generally to designs that are not among the simplest and most frequently used. This is apparent from the sample size and power capabilities of SAS/STAT 9.2 and is also apparent from the capabilities of Release 16 of MINITAB. Similarly, PASS 11 can be used to generate BIBs only, not solve for the number of blocks required or give the power for an entered number of blocks.

Lenth's applet also cannot handle BIB designs for sample size determination because whereas the number of blocks determines the error degrees of freedom, the number of blocks is not equal to the number of observations used in computing the mean for each level. Consequently, power would have to be computed manually by computing the value of the noncentrality parameter for the F-test and specifying the number of degrees of freedom for the error term and for the factor.

To illustrate, for simplicity we will again assume three levels of the factor, with the τ_i as given in Example 6.1, and also again assume that $\sigma^2 = 1$ and $\alpha = .05$. A very simple BIB design is obtained by starting with a RCBD in three blocks and then eliminating a different level from each block. Doing so produces the following BIB design with the columns being the blocks.

$$
\begin{array}{ccc}
A & C & B \\
B & A & C
\end{array}
$$

This satisfies the requirement that every treatment (i.e., level of the factor) occurs the same number of times (twice), and pairs of treatments occur together in the same block an equal number of times (once). The F-statistic has 2 degrees of freedom for the numerator since there are three levels, but the error term has only 1 degree of freedom since Blocks has 2 degrees of freedom. The expression for the noncentrality parameter is (Giesbrecht and Gumpertz, 2004, p. 219) $(t\lambda/m)\sum_{i=1}^{k}(\tau_i^2/\sigma^2)$, with t = number of treatments, k = number of levels, m = block size, r = number of replications, and $\lambda = [r(k-1)/(t-1)]$. Here $t = 3$, $m = 2$, $k = 3$, and $r = 2$, so $\lambda = 1$ and $(t\lambda/m) = 1.5$. The noncentrality parameter is then (1.5) $\sum_{i=1}^{3}(\tau_i^2/\sigma^2) = (1.5)[(1)^2 + 0^2 + (-1)^2]/1 = 3.0$. The power is very low at .081 because the denominator *d.f.* is only 1. If this design were replicated so that $r = 4$, the noncentrality parameter is then 6.0 and the denominator *d.f.* increases to 4 and the power increases to .31—still low. This low power relates to what is discussed in Section 6.2.7 on Latin square designs.

Although we can't determine sample size directly (or at least not easily) for a specified power, this is not a major problem because of the restrictions on sample size in order for the design to be balanced. Thus, it would be straightforward just to examine power for the feasible sample size; that is, the feasible number of blocks.

Partially balanced incomplete block (PBIB) designs present similar problems, but as with BIB designs, it is just a matter of computing the value of the non-centrality parameter and determining the appropriate numerator and denominator degrees of freedom for the *F*-statistic.

6.2.7 Latin Square Designs

A Latin square design is a design for a single factor of interest with two blocking factors. The layout of the design is a square with the number of cells in the square being the square of the number of levels, with each level appearing exactly once in each column and once in each row. The following is a 3×3 Latin square in standard order, so called because the first row and first column are in alphabetical order.

$$
\begin{array}{ccc}
A & B & C \\
B & C & A \\
C & A & B
\end{array}
$$

Ryan (2007) stated that a single Latin square should not be used because there is not sufficient power to detect a factor effect of moderate magnitude, such as equal to σ. Indeed, the average at each level is computed from only three observations, and the error term has only two degrees of freedom. (This is not a true error term because there is no replication, but rather results from the assumption of no interactions.)

For example, if we make the same assumptions regarding the values of σ^2, α, and σ_τ^2 that were made in Example 6.1, the power is only .1823 when a single Latin square design is used, but the power increases sharply to .5402 when two Latin squares are used, with the power being .8318 when three Latin squares are used. These are the numbers obtained by using the value of the noncentrality parameter and computing the power manually.

The noncentrality parameter for a single Latin square design is the same as for a CRD; namely, $\sum_{i=1}^{k}(n_i\tau_i^2/\sigma^2)$, for a Latin square of order k, as given at the start of this section, which simplifies to $\lambda = k\sum_{i=1}^{k}(\tau_i^2/\sigma^2)$. Thus, with a 3×3

Latin square and the assumptions of Exercise 6.1, the value of the noncentrality parameter is 6 and the probability of a noncentral-$F_{2,2}$ variate with $\lambda = 6$ exceeding its .05 critical value is .1823, as indicated in the preceding paragraph.

Because of the low power that will often occur when only a single Latin square design is used, Ryan (2007, p. 77) recommended the use of multiple Latin squares, and Giesbrecht and Gumpertz (2005, p. 126) indicated that this will often be desirable. When multiple Latin squares are used, the error degrees of freedom depends on the relationship between the squares, as illustrated in detail by Giesbrecht and Gumpertz (2005, pp. 127–130). The power is thus affected by this relationship, since it depends in part on the error degrees of freedom. If the squares are unrelated, the error degrees of freedom is $s(k-1)(k-2)$, with s denoting the number of squares, and as before, k denotes the order of each square. The noncentrality parameter is then $ks \sum_{i=1}^{k}(\tau_i^2/\sigma^2)$. This expression for the error degrees of freedom is based on the assumption that the model has square and the treatment $\times$ square interaction as model terms, in addition to the usual terms for treatment, row, column, and error. When this model is specified in Lenth's applet and square is treated as a fixed factor, the power for the treatment effect is .5402 and .8318 for two and three squares, respectively, in agreement with the numbers given previously in this section that were computed using the values of the noncentrality parameter for two and three unrelated squares, respectively.

Care should be exercised when using software to compute power for multiple Latin squares, as the results may not agree across different software because of different ways in which the error degrees of freedom is determined. For example, Lenth's applet only breaks out degrees of freedom for row, column, treatment, and error when the default model is used, although the user can specify a different model, if desired. Thus, multiple Latin squares will increase the error degrees of freedom, with the progression being 2, 11, 20, and 29, for a single Latin square, two, three, and four Latin squares, respectively. This is appropriate only if all the squares have common rows and columns and the effects due to squares and all interactions involving squares are not listed in an ANOVA table, with the degrees of freedom for these effects instead used to contribute to the error degrees of freedom.

If the squares are unrelated, the degrees of freedom for row and for column are the degrees of freedom for a single Latin square (the order of the square minus one) multiplied by the number of squares. Although certain terms might be combined to form the error term, the appropriate starting point should be the breakdown of degrees of freedom for each of the ways in which the multiple squares could be constructed (unrelated, common rows and columns, etc.), and then a decision made regarding the pooling of terms in forming the error term.

With experimental designs in general, it is not a good idea to assume that certain effects do not exist, as the existence of certain effects can constitute a violation of the model assumptions. Thus, appropriate checks should be performed.

Consider the following example.

■ **EXAMPLE 6.2**

Jaech (1969) gave a nuclear production reactor example that involved process tubes and positions on each tube. The experiment and data are apparently fictitious, which explains why the factor was not stated as being fixed or random. There was simply the statement: "Say there are five treatments to be evaluated in a given experiment." Presumably the dataset was based on the author's consulting experience. We will assume that the factor is fixed.

There were 10 tubes used and 20 positions on each tube for a total of 200 tube–position combinations. Eight 5×5 Latin squares were used to represent these combinations. The squares must obviously be related because if rows represented tubes, then 40 tubes would be required if different tubes were used for the Latin squares. Similarly, 40 tube positions would be required but only 20 were used. Thus, there were pairs of squares that used the same five tube positions (1 and 6, 2 and 7, 3 and 8, 4 and 9, and 5 and 10), with the five different tubes used in 1 and 6, but then repeated over 2 and 7, 3 and 8, and so on.

The key question is what is the *d.f.* for the error term, as that will determine the power? The degrees of freedom given by Jaech (1969), 164, does not result from a formula given for any of the ways of constructing the squares given by Giesbrecht and Gumpertz (2005). This is because of the pairing of squares for the experimental material. The pairing relative to tube position results in 4 *d.f.* for each group of 5 positions, and since there were 4 pairs of squares, there were thus 16 *d.f.* for positions. There were 8 *d.f.* for tubes, resulting from 4 *d.f.* each for tubes 1–5 and 6–10. With 7 *d.f.* for squares $(8 - 1)$ and 4 *d.f.* for treatments $(5 - 1)$, 164 *d.f.* for error is then obtained by subtraction.

If we still assume $\sigma_{\hat{\tau}}^2 = 1$ (so that $\sum_{i=1}^{5} \tau_i^2 = 4$), $\sigma^2 = 1$, and $\alpha = .05$, as in the previous examples, Power = 1 is the result, which is the same value obtained using the value of the noncentrality parameter in conjunction with the Power and Precision software. The atypical use of multiple Latin squares by Jaech (1969) results in an error degrees of freedom that apparently cannot be accommodated by Lenth's applet, so in this case computation of the power by using the value of the noncentrality parameter seems necessary.   ■

Such a high value of power results from the fact that so many Latin squares of a moderate size were used, combined with a sizable noncentrality parameter. For a 5×5 Latin square with $\sigma_{\hat{\tau}}^2 = \sigma^2 = 1$ and $\alpha = .05$, but now reducing the replications to 2 and assuming that the squares are unrelated results in a power of .9986 with Lenth's applet. This of course is the same value that is obtained by directly calculating the power from the noncentrality parameter and using 24 *d.f.* for the error term (not pooling the Treatment $\times$ Square interaction with the error term, although that could be done).

In this example it was assumed that the factor is fixed, whereas the power values will be different when the factor is random. For example, for this last scenario with $\sigma_{\hat{t}}^2 = \sigma^2 = 1$ and $\alpha = .05$ and the model as indicated previously, Lenth's applet gives power $= .2092$ for the treatment effect. Thus, the designation of the factor of interest as fixed or random makes a huge difference in the power in this example.

Since the Power and Precision software doesn't have Latin square as a menu item, power would have to be computed manually using the value of the non-centrality parameter. Obviously, it is preferable to use software with built-in capability for Latin square designs. PASS will not handle this and in general will handle only repeated measures designs and designs for clinical trials, such as crossover designs, in addition to fixed-effects Analysis of Variance with up to three factors with the software computing power after the user specifies the number of observations per cell. Thus, sample size is not determined directly with the latter.

As mentioned previously, sample size determination for designs with random factors is discussed in general in Section 6.13.

6.2.7.1 Graeco-Latin Square Designs

A Graeco-Latin square design is used when there are three extraneous factors that must be adjusted for, rather than two as in a Latin square design. The design is constructed by placing one Latin square on top of another Latin square. More formally, a pair of mutually orthogonal Latin squares are used, with Latin letters representing the factor levels in one of the squares and Greek letters used for the other square. Each combination of a Latin letter and a Greek letter occurs only once in the design.

A single Graeco-Latin square is plagued by low power in essentially the same way that a single Latin square is affected. For example, if we assume a 4×4 Graeco-Latin square design with a fixed factor of interest, $\sigma_{\hat{t}} = 1.5$ and $\sigma = 1$, so that we are trying to detect a 1.5-sigma effect, the power is only .613 for the F-test. The power is .834 when $\sigma_{\hat{t}} = 2.0$, but that isn't a very good power for detecting a 2σ effect. If the number of squares is increased to 2, then the power is essentially 1.0 for the 1.5-sigma effect and of course also virtually 1.0 for the 2σ effect. Thus, just using one additional Graeco-Latin square has a very profound effect. Note that the power with a single Graeco-Latin square is *less* than occurs with a 4×4 Latin square design, as the latter has power of .886 for detecting a 1.5-sigma effect. This can be explained by the difference in the degrees of freedom for the error term as the Latin square has more degrees of freedom (6 versus 3).

Thus, it is highly desirable to use multiple Graeco-Latin square designs, just as it is highly desirable to use multiple Latin square designs. Each Graeco-Latin square must be at least of order four because the degrees of freedom for the error term is $(t - 3)(t - 1)$, with t denoting the number of levels. Thus, a 3×3 Graeco-Latin square would not have any degrees of freedom for the error term.

As is true of Latin square designs, sample size determination for Graeco-Latin square designs thus amounts to determining how many squares to use.

6.3 TWO FACTORS

In this section we consider sample size determination when there are two factors, and we will highlight some input differences between some software for sample size determination. At the outset we will note that the "sample size" that the software computes is the number of replicates to use for each factor-level combination, not the total number of observations to obtain.

■ EXAMPLE 6.3

We will consider a factorial experiment with two factors, the first at three levels and the second at two levels. Thus, it is a 3×2 factorial design that can also be described as an example of two-way ANOVA. When Power and Precision is used, "Factorial analysis of variance (two factors)" is selected from the menu. The default option is to enter the effect sizes for each factor and the interaction. Although small, medium, and large are the options, alternatively a value can be entered for the effect size, which would certainly be preferable for the reasons discussed in Section 2.8. Alternative input options include the between-groups standard deviation for each factor and the mean for each level of the factor. (It should be noted that the divisor that is used for that standard deviation is the number of levels of the factor, not the number of levels minus one.) The other input option is to enter the range of the means (largest and smallest) and enter "the pattern of dispersion for remaining means," with the options being centered, uniform, and extreme. The within-cell standard deviation, σ, must also be specified.

As with sample size estimation in general, there is a burden on the software user to provide estimates that may not be easy to produce. Of course, this burden exists regardless of the software that is used. If PASS is used, very similar input options are available. First, assuming that the factors are fixed, the user would select Means > Many Means (ANOVA) > Fixed Effects ANOVA from the menu in the order indicated. The means for each level of each factor could be entered, or their standard deviation specified. Similarly, for the interaction effects, either the cell means or their standard deviation would be entered. For this example there are six cells (three times two).

Obviously, these input demands place a considerable burden on the user. If the user actually knew everything that has to be inputted, there would be no need to conduct the experiment since the magnitude of the main effects and interaction effect would be known. Of course, this information is not going to be known but past experimental data might enable a reasonable estimate of σ to be produced, and it is the relationship between the factor level means of each factor that determines the power for a given sample size, not the actual mean values. That is, the same power for a fixed sample size will result from specifying three factor-level means as 2, 4, and 6 as when 20, 40, and 60 are used, provided that σ is estimated appropriately. That is, σ would be larger by a factor of 10 if the true means were 20, 40, and 60 rather than 2, 4, and 6, and each data point that produced the latter were multiplied by 10. If, however, a constant (100) were added to the first set of factor-level means so as to produce 102, 104, and 106 for the second set, the power would be the same for this second set as for the first set with σ being the same for both sets. This is because a constant is being added, not multiplied, so there is no scale change.

Note that when PASS is used for a factorial design with two factors, the sample size cannot be solved for by specifying a desired value for the power. Rather, PASS provides an option for specifying the number of observations per cell (i.e., the number of replications), with the default option being the four values of 2, 4, 8, and 16. When this option is in force, the user can see the power values for each effect that is estimated and decide if the power is acceptable for one of these four values. If not, other values could be inputted, with the user perhaps deciding to enter more than four possible sample size values so that a finer grid of power values could be displayed.

MINITAB can be used to determine sample size for general full factorial designs. The user enters the number of levels for each factor, which for this example would be "3 2" or "2 3." Of course, this indirectly enters the number of factors. The user also inputs an estimate of the standard deviation and one or more values for the maximum difference between the main effect means, in addition to one or more target power values and a single significance level. A power curve is then generated for each combination, in addition to the numerical output.

For example, if the input is "3 2" for the levels, $\alpha = .05$, $\sigma = 2$, "2" for the highest-order term in the model, "4 5" for maximum difference between the main effect means, and ".90 .95" for the power values, the graph in Figure 6.3 is produced, in addition to the numerical output.   ■

Although such graphs are useful for determining the number of replicates to use, with the curves in Figure 6.3 for 3, 4, and 5 replicates, respectively, and the user having the option for displaying curves for other numbers of replicates, the user should keep in mind that these power figures are contingent on the condition $\sigma = 2$. Since σ almost certainly would not equal whatever value was specified, the power values will, technically, be incorrect. It would be helpful to construct

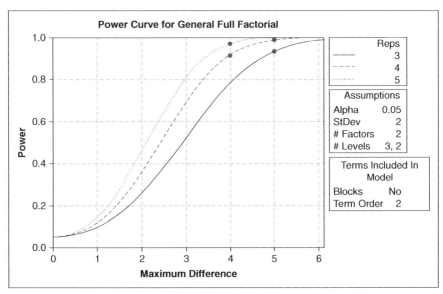

Figure 6.3 Power curves for determining number of replicates for a 3×2 factorial design.

an approximate confidence interval on the true power value, along the lines of the discussion in Section 3.3, but this would require a pilot study to estimate σ, which might not be possible or practical. Nevertheless, the concept is an important one but has not been addressed in the literature on sample size determination for experimental designs.

nQuery could also be used to determine the number of replicates to use for this 3×2 design, but the required inputs place more exacting demands on the user than is the case with MINITAB. Specifically, whereas MINITAB requires that the maximum difference between main effect means be specified, in addition to a value for σ, nQuery requires, in addition to σ, that the variance of the means for each of the two factors be specified, in addition to the variance of the means for the interaction term. Of course, this would require that each of the means be known, and if that were the case, there would be no point in conducting the experiment!

6.4 2^k DESIGNS

Two-level designs are the most commonly used factorial designs, with such full factorial designs designated as 2^k designs. These designs frequently have only one observation for each of the 2^k treatment combinations. When that is the case, the assumption of equal variances for all of the combinations cannot be tested. Consequently, experimenters routinely assume equal variances.

6.4.1 2^2 Design with Equal and Unequal Variances

We will first consider a replicated 2^2 design with levels of each factor fixed and the cell variances first considered to be equal and then assumed to be unequal.

For the equal variances case, Lachenbruch (1988) gave the sample size formula for each cell as

$$n = \frac{4\sigma^2 \left(Z_{\alpha/2} + Z_\beta\right)^2}{M^2}$$

with M defined as the contrast for the effect that is being tested. Specifically, with "R" denoting the row effect (and thus the effect of the factor that corresponds to the row), $M_R = \mu_{11} + \mu_{12} - \mu_{21} - \mu_{22}$, with μ_{ij} denoting the mean of the cell in the ith row and jth column. Similarly, the column effect is defined by the contrast $M_C = \mu_{11} - \mu_{12} + \mu_{21} - \mu_{22}$, and for the interaction effect, $M_I = \mu_{11} - \mu_{12} - \mu_{21} + \mu_{22}$.

For the unequal variances case, Guo and Luh (2010) gave the sample size formula for each cell, n_{ij}, as

$$n_{ij} = \frac{S_{ij} \left(S_{11} + S_{12} + S_{21} + S_{22}\right) \left(t_{\alpha/2,df} + t_{\beta,df}\right)^2}{M_R^2} \tag{6.4}$$

with the degrees of freedom, $d.f.$, defined as

$$d.f. = \frac{\left(s_a^2/n_a + s_b^2/n_b\right)^2}{\dfrac{\left(s_a^2/n_a\right)^2}{n_a - 1} + \dfrac{\left(s_b^2/n_b\right)^2}{n_b - 1}}$$

with $n_a = \sum_{j=1}^2 n_{1j}$, $n_b = \sum_{j=1}^2 n_{2j}$, $s_a = \sum_{j=1}^2 s_{1j}$ and $s_b = \sum_{j=1}^2 s_{2j}$ The s_{ij} are the estimates of the cell standard deviations, σ_{ij}. Equation (6.4) would of course have to be solved numerically for n_{ij} since there are terms involving t-values, which depend upon the sample size through the degrees of freedom.

6.4.2 Unreplicated 2^k Designs

When a 2^k design is unreplicated, the value of k must be determined carefully, in addition to using criteria that are different from the criteria that are normally used in solving for sample size. Indeed, the term "sample size" really doesn't have any meaning when only one observation is being used for each treatment combination.

Instead, the value of k must be determined such that it will be large enough so that the significant effects can be identified using any one of the methods that have been proposed and examined in the literature for identifying the significant effects with an unreplicated factorial. There are two things that must be considered: the value of k should be large enough so that each effect will be estimated using a reasonable number of observations so that the variance of the estimator will be tolerably small, and k must also be large enough so that the pseudo error term that is formed from high-order interactions will have a reasonable number of degrees of freedom.

Daniel (1976, p. 75) stated that, "as very crude guesses," approximately four real effects is average for a 2^4 design and seven for a 2^5 design. Therefore, it would be overkill and wasteful, especially when experimental runs are expensive, to use a 2^5 design, which would allow the estimation of all 31 effects when only a fraction of those effects will be real effects. Only when the cost of experimentation is extremely low, such as in computer simulation experiments, would it be practical to use a 2^k design when k is not small. Computer experiments are discussed in Section 6.15.

When a specific design is planned, Design-Expert can be used to determine the power for detecting effects of specified magnitudes, assuming that all effects will not be estimated, as would be impractical if $k > 3$. (Design-Expert is software solely for design of experiments.) This can be used as a guide for design selection.

■ **EXAMPLE 6.4**

Daniel (1976) gave an example of a 2^3 design used in a cement experiment for which σ was known to be about 12. Because of the latter, it is of interest to see the magnitude of effects than can be detected, relative to the effects that were declared significant using a normal probability plot approach.

If we solve for k in Eq. (6.2), with $n/2 = 4$, we obtain $k = 1.98$. Thus, an effect of magnitude 1.98σ is the smallest effect that could be detected with the design. With $\sigma = 12$, this is $1.98(12) = 23.78$. A normal probability plot leads to the identification of the B and C main effects and the BC interaction as being the real effects. The estimates of these effects are -132.75, -73.5, and 47.5, respectively. The next largest effect was the A effect, with an estimate of 15.5. Thus, the normal probability plot identifies the same effects as would be identified doing the hypothesis tests using the known value of σ.

A 2^3 design has rather limited practical value, however, because we would prefer to be able to detect effects smaller than 1.98σ. Furthermore, the latter is based on the assumption that σ is known. The typical scenario, however, is that σ is unknown. Table 3 of Lynch (1993) indicates that, assuming $\alpha = .05$ and σ to be estimated from the experimental data, a 2^3 design must be replicated in order to detect an effect of 2σ or smaller with power of at least $.80$. Specifically, two replications are needed to detect an effect of 1.8σ with power $.90$. Of course, it is somewhat easier to use software than to use statistical tables, and if we use

MINITAB (Release 16), we observe that the power is .88 for detecting an effect of 1.8σ. This disagrees slightly with the result in Lynch's table, with the difference apparently due to the fact that the Lynch tabular result is based on the assumption that 9 degrees of freedom are available for estimating σ (which would be the case if the *ABC* interaction were not estimated), whereas 8 degrees of freedom are available if all effects are estimated. Using MINITAB, we find that 3 replicates are necessary to detect an effect of 1.8σ if the power is to be at least .90, with the actual power being .985.

One complication relative to sample size determination for designs with two or more factors is that the denominator in the F-test for testing for effect significance is not the mean squared error (MSE) when there is a mixture of fixed and random factors. Although MSE will be a component of the denominator, it won't always be the only component. Similarly, the numerator of the statistic won't necessarily be represented by MSE plus a term for what is being tested, as the numerator can contain other terms. For this reason, some Java applets, such as http://www.math.yorku.ca/SCS/Online/power, will handle only fixed factors, as then all effects are tested against the error term.   ∎

6.4.3 Software for 2^k Designs

Although it is insightful and relatively important to see how power is computed, it is, of course, much easier to use software for this purpose.

In particular, we can use software such as Design-Expert to evaluate the power of 2^k designs, as indicated previously. For example, the software immediately warns the user who selects an unreplicated 2^3 design that "For this design, effects must be at least 2–3 standard deviations in size to be detected. Evaluate power for the expected number of effects. Do you want to continue with this design?"

Of course, the power depends on how many effects we wish to estimate with the 2^3 design. We cannot estimate all of them without an external estimate of error or a normal probability plot approach because there would be no degrees of freedom for error. Although mentioned in conjunction with Example 6.4, a normal probability plot approach would be somewhat shaky for a 2^3 design because, if we accept Daniel's rule-of-thumb, the number of real effects may render a normal probability plot useless as the pseudo error term that is created when such plots are used must be constructed using at least a moderate number of effects that are not likely to be significant.

The picture improves if we use two replicates of a 2^3 design, as then the power is .937 for detecting an effect of magnitude 2σ for any of the main effects or interactions. (The power is the same for each effect because each effect estimate is based on the difference of two averages that are each computed from 8 observations when a 2^3 design with two replicates is used.)

Of course, the experimenter must decide the minimum-size effect that is to be computed with high probability.

If a 1σ effect is deemed important to detect, then two replicates are not sufficient because the power is only .421 for detecting an effect of that magnitude, as obtained using MINITAB. If we use 3 replicates, the power increases to .633, to .775 for 4 replicates, and to .866 for 5 replicates. Thus, we would need 5 replicates in order for the power to be at least .80.

Thus, a 2^3 design is not a very good design unless replicates are inexpensive or we are interested in detecting large effects and would settle for an unreplicated design.

For a 2^4 design the picture is somewhat better, as the power of detecting a 2σ effect when the model contains only main effects and two-factor interactions is .887, but only .368 for a 1σ effect. If the design is replicated, the numbers improve to .999 and .769, respectively. With a 2^5 design, the first pair of numbers is .999 and .757, and the second pair of numbers is .999 and .975. (With more than five factors, a full factorial would generally be impractical, exceptions being experiments for which the experimental runs are very inexpensive, as mentioned previously in Section 6.4.2.)

By comparison with these results obtained using MINITAB, the tables of Lynch (1993) are not constructed in such a way that the power is given for 1σ or 2σ effects, nor can the tables be used to determine the effect size that can be detected with power .80, as there is a jump from .75 to .85. Power of .90 is included, however.

The picture that emerges when we put all of these numbers together is that a 2^3 or 2^4 design should be replicated if there is a need to detect effects smaller than 2σ.

6.5 2^{k-p} DESIGNS

Since 2^{k-p} designs are generally not replicated, sample size considerations would seem to be irrelevant since standard hypothesis tests cannot be performed. What is not irrelevant, however, is the determination of k and p, and the difference, $k - p$, for the size of the experiment is determined by the latter. Furthermore, k should be large enough that the percentage of real effects will be small and the pseudo error term that is used with a normal probability plot will be based both on a reasonable number of observations and real effects. Since every effect that is estimable with a particular 2^{k-p} design is computed as the difference of two averages, with each average based on 2^{k-p-1} observations, it is imperative that 2^{k-p-1} not be so small that each average has a large variance.

As indicated in Section 6.4, Daniel (1976, p. 75) stated that there are typically 7 significant effects when a 2^5 design is used. It follows that there would also be 7 significant effects when either a 2^{5-2} or a 2^{5-1} design is used because the real effects and the number of them are of course independent of the fractionalization. Therefore, an unreplicated 2^{5-2} design should generally not be used because we won't be able to identify 7 significant effects with only 8 design points because all normal probability plot methods fail if there is a very high percentage of significant effects, as is well known and has been discussed by, for example, Hamada and Balakrishnan (1998) and Ryan (2007, p. 136).

Would using a replicated 2^{5-2} design make any sense? Not really, as that would not only offset the savings that are gained by using a highly fractionated design, but with a few replicates there would not be enough observations at each design point to allow for good estimates of σ^2 at each point, so the estimate of σ^2 obtained from the average of the estimates over the design points could be an average computed from some large values. Carroll and Cline (1988) showed that at least 8–10 replications of a design point are necessary in order to obtain a good estimate of the variance at that point. Of course, it would be totally impractical to use at least 8 replicates of a 2^{5-2} design.

Thus, in selecting a particular 2^{k-p} design, the user should be guided by Daniel's rule-of-thumb and any other avilable empirical evidence regarding the number of significant effects that might be expected for a given value of k. If an experimenter wants to "push the limit" by using a highly fractionated design (i.e., using a small value of $k - p$), such experimenters should be guided by results given in the study of Hamada and Balakrishnan (1998) regarding the maximum number of real effects that can be handled with normal probability plot methods, and which normal probability plot methods should be used for various expected fractions of real effects.

6.6 DETECTING CONDITIONAL EFFECTS

The analysis of conditional effects (also called simple effects in the literature) was emphasized by Ryan (2007), and its use is imperative when there are large interactions. (A conditional effect is an effect computed by splitting the data and using part of it in computing each conditional effect.) Ryan (2007, pp. 113–114) briefly discussed sample size considerations in the estimation of conditional effects. For an unreplicated 2^k design, each conditional main effect and each conditional interaction effect is computed from the difference of two averages, with each average computed using 2^{k-2} observations, with the data split on one of the factors. Clearly, this can be a problem when k is small. In particular, each average is computed using only two observations when $k = 3$.

If a 2^k design is replicated so that an estimate of σ can be obtained, the tables of Lynch (1993) could *not* be applied for a given split of the data. To illustrate, assume that a 2^4 design with 2 replicates has been used. Each average computed to obtain a conditional effect estimate will be computed using 8 observations, which is the same number that would be used in computing each average that is used in obtaining a main effect estimate with an unreplicated 2^4 design. The error degrees of freedom doesn't match those given in Lynch's table, however.

Another problem that would complicate any inferential approach is that it would be logical to consider the *largest* conditional effect of a factor in trying to determine if the factor has a real effect. For example, with a 2^4 design and a desire to see if factor A has a real effect, considering all three two-factor interaction terms involving A, it would be logical to split the data on the factor that with A comprises the largest two-factor interaction. This selection process would have to be considered in determining an inferential procedure, as a routine approach (such as a two-sample t-test) won't work.

If a design is not replicated, a normal probability plot approach will generally be used in determining significant effects. Since conditional effects and regular effects have different variances, it is not possible to construct a normal probability plot that contains a mixture of the two, since variances of all of the plotted effect estimates must be equal. There is also the matter of having only one degree of freedom for regular effect estimates, and we don't generally split degrees of freedom to create fractional degrees of freedom.

One approach that might be used, however, when there are large two-factor interactions, would be to compute all the possible conditional main effects and conditional two-factor interaction effects, then compute the numerical difference between those numbers and the corresponding regular effect estimates. The largest difference for each factor and for two-factor interactions would then be used in a normal probability plot to try to identify significant effects. This is just an ad hoc approach, however, as the differences, while having the same variance, would be computed using different subsets of the data, so no formal inferential procedure could be used. Nevertheless, such a normal probability plot could be very illuminating for certain datasets.

Because of these complications, it would probably be best to view conditional effects analyses as an exploratory data analysis (EDA) tool, but to ensure that there is a sufficient number of observations for estimating both standard effects and conditional effects.

6.7 GENERAL FACTORIAL DESIGNS

Although full and fractional factorial two-level designs are the types of factorial designs that are most frequently used in practice, there is often a need to use a design that has more than two levels. Sample size determination for designs that have at least one factor with more than two levels can be performed using Lenth's applet or MINITAB.

To illustrate, with Release 16 of MINITAB the user specifies the number of levels for each factor, the maximum difference between main effect means that is to be detected with the desired power, α, a value for σ, and the highest-order term that is to be included in the model, and the software gives the number of replicates that is required.

■ EXAMPLE 6.5

For example, assume that a 3^2 design is to be used, $\alpha = .05$, the second-order term (the AB interaction) is to be included in the model, a term for replicates is *not* to be included in the model (there is an option for that), the maximum difference between treatment means is 4, σ is assumed to be 2, and the desired power is .90. MINITAB gives 3 as the number of replicates, with the assumed power value being .946. (This is not close to .90 because the error degrees of freedom jumps by 9 for every additional replicate, so the power numbers will also have large jumps.)

It should be noted that this result assumes fixed factors, and the power is for main effects, not the interaction term. In general, the power for main effects and interactions will differ for designs with more than two levels. When the number of levels differ, MINITAB determines the sample size based on the main effect (i.e., factor) with the largest number of levels, so as to provide conservative results. It is also important to note that the result for this example assumes that the two factors are fixed, as stated, and that F-tests are being performed to determine significance. The situation is more complex when at least one factor is random because then both factors are not tested against the error term, as they are when the factors are fixed.

When both factors in a two-factor design are random, the significance of each factor depends on both σ and the standard deviation of the interaction term, σ_{AB}, since each main effect is tested against the interaction term when the F-tests for the main effects are performed. In general, for fixed values of σ and σ_{AB}, the power is typically much less when both factors are random than when both factors are fixed. This is because power is determined in part by the denominator degrees of freedom for the F-test, and whereas replicates increase the degrees of freedom for the error term, they have no effect on the degrees of freedom for the interaction term.

Lenth's applet can also be used for determining sample size for a general factorial design, although the information that is inputted differs, as σ and the standard deviations of the effect estimators must be entered. ■

It will often be impractical to use very many replicates of a general $s \times t$ design unless s and t are small. In the preceding example, the number of design points increased by 9 for every additional replicate. For a 4×4 design, the number of design points will increase by 16 for every additional replicate, so an impractically large size for the experiment could easily be reached.

6.8 REPEATED MEASURES DESIGNS

Repeated measures designs are designs for which multiple measurements are made, over time, on the same subjects. Such designs have both advantages and disadvantages. Assume that the subjects are people. One advantage is that the people in the study serve as their own control, which permits the use of a smaller sample size than would otherwise be the case. A disadvantage is that there is the potential for carryover effects when two or more treatments are applied over time to the same people. When there is a strong possibility of carryover effects, designs for carryover effects should be used (see Ryan, 2007, p. 432).

Repeated measurements may be made over time without any treatments being applied, however. Vickers (2003) addressed the question of how many measurements to take in medical applications, such as how often patients should be evaluated after thoracic surgery.

Most sample size determination software and freeware will not handle repeated measures designs explicitly; that is, the design is not a design that is selected from a menu. PASS is an exception, however, as it has extensive capability for repeated measures designs. Specifically, if Means is selected from the menu, 67 procedures are listed, with two of them being Repeated Measures ANOVA and Tests for Two Means in a Repeated Measures Design.

"Before" and "after" measurements on the same subjects with the data analyzed as a test with paired (dependent) samples (Section 3.10) is a type of repeated measures design but a paired-t test is for only two levels of a single factor, so a more general method of analysis must be used for more levels and/or more factors.

We will first consider Example 3.5 that was used in Section 3.10. We will assume the same mean difference, correlation between the two measurements, and standard deviations, but that was a one-tailed test with $\alpha = .05$ whereas an F-test, as used with a repeated measures design, is a one-tailed test that sums the two tail areas for a t-test. Thus, we will need to convert Example 3.5 to a two-tailed test. Another necessary adjustment is that Example 3.5 used z-variates, whereas t-variates must be used in order to obtain the same sample size for an F-test since $(t_v)^2 = F_{1,v}$, with v denoting the degrees of freedom for the t-statistic and 1 and v denoting the numerator and denominator degrees of freedom, respectively, for the F-statistic. As in Example 3.5, we will let $\mu_d = 1$ and let $\sigma_1 = \sigma_2 = 5$, with the covariance being $\rho_{12}\sigma_1\sigma_2 = .8(5)(5) = 20$.

Using PASS and selecting Repeated Measures ANOVA with n-Regular F Test to be solved for and K (Means Multipliers) set to the default value of 1.0, entries would be made in the input section Within-Subject Repeated Factors, indicating, in turn, two levels for "W," $\alpha = .05$, power = .80, and any pair of mean values specified in the last part of that line such that the difference in the means is 1.0. The user would then click on the Covariance tab Covariance Matrix Columns and select 2) Covariance Matrix Columns and click the Input Spreadsheet icon at the bottom of the page after entering C1 C2 in that section to specify the columns that contain the covariance matrix. The 2×2 matrix would then be entered in the spreadsheet using the first two rows and first two columns, with the entries being 25, 20, 20, and

25 going across the two columns for the first row and then doing the same for the second row. Then specifying "Step 0 1" for `Time Metric` results in a sample size of 81, so that two measurements would be made on each of 81 subjects.

It may be instructive to see how this relates to Example 3.5. We will, however, need to make the adjustments mentioned earlier in this section. Specifically, $t_{80,.025} = 1.99006$ and $t_{80,.20} = 0.846137$. When these numbers are used in determining the sample size, as in Example 3.5, the result is $n = [(1.99006 + 0.846137)\sqrt{10}]^2 = 80.44$, so $n = 81$ would be used.

Determining sample size when there is more than one factor is potentially complicated because the user must decide what assumptions are tenable regarding error terms and correlations between factors within subjects and between subjects. The assumptions that can be made will determine how the data should be analyzed, and the method of analysis *should* determine the sample size, but the way to proceed may not be determinable until data have been obtained, which would then be used in testing certain assumptions.

A strategy for approaching the analysis of repeated measures data was given in Section 8.4 of Littell, Stroup, and Freund (2002). This section can be read online at `http://faculty.ucr.edu/~hanneman/linear_models/c8.html#8.4`.

Regardless of how one proceeds, the covariance structure must be specified and estimates of the variances and covariances must be provided, with the structure and estimates being factors that greatly influence the sample size, as the reader will see in working Exercise 6.12. See Littell, Pendergast, and Natarajan (2000) and Milliken (2004) for guidance in determining the covariance structure. The latter is a key step in determining both the sample size and how the data will be analyzed.

Repeated measurements are involved in pharmacokinetic and pharmacodynamic experiments and a moderate amount of research has been performed in determining sample size for such experiments. See, in particular, Ogungbenro and Aarons (2010a,b). Ogungbenro and Aarons (2008, 2009) and Ogungbenro, Aarons, and Graham (2006) may also be of interest in regard to such experiments.

Overall and Doyle (1994) provided sample size formulas for repeated measurement designs and Overall (1996) used simulation to examine the effects of different sample sizes. Other papers that may be of interest include the following. Lipsitz and Fitzmaurice (1994) considered sample size for repeated measures studies with a binary response variable and Jiang and Oleson (2011) considered sample size determination for repeated measures studies with multinomial outcomes. See also Muller and Barton (1989), Muller, LaVange, Ramey, and Ramey (1992), Lui and Cumberland (1992), Kirby, Galai, and Munoz (1994), Zucker and Denne (2002), Yi and Panzarella (2002), Jung and Ang (2003), and Liu and Wu (2005, 2008).

6.8.1 Crossover Designs

Crossover designs are a specific form of a repeated measures design. A crossover design, also called a changeover design, is one in which there is a switch, or changeover, in the treatments that the subjects receive, such as half of the subjects receiving, say, treatment A followed by treatment B, with the other half receiving treatment B followed by treatment A, with the subjects being randomly assigned to each of the two sequences.

The simplest type of crossover design is a 2×2 design—a design with two treatment sequences and two treatment periods, with the number of treatment periods equal to the number of treatments. Half of the subjects (i.e., one group) would logically receive one of the treatment sequences and the other half would receive the other treatment sequence.

Consider bioequivalence testing, as a 2×2 crossover design is often used in conjunction with bioequivalence testing. (Recall that equivalence testing was discussed briefly in Section 2.10.) Under the assumption that the upper bioequivalence limit is $0.2\mu_R$ (and the lower limit is $-0.2\mu_R$), with μ_R denoting the mean of a reference drug, Chow and Wang (2001) gave the necessary sample size for a two-period, two-sequence crossover design as

$$n = \frac{2 (CV)^2 \left(t_{\alpha,2n-2} + t_{\beta,2n-2} \right)^2}{(0.2 - |\theta|)^2} \tag{6.5}$$

Here $\theta = (\mu_T - \mu_R)/\mu_R$, with T and R denoting two treatments, such as a treatment drug (T) and a reference drug (R) in a drug study. The quantity CV, which represents "coefficient of variation," is defined as $CV = \sigma_e/\mu_R$ with σ_e denoting the intrasubject standard deviation. Obviously, an iterative solution for n is necessary since components of the fraction also contain n.

■ **EXAMPLE 6.6**

Assume that $\mu_T = 7$, $\mu_R = 6$, $\sigma_e = 3$, $\alpha = .05$, and power $= .90$, with upper bioequivalence limit $0.2\mu_R$ and lower limit $-0.2\mu_R$. Using Eq. (6.5) with the degrees of freedom for t set to infinity for illustration, we obtain

$$n = \frac{2 (CV)^2 \left(t_{\alpha,2n-2} + t_{\beta,2n-2} \right)^2}{(0.2 - |\theta|)^2}$$

$$= \frac{2 (0.5)^2 (1.64485 + 1.28155)^2}{(0.2 - 1/6)^2}$$

$$= 3853.72$$

so 3854 treatment subjects per group would be needed, and thus a total of $2(3854) = 7708$ subjects would be used. This is in agreement with the solution given by PASS, which uses the two one-sided tests of Schuirmann (1987).

If we just wanted to do a standard hypothesis test for the equality of two means using a 2×2 crossover design and still assuming $\mu_T = 7, \mu_R = 6, \sigma_e = 3$, $\alpha = .05$, and power $= .90$, but NOT in the context of equivalence testing, the required sample size will be much lower. Specifically, as can be obtained using PASS, $n = 192$ for a two-sided test with $\alpha = .05$ and power $= .90$ (actually .9014). Thus, the use of equivalence testing increases the required sample size greatly for this example.

There are other types of crossover designs, which we will designate as $k \times m$ designs, with k denoting the number of sequences and m denoting the number of periods.

Ahrens, Teresi, Han, Donnell, Vanden Burgt, and Lux (2001) discussed the determination of sample size when a crossover design is used, compared to what sample size would be needed if a parallel design had been used. (The latter is a design in which no subject is measured more than once. An analogy regarding the comparison of a crossover design and a parallel design would be a paired-t test vis-à-vis an independent sample t-test.) Fewer subjects are needed for a crossover design compared to a parallel design, as we would expect.

That advantage is offset somewhat, however, by the fact that crossover designs can be undermined by carryover effects, as stated previously. Specifically, the effect of a treatment in a previous time period can affect a measurement from a different treatment on the same subject in a subsequent time period. There are crossover designs that are balanced for carryover effects, however, so this is not an insurmountable problem. Whether or not there are likely to be carryover effects depends on what the treatments are and what is being measured. Of course, one way to try to prevent carryover effects is to have a substantial amount of time between treatments.

The Ahrens et al. (2001) paper contained a description of a study that involved a two-period crossover design. They gave the formula for sample size determination as $n = \sqrt{\text{mean squared error}}$/dose response slope, with estimates of the latter obtained using the definition: (change in response)/(change in $\log_{10}$ (dose)). Note that this approach determines the sample size for *each* efficacy variable outcome measure, not for a set of them. Of course, the idea would be to look at efficacy variables that do not require large sample sizes and the authors identified three such variables. The required sample sizes for the three were given by the authors as 23, 25, and 37, respectively, whereas the authors stated that corresponding sample sizes from "otherwise identical parallel studies" would be 657, 1438, and 2261—obviously orders of magnitude larger.

Chow, Shao, and Wang (2008) also discussed the problem more generally and gave the sample size for a crossover design relative to what the sample size would be for a parallel group design if the latter were used, keeping α and the power constant. That formula is

$$n_{\text{crossover}} = \frac{n_{\text{parallel}}}{2(1-\theta)}$$

with θ defined as

$$\theta = \frac{\gamma}{\left(z_{\alpha/2} + z_\beta\right)^2}$$

with γ defined as $\gamma = \sigma_p^2/\sigma^2$, with σ_p^2 denoting the variance of the random period effect and σ^2 being the variance of the response variable. Thus, the crossover design will require approximately half the sample size of a parallel group design when the period effect is negligible, but there might not be any reduction at all if there is a substantial period (carryover) effect. This shows mathematically one reason why it is desirable to avoid carryover effects when a crossover design is used, which can often be accomplished by allowing sufficient time between treatment periods.

See Chen, Chow, and Li (1997) and Qu and Zheng (2003) for information on sample size determination for higher-ordered crossover designs used in bioequivalence studies, and see also Potvin, DiLiberti, Hauck, Parr, Schuirmann, and Smith (2007), and Montague, Potvin, DiLiberti, Hauck, Parr, and Schuirman (2012), with the latter being a follow-up to the former. ■

6.8.1.1 *Software*

Software with capability for determining sample sizes for crossover designs include nQuery, SiZ, and PASS, with the latter having extensive capabilities and the user being able to specify one of the following crossover designs for sample size determination: 2×2, 2×3, 2×4, 4×2, and 4×4. By comparison, SiZ and nQuery can be used only for a 2×2 crossover design. Similarly, the user-written Stata command xsampsi can be used to determine sample size for a two-period, two-treatment crossover design. MINITAB does not have capability for a crossover design.

The advantage of using a 4×2 design (a Balaam design; Balaam, 1968) relative to a 2×2 design is that the two extra sequences of the former are sequences in which a subject receives the same treatment in the two time periods, which permits an assessment of within-subject variability, assuming no carryover effects. As with repeated measures designs, in general, a crossover design should be selected from the many that are available that perform well under a variety of conditions, including model misspecification.

We will consider a simple example to illustrate the use of PASS for a 2×2 crossover design. This will illustrate why caution should be used when using certain software.

■ **EXAMPLE 6.7**

When PASS is used for a 2×2 crossover design, the user specifies the difference between the two treatment means under the null hypothesis and must specify either the within-subject standard deviation (i.e., the standard deviation if repeated measurements were obtained when both the subject and treatment are constant) the standard deviation of paired difference or the standard deviation of the difference in the two treatments for a given subject.

If we specify the difference between means as 0.5, the within-subject standard deviation as 1.0, the power as .90, and $\alpha = .05$ for a two-sided test with the difference of the treatment means equal to zero under the null hypothesis, the required sample size is 88, as is obtained using PASS (Release 11).

For a difference, d, and within subject standard deviation S_w, the correct expression is $s_d^2 = 2s_w^2$, using the result that the variance of a difference of two independent random variables is the sum of the variances. Thus, for this example, $s_d^2 = 2s_w^2 = 2(1)^2 = 2$, so $s_d = \sqrt{2} = 1.414$. Therefore, if the user of PASS prefers to enter this standard deviation (which PASS labels "SdPaired = Std Dev of Paired Differences"), the value entered should be 1.414, after specifying that it is this type of standard deviation that will be entered. Doing so produces the same sample size, $n = 88$, as obtained previously when the within-subject standard deviation of 1.0 was specified.   ■

Other software that can be used for sample size determination includes Cytel Studio, Version 8. A user enters the treatment difference that is to be detected (δ), values for σ and α, whether the test is one-sided or two-sided, and the desired power, and the sample size is computed. For example, with $\delta = 1.5$, $\sigma = 4$, $\alpha = .05$, power $= .80$, and a two-sided test, the software gives 114 as the sample size. Alternatively, power can be examined for a range of sample sizes, such as 10 to 100 in increments of 1, or the necessary sample size could be displayed for a range of power values.

6.9 RESPONSE SURFACE DESIGNS

As stated near the beginning of the chapter, more than one design is generally used when a response surface analysis is performed, although Cheng and Wu (2001) and Bursztyn and Steinberg (2001) have proposed that the factor screening that is generally performed in the first stage be combined with the optimization that is used in the second stage and both be accomplished with a single design.

If a traditional approach were taken using two designs, the first design would be used to identify significant first-order effects; the second design would be used to identify the form of the response surface, which is one way of saying that the objective is to identify the form of a suitable model once the important factors have been identified; then the third stage would be to perform experiments to seek the optimum combinations of levels of the important factors that have been identified.

6.10   MICROARRAY EXPERIMENTS

Microarray experiments have been extremely popular for several years and are being performed in large numbers, so sample size determination is important, especially considering the cost of microarray experiments. These experiments present special experimental design challenges because classical experimental designs are not useful in microarray experiments.

Hwang, Schmitt, Stephanopoulos, and Stephanopoulos (2002) pointed out that there is a tendency to perform only a small number of microarray measurements because such measurements are costly, with the consequence that in many cases the number of measurements is inadequate. They addressed this problem by proposing a method that utilizes some discriminant analysis methodology. Their method does not involve a sample size expression, however, because the method is iterative, with the original sample size increased until the (retrospective) power is $1 - \beta$. Thus, it involves retrospective power, which has been criticized by Lenth (2001), in particular, as stated previously.

Lin, Hsueh, and Chen (2010) stressed the importance of using the correlation and effect size heterogeneity between genes in determining sample size and proposed a permutation method for determining sample size.

Dobbin and Simon (2005) stated that the complexity of microarray experiments and the large amount of data that they produce can make the sample size issue seem daunting and tempt researchers to use rules-of-thumb rather than formal calculations. They sought to overcome that problem by presenting formulas "for determining sample sizes to achieve a variety of experimental goals." Specifically, they presented eight formulas, with individual formulas for determining sample size for (1) the number of single-label microarrays to use, (2) the number of microarrays required when comparing two classes in a reference design with no technical replicates, (3) the number of samples required for dye-swap arrays, (4) the number of arrays required when m technical replicates of each sample are to be performed, (5) the number of arrays required for a balanced block design, (6) the number of arrays required for a balanced paired design with no dye-swap arrays, (7) the number of arrays required for a dye-swap paired design, (8) the number of arrays required for predictive and prognostic markers, and (9) the sample size for a reference design.

They emphasized that the sample size formulas that they presented are not for small samples. The reason for this, as they stated, is their formulas assume known parameter values and poor, unreliable estimates could result when small samples are used.

Their formulas are based on the assumption of a normal distribution but their simulations showed that the usefulness of their formulas is relatively insensitive to that assumption.

Because of the considerable research interest in microarray experimentation, many other papers have been written on sample size determination. See also Lee and Whitmore (2002), Pan, Lin, and Lee (2002), Wang and Chen (2004), Wei, Li, and Bumgarner (2004), Müller, Parmigiani, Robert, and Rousseau (2004), Tsai, Wang, Chen, and Chen (2005), Jung, Bang, and Young (2005), Pounds and Cheng (2005), Li, Bigler, Lampe, Potter, and Peng (2005), Pawitan, Michiels, Koscielny, Gusnanto, and Ploner (2005), Liu and Hwang (2007), Matsui, Zeng, Yamanaka, and Shaughnessy (2008), Matsui and Oura (2009), and Hirakawa, Hamada, and Yoshimura (2011) for additional information on determining sample sizes in microarray experiments.

6.10.1 Software

Software that can be used to determine sample size for microarray experiments includes PASS, which has capability for (1) a one-sample or paired-t test for microarray data, and (2) a two-sample t-test. A program in R for sample size estimation is described by Orr and Liu (2009).

6.11 OTHER DESIGNS

The sample size determination capability for experimental designs using Lenth's applet covers many other types of designs and generally covers any design for which the model can be written. This gives it greater capability than sample size determination software that has only programs for specific designs. We look at several other designs in the following sections, with Lenth's applet having a template for each of these designs.

6.11.1 Plackett–Burman Designs

Plackett–Burman (PB) designs are two-level designs with the number of runs not a power of two. More specifically, PB designs exist for 12, 20, 24, and 28 runs, up to 100 runs. MINITAB can be used to solve for the sample size for these designs. For example, assume a 12-point PB design for four factors, with $\sigma = 1.0$, $\alpha = .05$, power $= .80$, no center points, and it is desired to detect an effect of size 1.5. (Since there are multiple factors, "effect size" means the smallest effect size—the average response at the high factor level minus the average response at the low factor level—that one wishes to detect. For this example the effect size can be viewed as 1.5σ.) The solution will be in turns of the number of replicates and for this example two replicates are required, which gives a power of .936—much higher than requested. Of course, the jumps in power will be substantial for 2, 3, 4 reps, and so on, and are .936, .992, and .999, respectively.

MINITAB computes the power for a PB design as follows. The computation involves the noncentrality parameter when this design is used, which is $\lambda = rc\delta^2/4\hat{\sigma}_e^2$, with r = number of replicates, c = number of corner points in design, δ = effect, and $\hat{\sigma}_e^2$ is the estimated variance. The power is then computed as Power $= 1 - F(f_{\alpha,1,v}, 1, v, \lambda)$, with v denoting the error degrees of freedom and f_α denoting the value for the central F-distribution with 1 degree of freedom for the numerator and v for the denominator, and for which the right-tail area is α. Therefore, for a 12-point PB design with $\hat{\sigma}_e^2 = 1^2 = 1$, $\delta = 1.5$, $c = 12$, and $r = 1$, $\lambda = rc\delta^2/4\hat{\sigma}_e = (1)(12)(1.5)^2/4(1) = 6.75$. With all main effects assumed to be in the model, $v = 7$, so $f_{.05,1,7} = 5.59145$. If an unreplicated 12-point PB for four factors is used, the power is then $1 - F(f_{\alpha,1,v}, 1, v, \lambda) = 1 - F(5.59145, 1, 7, 6.75) = 1 - .3915 = .6085$. Thus, the unreplicated design has low power for detecting an effect of size 1.5σ. For two replicates, $\lambda = 13.50$, and $v = 19, f_{.05,1,19} = 4.38075$, so Power $= 1 - F(4.38075, 1, 19, 13.50) = 1 - .0639 = .9361$.

Thus, for a 12-point PB design for four factors, the power is too low for detecting a 1.5σ effect if the design is unreplicated, but there is a big jump in power to .936 when two replicates are used. This means that if we were to solve for the number of replicates needed to obtain power of .80, the answer would be close to 1.5. Although such a solution would not be of much practical value, the number of replicates in general would be obtained by iteratively solving for λ such that $F(f_{\alpha,1,v}, 1, v, \lambda) = .20$, then solving for r from the expression $\lambda = rc\delta^2/4\hat{\sigma}_e$. Although a closed-form solution for the number of replicates is not possible, Mathews (2010) gave a large-sample approximation, which is $r \geq (4/c)(z_{\alpha/2} + z_\beta)^2(\hat{\sigma}_e/\delta)^2$. For this example, this becomes $r \geq (4/12)(1.96 + 0.84)^2(10/15)^2 = 1.16$. Thus, the value of r is smaller than expected and certainly a large-sample approximation won't work very well when the necessary number of observations should be under 20, as is the case here.

Roughly, if r is estimated to be about 1.4, we then have $\lambda = 9.45$ and $f_{\alpha,1,v} = f_{.05,1,12} = 4.747$, so that $F(f_{\alpha,1,v}, 1, v, \lambda) = .19456$ and Power $= 1 - .19456 = .80544$ and is thus very close to the target value of .80. Of course, it is not possible to have 1.4 observations at each design point but it should be apparent that when we use a PB design we are seeking economy, so large sample approximations won't work very well. The approximation should work better when the required value of r is at least 2. For example, as stated previously, a 12-point PB design with 2 replicates for 4 factors with $\sigma = 1.0$ and $\alpha = .05$ has Power $= .936$ for detecting an effect of 1.5. Since we know the exact value of the power, we can give the approximation some help by using that value. Doing so gives $r \geq (4/12)(1.96 + 1.52)^2(1/1.5)^2 = 1.794$, so the approximation fares somewhat better this time but is still not close to the actual solution, although that is somewhat immaterial since only an integer number of replicates can be used.

Indeed, replicating PB designs practically defeats the purpose in using them, as they were designed to be used for studying up to k factors in $N = (k + 1)$ runs, and are thus meant to be economical designs.

Although replication will usually be necessary to achieve the desired power, fortunately that won't always be the case. For example, if a PB design with 20 runs is to be used for studying three factors, power = .8824 for detecting a minimum effect of size 1.5σ *without* the design being replicated.

This result should not be surprising, however, because the number of runs is more than the number of runs for a 2^3 design with two replicates. Interestingly, the power drops off slightly to .8796 when the design is used to study four factors and to .8763 and .8724 when the design is used to study five and six factors, respectively. Of course, eventually the power starts to drop off sharply as the number of factors is increased, but that doesn't happen until about 15 factors are used.

These designs can be useful although they have received some criticism (probably unwarranted) in the literature. [See the discussion in Ryan (2007, p. 490).] They have been used extensively in industry and biotechnology, in particular.

6.11.2 Split-Plot and Strip-Plot Designs

Lenth's applet has separate templates for split-plot designs and strip-plot designs, so we will consider both separately. The former might be labeled a split-unit design, which is a better descriptor because the term "split-plot" originated in agricultural applications of experimental designs, with a plot of land literally being split for the purpose of an experiment. Today, most applications of split-plot designs do not involve land. The simplest type of split-plot design is a design for an experiment with two fixed factors, each at two levels. One of these factors would be designated as the "whole-plot factor" and the other would be termed the "split-plot factor." It is necessary to make this identification, which determines the structure of the design, because the split-plot effect, also termed the subplot effect, will generally be estimated with greater precision than the whole-plot effect, although exceptions can occur (see Giesbrecht and Gumpertz, 2004, p. 169).

Consider an example with the design as explained in the preceding paragraph, with three replications to be used, which constitute the blocks for the experiment, which can be viewed as a random factor. We will use the default model given in Lenth's applet, which is, using the labels therein: Block + Whole + Block * Whole + Split + Whole * Split, with Block * Whole serving as the error term for testing the whole-plot effect and the residual serving as the error term for testing the split-plot effect.

Under the assumption that both σ and $\sigma_{\text{Block} * \text{Whole}} = 1$, Lenth's applet indicates that the power is only .237 for detecting a 1.5-sigma effect of the whole-plot factor, whereas the power is .783 for detecting a 1.5-sigma effect of the split-plot factor. Thus, there is an enormous difference for this simple example and the power is unacceptable for detecting the whole-plot factor effect. The power can be increased by increasing the number of blocks (replications), but it is necessary to use 8 blocks in order to have power of at least .80 for detecting a 1.5-sigma whole-plot factor effect. Using that many blocks of course drives the power for detecting a 1.5-sigma effect of the split-plot factor to virtually 1 (.9998).

Lenth's applet also has a template for a split-plot design with one whole-plot factor and two subplot factors, and for two whole-plot factors and one subplot factor. The addition of either one whole-plot factor or one subplot factor of course reduces the degrees of freedom for the error term, thus reducing the power. Letting W_1 and W_2 denote the first and second whole-plot factors, respectively, W_1 is tested against Block $* W_1$ and W_2 is tested against Block $* W_2$. Under the assumption that $\sigma = \sigma_{\text{Block} * W_1} = \sigma_{\text{Block} * W_2} = 1$ and three blocks are used, the power for detecting a 1.5σ effect is .213 for each of W_1 and W_2, with the power of .9946 of detecting a 1.5σ effect of the split-plot factor. Thus, the power for the whole-plot factors is slightly less than when there is a single whole-plot factor, but the power for the split-plot factor is much greater.

For the case of three blocks, one whole-plot factor and two split-plot factors, the whole-plot factor is tested against the Block $*$ Whole interaction, and the two split-plot factors are each tested against the error term, just as the single split-plot factor is tested against the error term when there is only one split-plot factor. Using the continuing assumption that both of these standard deviations are 1.0, the power for detecting a 1.5σ effect is .8881 for each of the two split-plot factors.

A strip-plot design is used when there are multiple stages involved, such as multiple stages in a production process. As such, it is a special case of a split-plot design, which is a design for two or more stages. Lenth's applet uses this name for the design, but since blocking is involved, a better name for the design would be either a strip-block or split-block design, these being two other names for the design that have been used in the literature. The components of the model for a strip-plot design are: blocks (replications), rows, columns, blocks $\times$ columns, blocks $\times$ rows, and rows $\times$ columns, with row and column each representing a factor of interest. [For more information about the design see Giesbrecht and Gumpertz (2004, Section 7.6), who also give two illustrative examples.]

For example, assume that four blocks are used and there are three levels of each of two factors, corresponding to rows and columns, respectively. The row effect is tested against the block $*$ row interaction and we will assume that the standard deviation of the latter is 1.0. Similarly, the column effect is tested against the block $*$ column interaction and we will assume that the standard deviation of the latter is also 1.0. With these assumptions, the power of detecting a 1.5σ row effect is .7129, which of course is the same for a 1.5σ column effect. That is a low power value, which can be increased by increasing the number of blocks (replications). Increasing the number of blocks from four to five increases each power to a much more acceptable .8615.

6.11.3 Nested Designs

A nested design is a design for which not all of the levels of the factors are crossed; that is, the number of treatment combinations is less than the product of all of the factor levels. A *nested factor* design has no factorial structure at all; that is, there is no crossing of levels of any of the factors. An example would be a design for three factors, A, B, and C, with B nested within A and C nested within B. The common notation for nesting is B(A), C((B|A)), and so on, and that notation will be used in this chapter.

A *nested factorial* design is a design for which there is some factorial structure within the design, such as when there are four factors at each of two levels and there is a full factorial structure in C and D at each level of B (so that the factorial structure exists for B, C, and D, but B_1 occurs only with A_1, and B_2 occurs only with A_2).

Lenth's applet handles both nested factor designs and nested factorial designs. For example, assume a single-stage nested design with two factors and factor B having four levels and each of two levels nested within A, with three replications of each factor combination. The power of detecting a 1.5σ effect of factor A is .894, and .774 for factor B(A). Both of these power values may be judged in a particular application setting, although the second number might be deemed too low. If so, the number of replications could be increased to four, which would raise the power for factor B to .924.

There is also a template for a nested design for three factors: A, B(A), and C((B|A)), with the latter denoting the levels of factor C nested within B nested within A. With three replications, there is a high power value for each of the three factors for detecting a 1.5σ effect, with the numbers being .998, .992, and .964 for A, B, and C, respectively. If two replications were used, however, the values would be .959, .883, and .723, respectively, with the last number likely being deemed too small.

Lenth's applet also has a template for a nested factorial design with one nested factor and two factors in a factorial arrangement, as well as templates for a nested factorial design with two whole-plot factors and one subplot factor and a nested factorial design with one whole-plot factor and two subplot factors.

The discussion in Section 6.5 regarding the need to have enough experimental runs so that conditional effects can be identified and estimated with reasonable precision applies to nested designs only if the design has factorial structure, as the investigation of conditional effects is motivated by large interactions, whereas nested designs without factorial structure do not have interactions.

Moerbeek, Van Breukelen, Berger, and Ausems (2003) gave an example of sample size determination for an experimental design in which individuals are nested within clusters.

6.11.4 Ray Designs

A ray design is a type of mixture design such that individual compounds are mixed together in amounts such that the proportion between them is constant. Casey, Gennings, Carter, Moser, and Simmons (2006) addressed sample size determination when such designs are used and the primary objective is to be able to detect interactions with reasonable power.

6.12 DESIGNS FOR NONNORMAL RESPONSES

Although the typical assumption is that the response variable is a continuous, normally distributed random variable, often this will not be the case. For example, the variable of interest may be the number of nonconforming units in a particular operation, with a desire to run an experiment to determine the primary causes of what might be an unacceptably high number or proportion of nonconforming units. Similarly, an experiment might be conducted to determine the causes of nonconformities, such as product blemishes.

In the first case, it would be reasonable to assume a binomial distribution for the response since there are two possible values for each unit, however defined, conforming or nonconforming, whereas a Poisson distribution might be appropriate in the second case.

Bisgaard and Fuller (1995) provided a table for determining sample size with a binary response when a 2^{k-p} design is to be used. They used the arcsin transformation, which is used in transforming binomial proportions to approximate normality. Other approximations were also involved, so the tabular values should be viewed as approximations, although probably good approximations. Indeed, the authors recommend that the table be used as a rough guide in determining the sample size. Of course, the cost of experimentation should also be considered. Readers interested in the theoretical development that led to the table are referred to Bisgaard and Fuller (1995).

For a given number of experimental runs, such as 16 (a common experiment size when a 2^{k-p} design is used), the number of units to be inspected at each of the 16 treatment combinations is determined so as to have a power of .90 of detecting a specified degree of improvement relative to the proportion nonconforming in the null hypothesis, p_0. To illustrate, if $p_0 = .05$ and it is desired to detect with probability .90 a 50% reduction to .025, Table A1 of Bisgaard and Fuller (1995) shows that 197 units would have to be inspected at each of the 16 combinations, for a total of 3152 units. (Note the very large sample size, which is caused by a small value of p_0.)

Of course, software is generally easier to use than tables and a Microsoft Excel spreadsheet that solves for the sample size given inputted values for p_0, Δ (the change from p_0), α, power, and the number of treatment combinations can be downloaded from www.statease.com/powercalc.html. To illustrate, assume that $p_0 = .20$ and a reduction of $\Delta = .06$ to $p = .14$ is desired to be detected with probability .90 when a 2^{k-p} design with 16 runs is to be used. Use of the spreadsheet shows that 117 units have to be inspected at each treatment combination. [This differs slightly from 116 units given in Table A1 of Bisgaard and Fuller (1995). This difference also occurs with other tabular entries and is caused by the spreadsheet rounding *up* the numbers, whereas the table apparently rounds *off* the numbers.] Although 117 may be an acceptable number, it should be kept in mind that this is the number of units *per run*, so with a 16-run design, the total number of units to be inspected is thus $16(117) = 1872$. Obviously, the total number of units to be inspected can be prohibitively large when the number of units to be inspected per run is large.

The spreadsheet is useful for various reasons, including the fact that the Bisgaard and Fuller (1995) table is only for a power of .90. Assume that 117 units in the previous example is more than can be afforded, so the experimenter is willing to settle for a power of .80. With this change 87 units would be inspected. The output from the program is given below.

```
p(bar) = 0.2 current proportion
Δ      = 0.06 minimum change in proportion

alpha (α is typically 0.05 or 0.10)   = 0.05 z-alpha/2 = 1.96
Power (1-b is typically 0.80 or more) = 0.80 z-beta    = 0.84

δ = 0.075190826 change in transformed scale

Design size                      N = 16 user input
                                     (number of runs)
Units per run for power            = 87
Units per run to avoid too many zeros = 25
Recommended Units per run;         n = 87

Total units = 1392
```

There have also been applications in which the response variable is the number of defects (e.g., Bisgaard and Fuller, 1994–1995) and the Poisson distribution will often be a logical choice for the distribution of the response variable. Unfortunately, there is apparently no software available for sample size determination for such experiments. The necessary theory would have to be developed and supported, as was done by Bisgaard and Fuller (1995) for the binomial case.

Once that was done, it would be simple and straightforward to develop an Excel spreadsheet or a MINITAB macro, for example, that would solve for the necessary sample size.

6.13   DESIGNS WITH RANDOM FACTORS

Sample size determination for designs with fixed factors is somewhat more straightforward and more intuitive than with random factors because it is easier to think in terms of effect sizes than sizes of variance components. Furthermore, there is very little software available for determining sample sizes with random factors. On the other hand, noncentrality parameters are not involved in testing for the effects of random factors, or, in general, testing for random effects, as interaction effects are considered to be random if at least one of the factors involved in the interaction is random.

As mentioned at the beginning of the chapter, Lenth's applet will also handle the random factor case. Specifically, the user can specify which factors are fixed and which are random for any balanced ANOVA model. The classification of a factor as fixed or random will often have a large effect on the sample size that is determined, so the classification should be done carefully and the experimenter must, of course, understand the definition of each type of factor. (A fixed factor is one for which the levels used in an experiment are the only levels of interest; a random factor is one for which interest centers on a range of possible levels, with the levels used in an experiment ideally randomly selected from the range of possible levels.)

For example, assume that there is a single factor with four levels and the factor is random. The model is then $Y_{ij} = \mu + \tau_i + \epsilon_{ij}$, with $\tau_i \sim N(0, \sigma_\tau^2)$ and $\epsilon_{ij} \sim N(0, \sigma^2)$. The null hypothesis is $H_0 : \sigma_\tau^2 = 0$. Note that since the factor is random, we are not interested in any particular τ_i, including the effects of the treatment levels used in the experiment. Rather, interest is in whether *any* τ_i in the population of possible treatment levels is nonzero. If $\sigma_\tau^2 = 0$ then all of the possible τ_i must be zero.

Assume that $\sigma_\tau^2 = \sigma^2 = 1, \alpha = .05$, and an equal number of observations will be used per level. Lenth's applet shows that eight observations must be used at each level in order to have a power of at least .80 (actually .8055) of having a significant F-test result, whereas only five observations are needed when the factor is fixed (power $= .8303$). Intuitively, this makes sense because stating significance for the population of treatment levels is a stronger statement than stating significance for the particular levels used in an experiment.

It can be shown (see, e.g., Sahai and Ageel, 2000, p. 60) that

$$P\left\{F\text{-statistic} > \frac{F_{a-1,a(n-1);\alpha}}{1 + n\sigma_\tau^2/\sigma^2}\right\} = 1 - \beta$$

where a denotes the number of levels and there are n observations per level. Note that the value of the denominator is 1 if the null hypothesis is true, and the probability is then .05.

We can't use this expression to obtain a closed-form solution for n because n is part of the denominator degrees of freedom for the F-variate, but it does allow us to "see" the solution, and of course the expression could be used to solve iteratively for n, if desired.

Specifically, with $a = 4$, $\sigma_\tau^2 = \sigma^2 = 1$, $\alpha = .05$, and, as stated, Lenth's applet giving $n = 8$, the fraction is then $2.947/(1 + 8(1)) = 0.3274$. $P(F\text{-statistic} > 0.3274) = 1 - .1945 = .8055$, as can be shown using MINITAB or other software. Thus, the solution given by Lenth's applet can be verified in this manner.

6.14 ZERO PATIENT DESIGN

Yazici, Biyikil, van der Linden, and Schouten (2001) proposed the idea of a "zero patient" design to compare the prevalences of rare diseases in different geographical regions, although the true prevalences may remain unknown. Their objective was to determine the size of a sample that can be expected to be free of a certain disease. Their sample size formula utilized the approximation, $\ln(1 - p) \approx -p$, which works well when p is small, such as $p < .02$. Utilizing this approximation, they obtained the required sample size as $n = -\ln(0.05)/p_0 = 3/p_0$, with p_0 denoting the hypothesized value of p. This is the required sample size for the 95% confidence bound $p < 3/n$. They showed by way of an example how their approach could be used in an hypothesis-testing framework to compare prevalences of a rare disease in different countries.

6.15 COMPUTER EXPERIMENTS

Computer experiments have become more popular during the past ten years or so, undoubtedly aided by the publication of books on the design of computer experiments such as Santner, Williams, and Notz (2003) and Fang, Li, and Sidjianto (2006). Guidance on sample size determination for such experiments has been lacking, however, as Loeppky, Sacks, and Welch (2009) stated: "Choosing the sample size of a deterministic computer experiment is important but lacks formal guidance."

Although computer experiments differ greatly from physical experiments since there are no experimental units to which treatments are assigned, there may nevertheless be constraints on the sample size in the former due to budgetary constraints that could limit the number of computer runs that could be made.

Chapman, Welch, Bowman, Sacks, and Walsh (1994) and Jones, Schonlau, and Welch (1998) used the rule-of-thumb that the number of runs being ten times the number of important input factors is a good initial guess. Loeppky et al. (2009) examined this recommendation and concluded that it is quite reasonable.

6.16   NONINFERIORITY AND EQUIVALENCE DESIGNS

This topic is covered last because although the terms *noninferiority design* and *equivalence design* are used in the literature, this is practically a misnomer. This is because these are not really types of experimental designs but rather "noninferiority" and "equivalence" refer to forms of hypothesis tests. Greene, Morland, Durkalski, and Frueh (2008) essentially indicated this as they stated: "Noninferiority designs are a one-sided test used to determine if a novel intervention is no worse than a standard intervention. Equivalence designs, a two-sided test, pose a similar question, but also allow for the possibility that the novel intervention is no better than the standard one." Thus, these are designs only if the term is used in a very broad sense and is not intended to refer to statistical designs. Even worse, Greene et al. (2008) stated that many studies in which noninferiority or equivalence was claimed were from studies that were not designed in such a way as to allow such conclusions to be drawn, such as claiming equivalence when a null hypothesis of superiority was not rejected.

6.17   PHARMACOKINETIC EXPERIMENTS

Pharmacokinetic experiments are performed to compare the effects of several drugs applied to several individuals. Aarons and Ogungbenro (2010) stated: "Despite the need to include sample size calculation in the design of population pharmacokinetic experiments . . . most population pharmacokinetic experiment designs still do not include a sample size calculation." There are various ways of determining sample size for such experiments and these are reviewed by Aarons and Ogungbenro (2010).

6.18   BAYESIAN EXPERIMENTAL DESIGN

Although Bayesian experimental design is a well-established field [see, e.g., the review paper by Chaloner and Verdinelli (1995)], with Kathryn Chaloner being one of the major contributors to the field, relatively little research has been published on sample size determination using Bayesian experimental design methods. One such paper is Goldstein and Wooff (1997), who used a Bayes linear approach for sample size determination.

6.19 SOFTWARE

Using Design-Expert to determine power for 2^k designs was discussed in Sections 6.4.2 and 6.4.3.

Although Power and Precision is useful for determining sample size and power, it has very limited capability for experimental designs, as its capability is limited to one-factor designs, with and without a covariate, and factorial designs with either two or three factors, with or without a covariate.

This contrasts sharply with the capability of Lenth's applet, which can handle any balanced ANOVA model, and has templates for nested factor and factorial designs, crossover designs, split-plot designs, randomized complete block designs, and Latin square and Graeco-Latin square designs. It is almost certainly the best freeware for determining sample size (meaning replicates, usually) for experimental designs.

In general, there are a variety of software from which to select for determining sample size and computing power for experimental designs. Capability varies greatly among freeware, however, with apparently no freeware coming close to the capability of Lenth's applet. For example, Web Power at `http://www.math.yorku.ca/SCS/Online/power` runs a SAS program for calculating power for factorial designs. There is some lack of flexibility, however, because all factors are assumed to be fixed and power can be calculated only for standardized effects sizes (effect size/σ) of 0.25, 0.50, 0.75, 1.00, and 1.25, with the program help file indicating that this choice of values (all of which could be specified, then the output would be a table) was influenced by Cohen (1988).

G*Power3 is downloadable freeware that has strengths in certain areas. Its capability for experimental design is somewhat limited, however, because it will handle only fixed effects. Furthermore, its default value for effect size is also obviously influenced by Cohen (1988), and it also restricts the user to the choice of 0.25, 0.50, 0.75, 1.00, or 1.25 for the standardized effect size. One potentially nice feature of the software is that it draws two curves for β and α, but this is shown as a function of values of the F-statistic, which means that someone learning the subject would have to convert the F-values to sample sizes.

MINITAB users may be interested in the MINITAB macro for computing power for fixed effects balanced designs given by Paul Mathews and available at `http://users.stargate.net/~pmathews/tot/source/power.mac`. This extends the capability of the MINITAB software, as in Release 16 the capability is limited to one-factor designs, replicated or unreplicated 2^k designs, replicated or unreplicated Plackett–Burman (PB) designs, and replicated or unreplicated general full factorial designs. Regarding the last three, there has to be some degrees of freedom for the error term, so if an unreplicated 2^k, PB, or general full factorial design is to be used, the user must specify the number of terms that are to be omitted from the model, thereby releasing degrees of freedom to be used for the error term. Of course, an estimate of the standard deviation must be provided in either case.

Thus, an estimate is needed for σ to be able to solve for the power. Since the sample size is fixed with an unreplicated 2^k, PB, or general full factorial design, there must be degrees of freedom for the error term so that hypothesis tests can be performed, with the software indicating the effect size that corresponds to the indicated power or the power for the indicated effect size.

In MINITAB, the effect size used with the PB design is the difference of means, so that the effect size is not standardized, with the user entering a value for σ. In general, the power depends only on (effect size/σ), so the specification of σ wouldn't be necessary for determining power for the standardized effect size if software permitted the input of a standardized effect size, such as G*Power permits, as mentioned previously. This is not how the sample size determination capability of MINITAB is constructed, however. The software can also be used for determining the minimum effect size that can be detected for a specified power. Given below is the output which illustrates this, as the output includes the effect size when the user inputs everything except the effect size.

Power and Sample Size

```
Plackett-Burman Design

Alpha = 0.05 Assumed standard deviation = 10

Factors:            15      Design: 20
Center pts (total): 0

Center          Total
Points  Reps   Runs    Power    Effect
     0     1     20      0.8   16.8200
```

It is also useful to see a graph of power plotted against effect size for the specified design, which is also part of the MINITAB output and is shown in Figure 6.4.

PASS is the most comprehensive sample size determination software and is also probably the easiest to use, although its capabilities for experimental designs are limited. (The software can be used to construct a variety of designs, but can be used to determine sample size for only a limited number of designs, as was noted in this chapter.)

nQuery is comparable in stature to PASS and has a large number of users, but it isn't quite as user friendly. For example, once a set of inputs has been entered, no component can be changed to see that effect without entering all of the components of the worksheet, or cutting and pasting. Like PASS, it really isn't software for determining sample size for experimental designs.

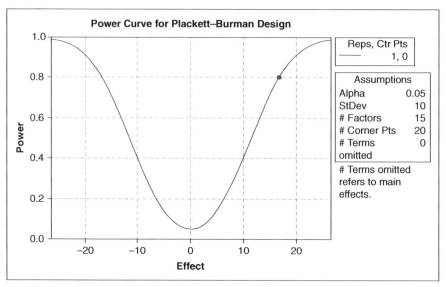

Figure 6.4 Power curve for 20-point Plackett–Burman design; effect size $= 1.5\sigma$.

This can undoubtedly be explained for PASS and nQuery and perhaps for other software as well by recognizing what the primary markets are for their software (e.g., pharmaceutical firms) and recognizing that these markets are not going to be interested in determining sample size for factorial designs or Taguchi designs, which are used in manufacturing applications. Rather, interest centers on a rather limited collection of designs.

Users of SAS Software can use **PROC GLMPOWER** for determining sample size for linear models. See http://support.sas.com/documentation/cdl/en/statug/63347/HTML/default/viewer.htm#statug_glmpower_a0000000154.htm. The output for, say, an ANOVA example with two factors has a realistic general form in that a single sample size is not given. Rather, as shown at http://support.sas.com/documentation/cdl/en/statug/63347/HTML/default/viewer.htm#statug_clientpss_sect025.htm for an example involving the two factors Drug and Gender the output states in part "You need a total sample size between 60 and 108 to yield a power of 0.9 for the Drug effect if the standard deviation is between 5 and 7. You need a sample size of half that for the Gender effect."

6.20 SUMMARY

Sample size determination for designed experiments deserves careful attention for the same reasons that sample size determination in general is important. Books on sample size determination in general have very little on sample size determination and the need to use multiples of certain designs, such as Latin square designs, is generally not stressed. More attention also needs to be devoted to sample size determination by statistical software companies. Until then, tables such as those given by Bratcher, Moran, and Zimmer (1970), which is for a single factor with and without blocking, can be useful, as can the tables of L. S. Nelson (1985), which are an extension of the Bratcher et al. (1970) tables. See also the extended tables in Diletti, Hauschke, and Steinjans (1992) for testing bioequivalence with a two-period crossover design. The tables provided in Hager and Möller (1986) may also be of interest. Odeh and Fox (1991) gave many charts to aid in sample size determination for experimental designs.

APPENDIX

Derivation of Eq. (6.1)

We will first derive the formula for a one-sided test, then arrive at the formula for the two-sided test using deduction. Assume that the alternative hypothesis is "greater than." Then

$$p(z < z_\alpha) = \Phi\left(z_\alpha - \frac{\Delta}{\sigma\sqrt{2/m}}\right) = \beta$$

with m denoting the common sample size and Δ denoting the difference between the two means, so

$$z_\alpha - \frac{\Delta}{\sigma\sqrt{2/m}} = \Phi^{-1}(\beta)$$

$$= z_\beta \quad \text{(since the subscript of } z \text{ denotes the right tail area)}$$

$$= -z_\beta$$

so

$$\frac{\Delta}{\sigma\sqrt{2/m}} = -z_\alpha - z_\beta$$

and thus

$$m = \frac{(z_\alpha + z_\beta)^2 2\sigma^2}{\Delta^2} = \frac{n}{2} \text{ in Eq. (6.1)}$$

The only component of this expression that is affected by whether the test is one-sided or two-sided is z_α, which is $z_{\alpha/2}$ if the test is two-sided. Therefore, that substitution gives the formula for m for a two-sided test.

REFERENCES

Aarons, L. and K. Ogungbenro (2010). Optimal design of pharmacokinetic experiments. *Basic and Clinical Pharmacology and Toxicology*, **106**(3), 250–255.

Ahrens, R. C, M. E. Teresi, S.-H. Han, D. Donnell, J. A. Vanden Burgt, and C. R. Lux (2001). Asthma stability after prednisone: A clinical model for comparing inhaled steroid potency. *American Journal of Respiratory and Critical Care Medicine*, **164**, 1138–1145.

Balaam, L. N. (1968). A two-period design with t^2 experimental units. *Biometrics*, **24**(1), 61–73.

Bang, H., S.-H. Jung, and S. George (2005). Sample size calculation for simulation-based multiple-testing procedures. *Journal of Biopharmaceutical Statistics*, **15**(6), 957–967.

Bisgaard, S. and H. T. Fuller (1994–1995). Analysis of factorial experiments with defects or defectives as the response. *Quality Engineering*, **7**(2), 429–443.

Bisgaard, S. and H. T. Fuller (1995). Sample size estimates for 2^{k-p} designs with binary responses. *Journal of Quality Technology*, **27**(4), 344–354.

Bishop, T. A. and E. J. Dudewicz (1978). Exact analysis of variance with unequal variances: Test procedures and tables. *Technometrics*, **20**, 419–430.

Borm, G. F., J. Fransen, and W. A. J. G. Lemmens (2007). A simple sample size formula for analysis of covariance in randomized clinical trials. *Journal of Clinical Epidemiology*, **60**, 1234–1238.

Box, G. E. P., W. G. Hunter, and J. S. Hunter (1978). *Statistics for Experimenters*. New York: Wiley. (The current edition is the 2nd edition, 2005.)

Bratcher, T. L., M. A. Moran, and W. J. Zimmer (1970). Tables of sample sizes in the analysis of variance. *Journal of Quality Technology*, **2**(3), 156–164.

Bursztyn, D. and D. M. Steinberg (2001). Rotation designs for experiments in high bias situations. *Journal of Statistical Planning and Inference*, **97**, 399–414.

Carroll, R. J. and D. B. H. Cline (1988). An asymptotic theory for weighted least squares with weights estimated by replication. *Biometrika*, **75**, 35–43.

Casey, M., C. Gennings, W. Carter, V. Moser, and J. Simmons (2006). Power and sample size calculations for linear hypotheses associated with mixtures of many components using fixed-ratio ray designs. *Environmental and Ecological Statistics*, **13**, 11–23.

Chaloner, K. and I. Verdinelli (1995). Bayesian experimental design: A review. *Statistical Science*, **10**(3), 273–304.

Chapman, W. L., W. J. Welch, K. P. Bowman, J. Sacks, and J. E. Walsh (1994). Arctic sea ice variability: Model sensitivities and a multidecadal simulation. *Journal of Geophysical Research*, **99**, 919–935.

Chen, K. W., S. C. Chow, and G. Li (1997). A note on sample size determination for bioequivalence studies with higher-order crossover designs. *Journal of Pharmacokinetics and Biopharmaceutics*, **25**(6), 753–765.

Cheng, S.-W. and C. F. J. Wu (2001). Factor screening and response surface exploration. *Statistica Sinica*, **11**, 553–580. Discussion: **11**, 581–604.

Chow, S.-C. and J. P. Liu (1999). *Design and Analysis of Bioavailability and Bioequivalence Studies*: New York: Marcel Dekker.

Chow, S.-C. and H. Wang (2001). On sample size calculation in bioequivalence trials. *Journal of Pharmacokinetics and Pharmacodynamics*, **28**(2), 155–169.

Chow, S.-C., J. Shao, and H. Wang (2008). *Sample Size Calculations in Clinical Research*, 2nd edition. Boca Raton, FL: Chapman & Hall/CRC.

Cohen, J. (1988). *Statistical Power Analysis for the Behavioral Sciences*, 2nd edition. New York: Routledge Academic.

Daniel, C. (1976). *Applications of Statistics to Industrial Experimentation*. New York: Wiley.

Diletti, E., D. Hauschke, and W. V. Steinjans (1992). Sample size determination: Extended tables for the multiplicative model and bioequivalence ranges of 0.9 to 1.11 and 0.7 to 1.43. *International Journal of Clinical Pharmacology, Therapy, and Toxicology*, **30**, Supplement 1, S59–S62.

Dobbin, K. and R. Simon (2005). Sample size determination in microarray experiments for class comparison and prognostic classification. *Biostatistics*, **6**(1), 27–38. (Available at http://biostatistics.oxfordjournals.Org/cgi/reprint/6/1/ 27.pdf.)

Fang, K.-T., R. Li, and A. Sudjianto (2006). *Design and Modeling for Computer Experiments*. New York: Chapman and Hall/CRC.

Geng, S. and F. J. Hills (1978). A procedure for determining numbers of experimental and sampling units. *Agronomy Journal*, **70**, 441–444.

Giesbrecht, F. G. and M. L. Gumpertz (2004). *Planning, Construction, and Statistical Analysis of Comparative Experiments*. Hoboken, NJ: Wiley.

Goldstein, M. and D. A. Wooff (1997). Choosing sample sizes in balanced experimental designs: A Bayes linear approach. *The Statistician*, **46**(2), 167–183.

Gravetter, F. J. and L. B. Wallnau (2009). *Statistics for the Behavioral Sciences*, 8th edition. Belmont, CA: Wadsworth.

Greene, C. J., L. A. Morland, V. L. Durkalski, and B. C. Frueh (2008). Noninferiority and equivalence designs: Issues and implications for mental health research. *Journal of Trauma Stress*, **21**(5), 433–439.

Guo, J. H. and W.-M. Luh (2010). On sample size calculation for 2×2 fixed effect ANOVA when variances are unequal. *British Journal of Mathematical and Statistical Psychology*, **62**, 417–425.

Hager, W. and H. Möller (1986). Tables for the determination of power and sample size in univariate and multivariate analyses of variance and regression. *Biometrical Journal*, **28**, 647–663.

Hamada, M. and N. Balakrishnan (1998). Analyzing unreplicated factorial experiments: A review with some new proposals. *Statistica Sinica*, **8**(1), 31–35.

Harris, M., D. G. Horvitz, and A. M. Mood (1948). On the determination of sample sizes in designing experiments. *Journal of the American Statistical Association*, **43**, 391–402.

Hirakawa, A., C. Hamada, and I. Yoshimura (2011). Sample size calculation for a regularized *t*-statistic in microarray experiments. *Statistics and Probability Letters*, **81**, 870–875.

Hwang, D., W. A. Schmitt, George Stephanopolous, and Gregory Stephanopolous (2002). Determination of minimum sample size and discriminatory expression patterns in microarray data. *Bioinformatics*, **18**(9), 1184–1193. (Available at http://bioinfor matics.oxfordjournals.Org/cgi/reprint/18/9/1184.pdf.)

Jaech, J. L. (1969). The Latin square. *Journal of Quality Technology*, **1**(4), 242–255.

Jiang, D. and J. J. Oleson (2011). Simulation study of power and sample size for repeated measures with multinomial outcomes: An application to sound direction identification experiments. *Statistics in Medicine*, **30**(19), 2451–2466.

Jones, D. R., M. Schonlau, and W. J. Welch (1998). Efficient global optimization of expensive black-box functions. *Journal of Global Optimization*, **13**, 455–492.

Jung, S.-H. and C. Ang (2003). Sample size estimation for GEE method for comparing slopes in repeated measurements data. *Statistics in Medicine*, **22**(8), 1305–1315.

Jung, S. H., H. Bang, and S. Young (2005). Sample size calculation for multiple testing in microarray data analysis. *Bioinformatics*, **6**(1), 157–169.

Keppel, G. (1991). *Design and Analysis: A Researcher's Handbook*, 3rd edition. Englewood Cliffs, NJ: Prentice Hall.

Kirby, A. J., N. Galai, and A. Munoz (1994). Sample size estimation using repeated measurements on biomarkers as outcomes. *Controlled Clinical Trials*, **15**(3), 165–172.

Lachenbruch, P. A. (1988). A note on sample size computation for testing interactions. *Statistics in Medicine*, **7**, 467–469.

Lee, M.-L. T. and G. A. Whitmore (2002). Power and sample size for DNA microarray studies. *Statistics in Medicine*, **21**(23), 3543–3570.

Lenth, R. V. (2001). Some practical guidelines for effective sample size determination. *The American Statistician*, **55**(3), 187–193. (Available at http://www.stat.uiowa.edu/techrep/tr303.pdf.)

Li, S. S., J. Bigler, J. W. Lampe, J. D. Potter, and Z. Peng (2005). FDR-controlling testing procedures and sample size determination for microarrays. *Statistics in Medicine*, **24**, 2267–2280.

Lin, W.-J., H.-M. Hsueh, and J. J. Chen (2010). Power and sample size estimation in microarray studies. *BMC Bioinformatics*, **11** (Supplement 1), S52.

Lipsitz, S. R. and G. M. Fitzmaurice (1994). Sample size for repeated measures studies with binary responses. *Statistics in Medicine*, **13**, 1233–1239.

Littell, R. C., J. Pendergast, and R. Natarajan (2000). Modeling covariance structure in the analysis of repeated measures data. *Statistics in Medicine*, **19**, 1793–1819.

Littell, R. C., W. W. Stroup, and R. J. Freund (2002). *SAS for Linear Models*, 4th edition. Cary, NC: SAS Institute, Inc.

Liu, P. and J. T. G. Hwang (2007). Quick calculation for sample size while controlling false discovery rate with application to microarray analysis. *Bioinformatics*, **23**(6), 739–746.

Liu, H. and T. Wu (2005). Sample size calculation and power analysis of time-averaged difference. *Journal of Modern Applied Statistical Methods*, **4**(2), 434–445.

Liu, H. and T. Wu (2008). Sample size calculation and power analysis of changes in mean response over time. *Communications in Statistics—Simulation and Computation*, **37**(9), 1785–1798.

Loeppky, J. L., J. Sacks, and W. J. Welch (2009). Choosing the sample size of a computer experiment: A practical guide. *Technometrics*, **51**(4), 366–376.

Luh, W.-M. and J.-H. Guo (2010). Developing the noncentrality parameter for calculating group sample sizes in heterogeneous analysis of variance. *The Journal of Experimental Education*, **79**(1), 53–63.

Lui, K-.J. and W. G. Cumberland (1992). Sample size requirement for repeated measurements in continuous data. *Statistics in Medicine*, **11**, 633–641.

Lynch, R. O. (1993). Minimum detectable effects for 2^{k-p} experimental plans. *Journal of Quality Technology*, **25**(1), 12–17.

Mathews, P. (2010). *Sample Size Calculations: Practical Methods for Engineers and Scientists.* Harbor, OH: Mathews, Malnar, and Bailey, Inc.

Matsui, S. and T. Oura (2009). Sample sizes for robust ranking of genes in microarray experiments. *Statistics in Medicine*, **28**, 2617–2638.

Matsui, S., S. Zeng, T. Yamanaka, and J. Shaughnessy (2008). Sample size calculations based on ranking and selection in microarray experiments. *Biometrics*, **64**, 217–226.

Milliken, G. A. (2004). Mixed models and repeated measures: Some illustrative industrial examples. In *Handbook of Statistics, Vol. 22: Statistics in Industry*, Chap. 5 (R. Khattree and C. R. Rao, eds.). Amsterdam, The Netherlands: Elsevier Science B.V.

Moerbeek, M., G. J. P. Van Breukelen, M. P. F. Berger, and M. Ausems (2003). Optimal sample sizes in experimental designs with individuals nested within clusters. *Understanding Statistics*, **2**(3), 151–175.

Montague, T. H., D. Potvin, C. E. DiLiberti, W. W. Hauck, A. F. Parr, and D. J. Schuirman (2012). Additional results for "Sequential design approaches for bioequivalence studies with crossover designs." *Pharmaceutical Statistics*, **11**(1), 8–13.

Muller, K. E. and C. N. Barton (1989). Approximate power for repeated measures ANOVA lacking sphericity. *Journal of the American Statistical Association*, **84**(406), 549–555.

Muller, K. E., L. E. LaVange, S. L. Ramey, and C. T. Ramey (1992). Power calculations for general linear multivariate models including repeated measures applications. *Journal of the American Statistical Association*, **87**(420), 1209–1226.

Muller, P., G. Parmigiani, C. Robert, and J. Rousseau (2004). Optimal sample size for multiple testing: The case of gene expression micoarrays. *Journal of the American Statistical Association*, **99**(468), 990–1001.

Nelson, L. S. (1985). Sample size tables for analysis of variance. *Journal of Quality Technology*, **17**, 167–169.

Nelson, P. R. (1983). A comparison of the sample sizes for the Analysis of Means and the Analysis of Variance. *Journal of Quality Technology*, **15**(1), 33–39.

Nelson, P. R. (1985). Power curves for the Analysis of Means. *Technometrics*, **27**, 65–73.

Nelson, P. R., P. S. Wludyka, and K. A. F. Copeland (2005). *The Analysis of Means: A Graphical Method for Comparing Means, Rates and Proportions*. ASA-SIAM Series on Statistics and Applied Probability. Philadelphia, PA: Society for Industrial and Applied Mathematics.

Odeh, R. E. and M. Fox (1991). *Sample Size Choice: Charts for Experiments with Linear Models*, 2nd edition. Boca Raton, FL: CRC Press.

Ogungbenro, K. and L. Aarons (2008). How many subjects are necessary for population pharmacokinetic experiments? Confidence interval approach. *European Journal of Clinical Pharmacology*, **64**(7), 705–713.

Ogungbenro, K. and L. Aarons (2009). Sample-size calculations for multi-group comparison in population pharmacokinetic experiments. *Pharmaceutical Statistics*, **9**(4), 255–268.

Ogungbenro, K. and L. Aarons (2010a). Sample size/power calculations for repeated ordinal measurements in population pharmacodynamic experiments. *Journal of Pharmacokinetics and Pharmacodynamics*, **37**(1), 67–83.

Ogungbenro, K. and L. Aarons (2010b). Sample size/power calculations for population pharmacodynamic experiments involving repeated-count measurements. *Journal of Biopharmaceutical Statistics*, **20**(5), 1026–1042.

Ogungbenro, K., L. Aarons, and G. Graham (2006). Sample size calculations based on generalized estimating equations for population pharmacokinetic experiments. *Journal of Biopharmaceutical Statistics*, **16**(2), 135–150.

Orr, M. and P. Liu (2009). Sample size estimation while controlling false discovery rate for microarray experiments using the ssize.fdr Package. *The R Journal*, **1**(1), 47–53.

Overall, J. E. (1996). How many repeated measurements are useful? *Journal of Clinical Psychology*, **52**(3), 243–252.

Overall, J. E. and S. R. Doyle (1994). Estimating sample sizes for repeated measurement designs. *Controlled Clinical Trials*, **15**(2), 100–123.

Pan, W., J. Lin, and C. T. Lee (2002). How many replicates of arrays are required to detect gene expression changes in microarray experiments? A mixture model approach. *Genome Biology*, **3**, 0022.1–0022.10.

Pan, Z. and L. Kupper (1999). Sample size determination for multiple comparison studies treating confidence interval width as random. *Statistics in Medicine*, **18**(12), 1475–1488.

Pawitan, Y., S. Michiels, S. Koscielny, A. Gusnanto, and A. Ploner (2005). False discovery rate, sensitivity and sample size for microarray studies. *Bioinformatics*, **18**(9), 1184–1193.

Pounds, S. and C. Cheng (2005). Sample size determination for the false discovery rate. *Bioinformatics*, **21**(3), 4263–4271. Erratum: **25**(5), 698–699.

Potvin, D., C. E. DiLiberti, W. W. Hauck, A. F. Parr, D. J. Schuirmann, and R. A. Smith (2007). Sequential design approaches for bioequivalence studies with crossover designs. *Pharmaceutical Statistics*, **7**, 245–262.

Qu, R. P. and H. Zheng (2003). Sample size calculation for bioequivalence studies with high-order crossover designs. *Controlled Clinical Trials*, **24**(4), 436–439.

Ryan, T. P. (2007). *Modem Experimental Design*. Hoboken, NJ: Wiley.

Sahai, H. and M. I. Ageel (2000). *The Analysis of Variance: Fixed, Random and Mixed Models*. Boston: Birkhaüser.

Santner, T. J., B. J. Williams, and W. Notz (2003). *The Design and Analysis of Computer Experiments*. New York: Springer.

Schuirmann, D. (1987). A comparison of the two one-sided tests procedure and the power approach for assessing the equivalence of average bioavailability. *Journal of Pharmacokinetics and Biopharmaceutics*, **15**(6), 657–680.

Schwertman, N. C. (1987). An alternative procedure for determining analysis of variance sample size. *Communications in Statistics—Simulation and Computation*, **16**(4), 957–967.

Senn, S. (2002). *Cross-over Trials in Clinical Research*. New York: Wiley.

Simon, R. M., E. L. Korn, L. M. McShane, M. D. Radmacher, G. W. Wright, and Y. Zhao (2004). *Design and Analysis of DNA Microarray Investigations*. New York: Springer.

Tsai, C.-A., S- J. Wang, D.-T. Chen, and J. J. Chen (2005). Sample size for gene expression microarray experiments. *Bioinformatics*, **21**(8), 1502–1508.

Vickers, A. J. (2003). How many repeated measures in repeated measures designs? Statistical issues for comparative trials. *BMC Medical Research Methodology*, **3**, 1–22.

Wang, S. J. and J. J. Chen (2004). Sample size for identifying differentially expressed genes in microarray experiments. *Journal of Computational Biology*, **11**(4), 714–726.

Wei, C., J. Li, and R. E. Bumgarner (2004). Sample size for detecting differentially expressed genes in microarray experiments. *BMC Genomics*, **5**(1), 87. (Electronic resource, paper available at www.biomedcentral.com/1471-2164/5/87.)

Witte, J. S., R. C. Elston, and L. R. Cardon (2000). On the relative sample size required for multiple comparisons. *Statistics in Medicine*, **19**, 369–372.

Yazici, H., M. Biyikil, S. van der Linden, and H. J. A. Schouten (2001). The "zero patient" design to compare the prevalences of rare diseases. *Rheumatology*, **40**(2), 121–122.

Yi, Q. and T. Panzarella (2002). Estimating sample sizes for tests on trends across repeated measurements with missing data based on the interaction term in a mixed model. *Controlled Clinical Trials*, **23**(5), 481–496.

Zucker, D. M. and J. Denne (2002). Sample size redetermination for repeated measures studies. *Biometrics*, **58**(3), 548–559. Discussion: **60**, 284–285.

EXERCISES

6.1. Assume that you wish to detect a difference between means of two populations of 2.0 when the standard deviation of each population is assumed to be 6, $\alpha = .05$, and the power is to be .90. How large should the common sample size be? If software is to be used to determine the sample size, is it necessary to use software with experimental design capability? Explain.

6.2. Consider a 4×4 Latin square design with, as in Example 6.1, $\sigma^2 = \sigma_{\hat{t}}^2 = 1$ and $\alpha = .05$. Determine the power figures for 1, 2, and 3 Latin squares, with each member of each set of multiple Latin squares being unrelated to the other members of the set.

6.3. Assume that six 4×4 Latin squares are to be used and that $\alpha = .05$ and $\sigma^2 = 1$. How large a value of $\sigma_{\hat{t}}^2$ (or equivalently, a value for $\sum_{i=1}^{4} \tau_i^2$) can be detected with a power of .90? If we wanted to detect that value with a power of .80, how many Latin squares should be used?

6.4. Assume that an experiment is to be conducted using three levels of a single factor, with these levels being the only ones of interest, so that the factor is fixed. If you have no idea of the effect that each level will have, what complications, if any, does this present? Explain.

6.5. Consider designs for nonnormal responses, as discussed in Section 6.12. Determine the sample size that would be needed to detect a reduction from $p_0 = .10$ to $p = .05$ with a two-tailed test with $\alpha = .05$ and power $= .90$ when a 2^4 design is used.

6.6. Assume that a 20-run Plackett–Burman design is to be used for 14 factors. What is the power for detecting a 1σ effect if the design is not replicated? Would you suggest that such a design be used, or would you prefer to have two replicates and accept the power that is obtained using two replicates? In particular, does using two replicates instead of one help very much? Explain.

6.7. Assume that a one-way ANOVA is to be used with three levels of the factor. With $\alpha = .05$, $\sigma^2 = 1$, and $\sigma_\tau^2 = 2$, how many observations should be used with each level in order to have power $= .90$?

6.8. Consider the standardized effect sizes used by Cohen (1988) that were listed in Section 6.2. If you wanted to design software to make it as simple as possible for the user and decided to select six standardized effect sizes from which the user would select and thus avoid having to estimate σ, which six values would you select? Do they differ considerable from those given by Cohen? If so, explain why.

6.9. When will the desired power for a particular experimental design not be at least approximately met?

6.10. Regarding Exercise 6.1, if one of the standard deviations was believed to be 9 and the other two 6, how would you proceed in determining sample size? In particular, would you use different sample sizes? Explain.

6.11. Geng and Hills (1978) considered the determination of sample size for certain experimental designs. In one example that they cited from the literature, a replicated 6×6 Latin square design was used. This study was used to provide necessary parameter estimates for another study in which the same design is to be used. The experimenter wanted to detect one mean being 10% greater than the overall mean, assumed to be 13.5. They computed the noncentrality parameter to be 2.24. This should apparently be 2.40, although they define the noncentrality parameter as some writers have done, by taking the square root of the expression used in this chapter. Since software for computing power for experimental designs was not readily available in the mid-1970s, they used a Pearson and Hartley chart and concluded that the power would be greater than .90. For either definition of the noncentrality parameter, do you agree that the power is greater than .90? Explain. From a practical standpoint, if five of the six treatment means are equal to the hypothesized average value and only one mean differs from the average, and it differs by only 10%, would we expect an F-test, thinking about what the test is designed to detect, to be able to detect this difference with high power without using a very large number of observations?

6.12. Consider Example 3.5, which was analyzed as a repeated measures design in Section 6.8. Use PASS or other software and enter the covariance matrix as 25, a, a, 25, with $a = 19$ and 22, in addition to the $a = 20$ in that example.

(a) What effect do these changes in the value of a have on the sample size?

(b) Considering the definition, $\rho_{XY} = \text{Cov}(X, Y)/(\sigma_X \sigma_Y)$, with ρ_{XY} denoting the correlation between X and Y and $\text{Cov}(X, Y)$ denoting the covariance between X and Y, with σ_X and σ_Y fixed in this example, what is happening to the correlation between the two factor levels as a is increased? Does the change in the sample size relative to the change in the correlation make sense intuitively? What does this tell you?

(c) Although negative correlations generally do not occur with repeated measures designs, now let $a = -19, -20$, and -22 and determine the sample size for each of these values. Comment relative to what you saw using positive values of a.

CHAPTER 7

Clinical Trials

As indicated at the beginning of Chapter 2, some strange statements and strange ad hoc sample size determination formulas can be found in the literature. The medical literature is not immune to such problems, as Sathian, Sreedharan, Baboo, Sharan, Abhilash, and Rajesh (2010) used the words "proved" and "proven" in their article. In particular, they stated: "Thus, the study has to be repeated on a larger sample so that the real difference can be statistically proved." Nothing can ever be *proved* using statistics as there will always be an element of doubt since samples are taken from populations, rather than entire populations used (which would be highly impractical), so statements of that strength are improper. Such misstatements undoubtedly occur in many fields of application, however.

As the list of papers in the References at the end of this chapter indicates, a very large number of papers have been written on sample size determination for clinical trials. Some of these are tutorial-type papers that constitute recommended reading as supplements to this chapter and the books that have been written on the subject. For example, Thabane, Ma, Chu, Cheng, Ismalia, Rios, Robson, Thabane, Giangregorio, and Goldsmith (2010), Julious (2004), and Wittes (2002) are papers in this category. They can be useful supplements to the books that are listed in Section 7.1. Although not a tutorial paper on methodology, Bacchetti (2002) makes some important points about the refereeing of papers on sample size determination, suggesting that some research is not being published that should be published. Specifically, he stated: "Peer reviewers often make unfounded statistical criticisms, particularly in difficult areas such as sample size determination and power." These thoughts are echoed by Zwarenstein (2002) and others.

Lan and Shun (2009) discussed some important practical issues regarding clinical trials. In particular, they pointed out that the typical approach to sample size determination by solving for *n* such that there is the desired power of rejecting the

Sample Size Determination and Power, First Edition. Thomas P. Ryan.
© 2013 John Wiley & Sons, Inc. Published 2013 by John Wiley & Sons, Inc.

null hypothesis when the true state of affairs is a specified alternative hypothesis is not necessarily what should be done. If two treatments are being compared, the null hypothesis is typically that their effects are equal; this being what the experimenter wants to reject. If that is done, however, the conclusion is that the new treatment is superior to the old treatment if the test is one-sided, or that the effects of the two treatments are unequal if the test is two-sided.

One interesting question is how much clinicians' beliefs should influence the sample size calculation. That is, should a trial committee include only people who are enthusiastic about a forthcoming trial or should the committee include a larger community of experts, including both enthusiasts and skeptics? This issue, which will likely influence sample size, was addressed by Fayers, Cushieri, Fielding, Uscinska, and Freedman (2000).

Simple superiority will generally be an inadequate conclusion, however, as the experimenter would like to conclude, with some high probability, that the true difference is at least equal to Δ_m, using the Lan and Shun (2009) terminology. Just setting the alternative hypothesis equal to Δ_m will not accomplish that, however. This problem can be remedied by simply setting the null and alternative hypotheses equal to $H_0: \Delta \leq \Delta_m$ and $H_a: \Delta > \Delta_m$, respectively, but the specification of such hypotheses seems to be uncommon in the medical literature, as well as in the applied literature, in general, although it is an established part of the theory of hypothesis testing.

In a relatively recent article that should be read by anyone involved in clinical trials and medical research, in general, as well as reading certain cited references, Bacchetti (2010) stated the following.

> Early in my career, an epidemiologist told me that dealing with sample size is the price one has to pay for being a biostatistician. Since then, I have spent untold time and effort paying this price, while also coming to realize that such effort produces no real scientific benefit. Unfortunately, widespread misconceptions about sample size hurt not only statisticians, but also the quality of medical science generally .... I present here a wider challenge to current conventions, including how they cause serious harm .... Reports of completed studies should *not* [emphasis mine] include power calculations, and guidelines requiring them should be changed to instead discourage them.

In previous chapters, the difficulty of providing reasonable necessary input values was stressed, and this difficulty was especially apparent in Chapter 5 because of what had to be inputted. This is one of Bacchetti's main points, in addition to stating that the current approach "assumes a meaningful boundary between adequate and inadequate sample sizes that does not actually exist, not even approximately." He also pointed out that there is no indication of how a completed study's information should actually be used.

So what should be done instead? Bacchetti (2010) obviously feels that there should be a shift toward reporting point estimates and confidence intervals.

(Of course, many others feel the same way.) As he stated, "power is irrelevant for interpreting completed studies." Indeed, power is never really known because it depends on parameter values that are never known. This means, in turn, that sample sizes that are used are never known to be "correct."

Beyond that, Bacchetti (2010) stated: "A common pragmatic strategy is to use the maximum reasonably feasible.... When constraints imposed by funders determine feasibility, doing the maximum possible within those constraints is a sensible choice." The author also suggested considering the use of sample sizes that have worked well in the past for similar studies, pointing out that power calculations are frequently based on such studies anyway since preliminary data are frequently unavailable.

There are special considerations that must be made in determining sample size when the subjects are people, including the dropout rate and ethical considerations. These are discussed in Sections 7.1 and 7.2.

7.1 CLINICAL TRIALS

The determination of an appropriate sample size is especially important when the sample units are people. As discussed in Section 2.3, there are ethical considerations as it is important that a clinical study have sufficient power to detect an effect that would be deemed significant, as it would be unethical to expose the subjects to risks if a study was not likely to have a significant outcome.

There are various other factors that should be considered, including the dropout rate and time and resource constraints. Because of the considerable importance of determining an appropriate sample size when people are involved, more than a few books have been written on sample size determination for clinical trials, including Machin, Campbell, Tan, and Tan (2009), Julious (2009), Chow, Shao, and Wang (2008), and Lemeshow, Hosmer, Klar, and Lwanga (1990). See also Shuster (1992), Senn (2002), Kenward and Jones (2003) and the tables provided by Machin, Campbell, Fayers, and Pinol (1997), in addition to the material on sample size determination in Peace (2009).

The latter explained that although the FDA requires two clinical trials before approval of a new drug can be granted, under certain conditions a single clinical trial will suffice. Indeed, Darken and Ho (2004) argued for a single confirmatory trial and pointed out that use of a single trial has been gaining acceptance. If only one trial is used, it is obviously imperative that the trial be well designed, and of course the trial must show statistical significance. It is also highly desirable if only one trial is used for the p-value for the test of a new drug be extremely small, much less than what is needed to show statistical significance if $\alpha = .01$ or .05 is used. This is because of the reproducibility probabilities given in Table 1.12 of Chow et al. (2008, p. 6), which shows that there is approximately a 90% chance of a p-value less than .001 being observed in future clinical trials if the

p-value was .001 for the single clinical trial that was conducted. This contrasts with having only about a 50-50 chance of reproducing a p-value of .05 if that number was observed in the trial.

There are actually multiple sample sizes that need to be determined in clinical trials because there are multiple phases. Specifically, a Phase I study is a preliminary study that generally uses only a few patients (such as 5 or 6) at each dose level, with one of the objectives being to determine dosage level to be used in a later phase, such as the maximum tolerated dose levels; Phase II involves a moderate number of patients with an eye toward a preliminary assessment of new drug efficacy (without the use of a control group); and Phase III is intended to provide a definitive assessment of efficacy, often involving thousands of patients. There is usually a progression from Phase I to Phase II if only a specified minimum number of patients respond favorably to the drug. There can also be multiple stages within Phase II, with the outcome at each stage determining whether or not the next stage is reached. This is illustrated in Section 7.8.

As we would expect, Phase I and Phase II studies predominate because of the cost and effort involved in Phase III studies.

Parker and Berman (2003) described a clinical study in which one of them was involved that illustrates what often happens in the real world versus what happens in statistics books. In particular, they pointed out that the "variability known" assumption is frequently unfounded. Even if prior data exist, which will often not be the case, it may not be possible, or at least defensible, to use the estimate of σ from that data because that population may differ from the population under study, and different times and different conditions may also be important factors. The expected dropout rate must also be considered, and this may be difficult to estimate.

General considerations that should be made in determining sample size for clinical trials were given by Kirby, Gebski, and Keech (2002) and Eng (2003) is also an instructional article, written by an M.D., which mentions that many published clinical studies have suffered from low power. In an early paper, George and Desu (1974) considered the dual problem of determining sample size and the required duration of a trial for a fixed sample size. Makuch and Simon (1982) generalized those results.

An indirect way of determining sample size for clinical trials, by using simulation to determine the probability of observing a significant result for a given sample size and a given degree of superiority of the treatment relative to the control, was given by Allen and Seaman (2009). They approached this from a standpoint of both "noninferiority" and superiority, with the former defined as the absolute value of the control minus the new treatment being inside the confidence interval of $\pm k\%$, with k being the number that is judged to signify an important clinical difference. This simply means that the proposed treatment is not grossly inferior, if inferior at all, to the control. Of course, superiority would be signaled by the absolute difference of control minus treatment being greater than $k\%$, with the outcome variable being such that a small percentage is desirable. Certainly simulations are only as good as the assumptions upon which they are based, but the charts and tables that the authors provided might be used as an aid in determining sample size. Eng (2004) also discussed the use of simulation to determine sample size, especially for complex designs. Similarly, Landau and Stahl (2013) also discussed the use of simulation for determining sample size, as they pointed out that complex modeling techniques might be used for which power formulas do not exist.

7.1.1 Cluster Randomized Trials

Cluster randomized trials, in which groups of individuals are randomized, are often used in the health field. Sample size determination must incorporate the effect of the clustering, which requires good estimates of intracluster correlation coefficients (ICCs). Campbell, Grimshaw, and Steen (2000) considered sample size determination for such studies and generated estimates of ICCs. You, Williams, Aban, Kabagambe, Tiwari, and Cutter (2011) considered sample size and power in the presence of variable cluster sizes.

7.1.2 Phase II Trials

Chang, Shuster, and Kepner (2004) considered Phase II clinical trials for which a binomial proportion was tested. They determined sample size for an exact unconditional test when the control group information has already been collected. Simon (1989) presented optimal two-stage designs for Phase II trials that were optimal in terms of minimizing the expected sample size for a given response probability, subject to certain constraints.

7.1.2.1 Phase II Cancer Trials

As explained by Chen (1997), the objective of a Phase II cancer clinical trial is to screen a treatment that can produce a similar or better response rate as can be achieved using standard methods. The screening is generally performed in two stages but Chen (1997) extended the procedure to three stages and considered sample size for each stage.

7.1.3 Phase III Trials

Gittins and Pezeshk (2002) discussed a "Behavioral Bayes" approach to sample size determination for Phase III clinical trials and for which a normal distribution is assumed. The optimal sample size is determined by minimizing the expected net cost as a function of the sample size. Chuang-Stein and Yang (2010) considered sample size decisions in the design of a Phase III superiority trial and argued that it is better to base the sample size decision for a confirmatory trial on the probability that the trial will produce a positive outcome rather than use the traditional power approach. In an earlier, related paper, Chuang-Stein (2006) discussed the distinction between statistical power and the probability of having a successful trial and proposed an "average success probability." Richardson and Leurgans (1998) advocated a very reasonable approach for Phase III/IV clinical trials that clinical personnel and other professionals would do well to adopt. Specifically, they advocated doing a power analysis using a range of reasonable values or parameters that must be specified in order to determine sample sizes. Note that this is very similar to using the endpoints of a confidence interval for such parameters, as discussed in Section 2.1. De Martini (2010) considered the estimation of sample size for a Phase III trial based on Phase II data and De Martini (2011) considered the robustness of this approach when the effect size is lower in Phase III than in Phase II. Jiang (2011) considered optimal sample sizes for Phase II and Phase III work when decisions to move forward or not are based on probability of success.

7.1.4 Longitudinal Clinical Trials

Galbraith and Marschner (2002) considered longitudinal clinical trials and how to choose the sample size and frequency of measurement, with the objective being to minimize either the total number of measurements or the cost of the study. They proposed general design guidelines when there is dropout. See also Heo, Kim, Xue, and Kim (2010), who considered sample size for a longitudinal cluster randomized clinical trial.

7.1.5 Fixed Versus Adaptive Clinical Trials

In recent years there has been a push toward increased usage of adaptive clinical trials. That is, let the sample size be determined by results of a clinical trial as it progresses. Since sample size calculations can be a problem, one possibility would be to use adaptive trials rather than fixed trials. It is claimed that this reduces both the number of patients required and the length of time required for the trial. [See, for example, http://pharmexec.findpharma.com/pharmexec/article/articleDetail.jsp?id=352793 and Jennison and Turnbull (2010).]

Adaptive designs are not without shortcomings, however. Chow and Chang (2008) provided a good review article of adaptive designs, presenting both the strengths and weaknesses and covering various types of adaptive designs. One of the weaknesses is that adaptive designs complicate matters somewhat and make the proper application of statistical methods more difficult. Another concern is that the actual patient population after the adaptations may differ from the original target population and the Type I error rate may not be controlled. Jahn-Eimermacher and Hommel (2007) indicated that an adaptive design won't always be the best approach. Nevertheless, Tracy (2009, p. 117) stated that the use of adaptive designs is a "growing trend." Orloff, Douglas, Pinheiro, Levinson, Branson, Chaturvedi, Ette, Gatto, Hirsch, Mehta, Patel, Sabir, Springs, Stanski, Evers, Fleming, Singh, Tramontin, and Golub (2009) urged a move away from the traditional clinical development approach and toward an integrated approach that uses adaptive designs.

Software appropriately designed can facilitate the use of adaptive designs and make the use of such designs less difficult, thus overcoming the weakness stated by Chow and Chang (2008). Adaptive designs are in the same general spirit as pilot studies that were discussed in Section 2.1, which should be viewed positively, not negatively. Other papers on adaptive designs include Lehmacher and Wassmer (1999), Posch and Bauer (2000), Morgan (2003), Mehta and Patel (2006), Gao, Mehta, and Ware (2008), Coffey and Kairalla (2008), Bartroff and Lai (2008), Bretz, Koenig, Brannath, Glimm, and Posch (2009), and Lu, Chow, Tse, Chi, and Tang (2009), Mehta and Pocock (2011), and Wassmer (2011).

Sample size reestimation is possible as the clinical trial progresses, as discussed by Jennison and Turnbull (2003). There is a moderate amount of information on sample size reestimation in the literature, including review articles by Gould (2001), Chuang-Stein, Anderson, Gallo, and Collins (2006), and Proschan (2009). See also Gould (1995) and Herson and Wittes (1993).

7.1.6 Noninferiority Trials

Noninferiority trials are frequently conducted to justify the development of new drugs and vaccines. Chan (2002) developed a method for sample size and power calculations based on an exact unconditional test of noninferiority for testing the difference of two proportions. Friede and Stammer (2010) considered noninferiority clinical trials and presented a case study of a completely randomized active controlled trial in dermatology. Dann and Koch (2008) discussed methods that have been popular in the literature on noninferiority and discussed sample size considerations. Schwartz and Denne (2006) described a two-stage approach for sample size recalculation in noninferiority trials.

7.1.7 Repeated Measurements

Repeated measurements are often made in clinical trials. Sample size determination when there are repeated measurements has been addressed by Bloch (1986), Ahn, Overall, and Tonidandel (2001), Zhang and Ahn (2011), and Peters, Palmer, den Ruitjer, Grobbee, Crouse, O'Leary, Evans, Raichlen, and Bots (2012). Ahn and Jung (2005) investigated the implications of dropouts for the sample size estimates when a ramdomized parallel-groups repeated measurement design is used to compare two treatments. Lu, Luo, and Chen (2008) recognized subject attrition and proposed formulas for sample size estimation that take this into consideration.

Frison and Pocock (1992) considered, in particular, how to choose the number of baseline and post-treatment measurements. [Stata users may be interested in the command `sampsi2` for repeated measurement data, which implements the formulas in Frison and Pocock (1992).] See also Jung and Ahn (2003), who considered sample size determination with repeated measurements data when a generalized estimation equation approach is to be used for analysis. Dawson and Lagakos (1993) examined extensions of the approach of using a single summary statistic for each subject when there are repeated measures. Schouten (1999) also addressed the question of what statistics should be used when clinical trials have repeated measures.

7.1.8 Multiple Tests

There is often a need to perform multiple comparison tests with clinical trials data, such as when clinical trials are designed with multiple endpoints. Bang, Jung, and George (2005) presented a simple method for calculating sample size and power for a simulation-based multiple testing procedure that could be used in such situations. Senn and Bretz (2007) also considered sample size determination when there are multiple endpoints and multiple tests.

7.1.9 Use of Internal Pilot Studies for Clinical Trials

The general use of internal pilot studies as an aid in sample size determination was discussed in some detail in Section 2.1. The use of internal pilot studies in clinical trials work has been covered by Wittes and Brittain (1990), Birkett and Day (1994), and Proschan (2005), with the latter reviewing previous work. Kraemer, Mintz, Noda, Tinjlenberg, and Yesavage (2006) did urge caution in the use of pilot studies in clinical trials for guiding power calculations. Friede and Kieser (2003) discussed sample size reassessment in noninferiority and equivalence trials when an internal pilot study is used and Friede and Kieser (2011) considered an internal pilot study when an analysis of covariance is applied.

7.1.10 Using Historical Controls

Makuch and Simon (1980) developed a sample size formula for historical clinical trials, with the true control treatment effect considered to be equal to the observed effect from the historical control group. Many researchers subsequently pointed out, however, that the Makuch–Simon approach does not preserve the nominal power and Type I error due to the uncertainty in the true historical control treatment effect. This problem was addressed by Zhang, Cao, and Ahn (2010), who developed a sample size formula that properly accounts for the randomness in the observations from the historical control group. O'Malley, Norman, and

Kuntz (2002) used a Bayesian approach to determine the optimal sample size for a trial with a historical control.

7.1.11 Trials with Combination Treatments

Wolbers, Heemskerk, Chan, Yen, Caws, Farrar, and Day (2011) considered how best to separate the effects of combination treatments, as they compared a simple randomized trial of combination versus treatment with the use of a 2^2 factorial design. They concluded that, in the absence of interaction, an adequately powered 2^2 factorial design would require eight times as many observations as the combination trial.

7.1.12 Group Sequential Trials

A group sequential trial is a trial that allows for premature stopping due to safety, futility/efficacy, or both with options of additional adaptations based on results of an interim analysis. Jiang and Snapinn (2009) investigated the impact of nonproportional hazards on the power of group sequential methods. Chi, Hung, and Wang (1999) proposed a new group sequential test procedure that they claimed preserved the Type I error probability when there is sample size reestimation. Kim and DeMets (1992) considered sample size determination for group sequential trials when there is an immediate response and He, Shun, and Feng (2010) considered sample size when predefined group sequential stopping boundaries have to be adjusted. See also Mehta and Tsiatis (2001), Lai and Shih (2004), Jennison and Turnbull (2003, 2010), and, in particular, Chapter 8 of Chow et al. (2008).

7.1.13 Vaccine Efficacy Studies

Chan and Bohidar (1998) considered sample size determination for vaccine efficacy studies and compared the results obtained using two exact methods with the results obtained using a method based on a normal approximation.

7.2 BIOEQUIVALENCE STUDIES

Bassiakos and Katerelos (2006) proposed a sample size calculation for the case of therapeutic equivalence of two pharmaceuticals and Blackwelder (1993) addressed sample size and power for an equivalence trial of vaccines when there is interest in the relative risk of disease. Chow and Wang (2001) also considered sample size calculation for bioequivalence studies. They developed formulas for use with a crossover design and a parallel-group design with either raw data or log-transformed data. Siqueira, Whitehead, Todd, and Lucini (2005) compared sample size formulas for a 2×2 crossover design applied to bioequivalence studies. See also Hauschke, Steinjans, Diletti, and Burke (1992).

7.3 ETHICAL CONSIDERATIONS

Ethical considerations were discussed generally in Section 2.3. This is especially important in clinical trials since people are involved, who should of course not be subjected to undue risks.

7.4 THE USE OF POWER IN CLINICAL STUDIES

Although Bacchetti (2010) decried the use of the word "power" in research articles describing the results of clinical trials, it is very unlikely that this practice will change anytime soon. It is often pointed out that trials involving human subjects could be considered unethical if the study is underpowered and there is some risk in participating in the clinical trial. This would especially be of concern with rapidly lethal diseases, with people participating in a trial for partly altruistic reasons. Horrobin (2003) discussed this scenario.

Bedard, Krzyzanowska, Pintillie, and Tannock (2007) surveyed all papers on two-arm Phase III randomized control trials presented at annual meetings of the American Society of Clinical Oncology during 1995–2003 and concluded that more than half of the randomized control trials with negative results did not have an adequate sample size to detect a medium-size treatment effect. [See also the discussion of this topic in Fayers and Machin (1995).]

Vickers (2003) investigated whether standard deviation values used in sample size calculations are smaller than those in the resulting study sample. The author concluded that there seems to be insufficient understanding that the standard deviation of a sample is a random variable and thus has variability and that standard deviations cannot easily be extrapolated from one population to another.

Obviously the results of Bedard et al. (2007) indicate a poor choice of sample size but Bacchetti (2010) takes issue with the position that such underpowered studies are unethical in stating: "The contention that inadequate power makes a study unethical . . . relies entirely on the threshold myth, a false belief that studies with less than 80% power cannot be expected to produce enough scientific or practical value to justify the burden imposed on participants. Because larger studies burden more participants, the fact of diminishing marginal returns implies that the ratio of projected value to total participant burden can only get worse with larger sample sizes. The risk of inadequate projected value relative to participant burden therefore applies to studies that are too large, not too small." [See Bacchetti, Wolf, Segal, and McCulloch (2005) for elaboration on this viewpoint.]

Bacchetti's position on power stands in stark contrast to the tenor of other articles, such as Whitley and Bell (2002), who were specifically concerned with the "hazard of under-powered studies," lamenting the fact that a study by Moher, Dulberg, and Wells (1994) revealed that for the results of 383 randomized controlled trials published in the *Journal of the American Medical Association, New England Journal of Medicine*, and *Lancet*, of the 102 null trials, only 16% had 80% power to detect a 25% relative difference between groups. Similarly, Freedman, Back, and Bernstein (2001) reviewed 717 manuscripts published in certain British and American orthopedic journals in 1997, from which 33 randomized, controlled trials were identified. Of the 25 studies which did not have an adequate sample size to detect a small effect (defined as 0.2 times the standard deviation), the average sample size used was only 10% of the required number. Thus, they concluded that inadequate sample sizes were being used in clinical orthopedic research.

Both positions have some merit. Clearly, power will always be unknown, both before and after a study has been conducted, and certainly some important information can still be gleaned from null studies. Not paying attention to power would certainly be unwise, however, as sample sizes should be large enough that there is a high probability of detecting an effect of such a magnitude that a scientist would want to detect.

7.5   PRECLINICAL EXPERIMENTATION

Tan, Fang, and Tian (2009) presented an experimental design for detecting departures from additivity of multiple drugs in preclinical studies and discussed sample size determination for their design.

7.6   PHARMACODYNAMIC, PHARMACOKINETIC, AND PHARMACOGENETIC EXPERIMENTS

Pharmacodynamic experiments are experiments involving test drugs that produce count measurements. Sample size determination for these and pharmacokinetic experiments have been addressed by Ogungbenro and Aarons (2010a,b) and Ogungbenro, Aarons, and Graham (2006). Pharmacogenetic experiments seek to identify the genetic factors that influence the intersubject variation in drug response. Tseng and Shao (2010) considered sample size determination for such studies. Sethuraman, Leonov, Squassante, Mitchell, and Hale (2007) gave sample size derivations for various designs that might be used in assessing or demonstrating pharmacokinetic dose proportionality.

7.7   METHOD OF COMPETING PROBABILITY

The method of competing probability, as introduced by Rahardja and Zhao (2009), was mentioned somewhat briefly in Section 2.2.4. The general idea is to determine sample size using this approach. For random variables X and Y chosen from the control and experimental treatments, respectively, the competing probability (CP) was defined by the authors as

$$\pi = \Pr(X < Y) + 0.5\Pr(X = Y)$$

Rahardja and Zhao (2009) stated that Bamber (1975) showed that the CP is equal to the area under the curve of the Receiver Operating Characteristics (ROC) curve, which is used in medical diagnostic testing.

Recall Eq. (3.6), which for a two-sided test would be

$$
\begin{aligned}
n &= \frac{(\sigma_1^2 + \sigma_2^2)(Z_{\alpha/2} + Z_\beta)^2}{(\Delta - \Delta_0)^2} \\
&= \frac{(2\sigma^2)(Z_{\alpha/2} + Z_\beta)^2}{(\Delta - \Delta_0)^2}
\end{aligned}
\tag{7.1}
$$

under the assumption that $\sigma_1^2 = \sigma_2^2 = \sigma^2$ and assuming that $n_1 = n_2 = n$, with Δ denoting $\mu_2 - \mu_1$ and Δ_0 denoting the value of $\mu_2 - \mu_1$ under the null hypothesis, which is typically zero.

Following Rahardja and Zhao (2009), the sample size can be written in terms of CP by first writing

$$
\begin{aligned}
\pi &= P(X < Y) + 0.5\,\Pr(X = Y) = \Pr(X - Y < 0) \\
&= P\left(\frac{X - Y - (-\Delta)}{\sigma\sqrt{2}} < \frac{\Delta}{\sigma\sqrt{2}}\right)
\end{aligned}
$$

with $\Delta/\sigma\sqrt{2}$ playing the role of $Z_{1-\pi}$ in terms of the general form of such probability statements Since the (standardized) effect size can be viewed as Δ/σ, it follows that $\Delta/\sigma = Z_{1-\pi}\sqrt{2}$. Letting Δ_0 in Eq. (7.1) $= 0$, the sample size formula in Eq. (7.1) can then be written as a function of $Z_{1-\pi}$:

$$n = \frac{(Z_{\alpha/2} + Z_\beta)^2}{Z_{1-\pi}^2} \tag{7.2}$$

Rahardja and Zhao (2009) stated that this formula would be used in conjunction with the question: "What is a clinically meaningful probability that the experimental treatment is better than the control?" The answer to that question would determine $Z_{1-\pi}$ and thus determine n.

To illustrate their proposed approach, the authors gave an example in which a clinical trial was to be used to compare the drug duloxetine with a placebo for the treatment of patients with diabetic peripheral neuropathic pain, with the measurement variable being the average weekly score of 24-hour average pain severity on an 11-point Likert scale. They referred to this study as described in Wernicke, Pritchett, D'Souza, Waninger, Tran, Iyengar, and Raskin (2006). Rahardja and Zhao (2009) stated that "it may be difficult to understand how an effect size of 0.545, as used by Wernicke et al. (2009), can be translated into the benefit that a patient may receive from duloxetine." With $\Delta/\sigma = Z_{1-\pi}\sqrt{2} = 0.545$, it follows that $Z_{1-\pi} = 0.385373$. Thus, $\Phi(0.385373) = \pi = .65$. With $\alpha = .05$ and a desired power of .90, the use of Eq. (7.2) produces

$$n = \frac{(1.95996 + 1.28155)^2}{(0.385375)^2}$$

$$= 70.75$$

so $n = 71$ would be used for each of the two groups.

7.8 BAYESIAN METHODS

As in other applications of sample size determination methods, there are Bayesian approaches that have been proposed for use in clinical trials, such as the methods proposed by Sahu and Smith (2006), Gajewski and Mayo (2006), Grouin, Coste, Bunouf, and Lecoutre (2007), Wang (2007), Patel and Ankolekar (2007), Brutti and De Santis (2008), Brutti, De Santis, and Gibbiotti (2008), Kikuchi, Pezeshk, and Gittins (2008), Whitehead, Valdés-Márquez, Johnson, and Graham (2008), Kikuchi and Gittins (2009), Cheng, Branscum, and Stamey (2010), and Zaslavsky (2009, 2012). Willan (2008) proposed a Bayesian approach that was designed to maximize expected profit, contingent upon the validity of the assumed model for expected total profit, and the method depending on the Central Limit Theorem. Two examples were given that illustrated the approach. Pezeshk (2003) gave a short review paper on Bayesian sample size determination techniques in clinical trials. See also Lan and Wittes (2012). Yin (2002) used a Bayesian approach for determining sample size for a proof of concept study, this being a study conducted by a pharmaceutical company for internal decision making.

Wang, Chow, and Chen (2005) proposed a Bayesian approach using a non-informative prior. It is obviously desirable to incorporate uncertainty into the parameter estimates that must be specified in sample size determination and from a practical standpoint an important question is how much difference this will make in the sample size. Wang et al. (2005) gave an example in which they compared the sample sizes obtained using their approach with the sample sizes obtained using the standard frequentist formulas for testing equality, superiority, and equivalence. The standard formulas gave sample sizes of 273, 628, and 181, respectively, whereas their Bayesian approach produced corresponding sample sizes of 285, 654, and 188, respectively. Of course, the sample sizes using a Bayesian approach should be larger and here the percentage increases are 4.40, 4.14, and 3.87, respectively, so the percentage increases differ only slightly. Clearly, parameter estimate uncertainty should be incorporated in some manner and a Bayesian approach is one way to accomplish that.

7.9 COST AND OTHER SAMPLE SIZE DETERMINATION METHODS FOR CLINICAL TRIALS

Other nontraditional methods of sample size determination have been proposed for clinical trials. For example, Bacchetti, McCulloch, and Segal (2008) considered sample sizes based on cost efficiency. Bloch (1986) also considered cost, as did Briggs and Gray (1998), Kikuchi, Pezeshk, and Gittins (2008), Boyd, Briggs, Fenwick, Norrie, and Stock (2011), and Zhang and Ahn (2011). Cheng, Su, and Berry (2003) used decision analysis methods to arrive at sample sizes in each stage when a clinical trial is to be performed in two stages.

Another approach is the expected value of the information produced minus the total cost of the study. These are referred to as value of information (VOI) methods designed to determine the sample size so as to maximize the expected net gain. Such methods are described by Willan and Eckermann (2010). See also Willan and Pinto (2005) and Willan and Kowgier (2008).

7.10 META-ANALYSES OF CLINICAL TRIALS

Within the past 25 years, there has been much interest in meta-analysis, by which is meant combining data from individual studies and analyzing the data as if they had come from one huge study. This has been especially popular in clinical trials work, but the approach does have some limitations. DerSimonian and Laird (1986) examined eight published review articles, each of which reported results from several related trials. Clinical trials performed at different locations, under different conditions, and with differing numbers of subjects can't simply be merged in an unthinking manner. DerSimonian and Laird (1986) reported that Halvorsen (1986) found that only one article out of 589 examined considered combining results using formal statistical methods. DerSimonian and Laird (1986) proposed a random effects model for combining results from a series of experiments comparing two treatments. Jackson, Bowden, and Baker (2010) found, however, that it is inefficient for estimating the between-study variance unless all of the studies that are combined are of similar size, but they did find that it is quite efficient for estimating the treatment effect. The DerSimonian and Laird model was extended by Jackson, White, and Thompson (2010). See also Shuster (2010) and the discussion of that paper.

7.11   MISCELLANEOUS

Internal pilot studies can certainly be useful but using results from other populations may not be helpful at all. Nevertheless, Yan and Su (2006) gave sample size formulas for a long-term trial involving patients with chronic disease by using results from existing short-term studies, as these may predict long-term disease progression patterns. Chen, DeMets, and Lan (2004) discussed the effect on the Type I error rate when the sample size is increased based on interim results and the study is unblinded. In contrast, Gould and Shih (1992) considered sample size reestimation *without* unblinding, but Waksman (2007) pointed out that some have claimed that the method can result in a severe underestimation of the within-group standard deviation.

Li, Shih, Xie, and Lu (2002) considered sample size adjustment in clinical trials based on conditional power and modified the procedure of Proschan and Hunsbarger (1995). Lachin (2005) reviewed methods for futility stopping based on conditional power. Lan, Hu, and Proschan (2009) discussed the use of conditional power and predictive power for early termination of a clinical trial. Spiegelhalter, Freedman, and Blackburn (1986) considered using interim results to obtain the predictive power of a trial, which would be obtained by averaging the conditional power (conditioned on the interim results) with the current belief about the unknown parameters. Dallow and Fina (2011), however, were critical of the use of predictive power and pointed out that the use of predictive power can lead to much larger sample sizes than either conditional power or standard sample size calculations. Wüst and Keiser (2003) considered possible adjustment of the sample size based on the value of the sample variance computed at an interim step. Xiong, Yu, Yan, and Zhang (2005) considered sample size for a trial for which the efficacy of a treatment is required for multiple primary endpoints. Liu and Dahlberg (1995) considered sample size requirements for K-sample trials with survival endpoints and $K = 3$ or 4. Wang, Chow, and Li (2002) derived sample size formulas for testing equality, noninferiority, superiority, and equivalence based on odds ratio for both parallel and crossover designs. Tango (2009) proposed a simple sample size formula for use with randomized controlled trials in which the endpoint is the count of recurrent events.

As a response to the question of whether a one-sided or two-sided test should be used, Dunnett and Gent (1996) proposed an alternative approach that tests simultaneously for a positive difference and for equivalence. Shen and Cai (2003) considered sample size reestimation for clinical trials that involve censored survival data. Lin, Parks, Greshock, Wooster, and Lee (2011) focused on sample size calculations for clinical trial studies with a time-to-event endpoint in the presence of predictive biomarkers. Maki (2006) considered sample size determination when subjects are at risk for events other than the one of interest. Su (2005) determined sample size for endometrial safety studies that satisfies an FDA requirement and a requirement of the Committee on Proprietary Medicinal Products. Stalbovskaya, Hamadicharef, and Ifeachor (2007) presented an approach to sample size determination that involved estimation of probability density functions and confidence interval of parameters of a ROC (receiver operating characteristics) curve. Sozu, Sugimoto, and Hamasaki (2010, 2011, 2012) considered sample size determination when a trial has multiple co-primary endpoints. Fang, Tian, Li, and Tang (2009) considered sample size determination for trials with combinations of drugs. Sample size determination can be complicated by drug doses having different effects over populations in different regions. Zhang and Sethuraman (2010) considered this issue. Friede and Schmidli (2010a) developed a sample size reestimation strategy for count data in superiority and noninferiority trials that maintains the blinding of the trial. Friede and Schmidli (2010b) also considered sample size reestimation with count data with application to multiple sclerosis studies. Shun, He, Feng, and Roessner (2009) focused attention on sample size adjustment so as to maintain the Type I error rate. Shih (1993) and Shih and Zhao (1997) considered sample size reestimation for double-blinded trials with binary data. Shih (2009) devised a "perturbed unblinding" approach to sample size reestimation that keeps the treatment effect masked but allows an estimate of the variance using data from an interim stage. Hosmane, Locke, and Chiu (2010) considered power and sample size determination in QT/QTc studies.

McMahon, Proschan, Geller, Stone, and Sopko (1994) considered sample size determination relative to entry criteria for clinical trials that involve chronic diseases. Huang, Woolson, and O'Brien (2008) presented a sample size computation method for clinical trials with multiple outcomes and either O'Brien's (1984) test or its modification (Huang, Tilley, Woolson, and Lipsitz, 2005) is used for the primary analysis. Ivanova, Qaqish, and Schoenfeld (2011) gave a sample size formula for a sequential parallel comparison design. Kwong, Cheung, and Wen (2010) considered sample size determination when multiple comparisons of treatments are to be made with a control. Lakatos (1986) considered sample size determination when there are time-dependent rates of losses and noncompliance. Wu, Fisher, and DeMets (1980) considered sample size determination for long-term medical trials when there is time-dependent dropout.

Nomograms do not, in general, have the utility for sample size determination that they had 20 years ago because of current software capability. Software doesn't cover everything, however, so some researchers may find the nomogram of Malhotra and Indrayan (2010) useful, as it is for determining sample size for estimating sensitivity and specificity of medical tests.

7.12 SURVEY RESULTS OF PUBLISHED ARTICLES

The difficulties faced in trying to determine sample size have been discussed in previous chapters. This raises the question of how researchers actually arrive at sample size determinations, in clinical trials and in other types of studies.

Unfortunately, a recent study shows some serious problems and shortcomings. Specifically, Charles, Giraudeau, Dechartes, Bacon, and Ravaud (2009) "searched MEDLINE for all primary reports of two arm parallel group randomised controlled trials of superiority with a single primary outcome published in six high impact factor general medical journals between 1 January 2005 and 31 December 2006." The authors studied 215 articles, of which 5% did not report any sample size computation and 43% did not report all the parameters necessary for performing the computation.

Certain results from the study are somewhat distressing. For example, for the 157 reports that provided enough information for the sample size to be computed, the researchers found that their computed sample size and the reported sample size differed by more than 10% in 47 (30%) of the reports. Also disturbing was the fact that the difference between the assumptions for the control group and the observed data differed by more than 30% in 31% of the articles, and was greater than 50% in 17% of the articles. Only 34% of the articles reported all data that were necessary to compute the sample size, had an accurate sample size calculation, and used assumptions that were not refuted by the data. There was some guesswork done by the authors, however, as they assumed $\alpha = .05$ and a two-tailed test if the only missing information was the α-value and whether the test was one-sided or two-sided.

Of course, what would be most interesting would be an assessment of the proportion of studies with significant results that had these types of problems, and similarly for the proportion of studies that had nonsignificant results. For example, were nonsignificant results reported because errors resulted in a sample size being used that was too small (i.e., the study was underpowered)? This was not covered in the paper but it was covered in an online response by the first author. That author indicated that the results were similar for significant and nonsignificant results, with 55% of the studies with nonsignificant results reporting all the parameter values necessary for computing the sample size and this being done in 50% of the studies with significant results. The percentages with sample size computations that could be replicated were 80% and 73%, respectively. There is no indication of whether the authors were able to replicate the same numbers, however.

These results, although disturbing, should not be surprising in view of the difficulties noted in previous chapters. The numbers might actually be worse, however, as Charles et al. (2009) stated: "An important limitation of this study is that we could not directly assess whether assumptions had been manipulated to obtain feasible sample sizes because we used only published data." Such (possible) manipulation was called "sample size samba" by Schulz and Grimes (2005). The need to report sample size calculations seems clear and has been urged by Sjögren and Hedström (2010).

7.13 SOFTWARE

The N Solution 2008 software (http://www.pharmasoftware.net/pro ducts/n-solution) is based on Chow, Shao, and Wang (2008). Java applets for Phase I and Phase II clinical trials are available at http://biostats. upci.pitt.edu/biostats/ClinicalStudyDesign. The latter is intended for use by the University of Pittsburgh Cancer Institute Biostatistics Facility only, but is also available for external users. See also the free software for clinical trials available at http://www.cancerbiostats.onc.jhmi. edu/software.cfm and the applet for a two-treatment crossover design or parallel design clinical trial at http://hedwig.mgh.harvard.edu/sample _size/size.html. (That applet can also be used to detect a relationship between a dependent variable and an independent variable, although the type of relationship to be detected is not clear.)

In addition to the software mentioned in this chapter, another prominent software package specifically for clinical trials is East by Cytel Software Corporation, which is apparently the most widely used clinical trial software system and has greater capabilities than other general-purpose commercial sample size determination software that is not just for clinical trials. The East-Adapt option permits midcourse sample size corrections, in the spirit of adaptive clinical trial designs. East 5 has considerable capabilities, as should be apparent from www.cytel.com/pdfs/East_5_brochure_webFINAL.pdf.

ExpDesign Studio is used for classical and adaptive clinical trial designs; its use is explained by Chang (2008).

Some of the popular sample size determination software mentioned repeatedly in previous chapters can also be used for clinical trials work. For example, PASS 11 has the capability for sample size determination for Phase II clinical trials: single-stage, two-stage, or three-stage.

For a single-stage Phase II clinical trial, PASS 11 determines sample size based on the work of A'Hern (2001), who provided tables for single-stage Phase II designs based on an exact test of proportions using the binomial distribution. To illustrate, the user would enter α and the desired power and enter the "maximum response rate of a poor treatment" (p_0, the null hypothesis) and the "minimum response rate of a good treatment" (p_1, the alternative hypothesis). For example, with $\alpha = .05$ and power $= .90$ for the one-sided test and $p_0 = .10$ and $p_1 = .20$, the software gives $n = 109$.

The algorithm that PASS 11 uses for two-stage Phase II clinical trials is based on and extends the work of Simon (1989). The algorithm will generally take quite a while to run since it is a brute force search procedure. The output is far more extensive than the output for the single-stage case, as would be expected. To illustrate, again assume $p_0 = .10$, $p_1 = .20$, $\alpha = .05$, and power $= .90$. The detailed output is given below.

```
Two-Stage Clinical Trials Sample Size
Possible Designs For P0 = 0.100, P1 = 0.200, Alpha =
0.050, Beta = 0.100
```

								Constraints
N1	R1	PET	N	R	Ave N	Alpha	Beta	Satisfied
109	16	0.000	109	16	109.00	0.043	0.099	Single Stage
70	6	0.442	109	16	91.77	0.043	0.100	Minimax
42	4	0.588	121	17	74.56	0.049	0.099	Optimum

References

```
Simon, Richard. 'Optimal Two-Stage Designs for Phase II
Clinical Trials',Controlled Clinical Trials, 1989,
Volume 10, pages 1-10.
```

Report Definitions
N1 is the sample size in the first stage.
R1 is the drug rejection number in the first stage.
PET is the probability of early termination of the study.
N is the combined sample size of both stages.
R is the combined drug rejection number after both stages.
Ave N is the average sample size if this design is repeated
many times.
Alpha is the probability of rejecting that P<=P0 when this
is true.
Beta is the probability of rejecting that P>=P1 when this
is true.
P0 is the response proportion of a poor drug.
P1 is the response proportion of a good drug.

Summary Statements
The optimal two-stage design to test the null hypothesis
that P<=0.100 versus the alternative that P>=0.200 has an
expected sample size of 74.56 and a probability of early
termination of 0.588. If the drug is actually not
effective, there is a 0.049 probability of concluding that
it is (the target for this value was 0.050). If the drug is

```
actually effective, there is a 0.099 probability of
concluding that it is not (the target for this value was
0.100). After testing the drug on 42 patients in the first
stage, the trial will be terminated if 4 or fewer respond.
If the trial goes on to the second stage, a total of 121
patients will be studied. If the total number responding
is less than or equal to 17, the drug is rejected.
```

The symbols are defined in the section "Report Definitions." The program inputs should be made judiciously so that the output is not voluminous and the algorithm does not run for a long time—like for hours. (The latter can easily happen, as explained in the program's help file.)

For example, it will usually be desirable to use the "optimum designs" selection so that a large number of other designs that satisfy the constraints are not additionally printed out. When that selection is made, the output includes the single-stage design and the minimax design, in addition to the optimum design. The latter is the design that minimizes the expected sample size, $E(N)$, which is denoted in the output as "Ave N." This design is found through an exhaustive search of all possible designs. The minimax design is the design with the smallest total sample size. The reason there is an expected sample size rather than a known total sample size is the trial could terminate early after the first stage, and in this example that would happen if fewer than five patients responded to the drug. The expected sample size is computed, as would be expected, as $E(N) = N1 + (1 - PET)(N - N1)$. That is, it is the sample size in the first stage plus the second-stage sample size times the probability that the second stage is reached.

PASS 11 also has the capability for three-stage Phase II sample size determination, which is listed under "Proportions" in their menu. This is just an extension of a two-stage Phase II clinical trial, with a decision made at the end of the second stage as to whether or not to proceed to the third stage. Judicious choice of input selections is, of course, even more important for three stages than it is for two stages, so that the program doesn't run for hours and produce output that might be deemed unnecessary.

Stata 12 has the capability for sample size determination for clinical trials through various programs, including the menu-driven program of Royston and Babiker (2002), with this updated by Barthel, Royston, and Babiker (2005). See also Barthel, Royston, and Parmar (2009), who gave both menu and command-driven Stata programs for a time-to-event outcome with two or more experimental arms. A user-written command, `sampsi_fleming`, will determine sample size for a Fleming design (Fleming, 1982), which is a design for a Phase II clinical trial. For example, if the null hypothesis of $p_0 = 0.2$ is tested against an alternative of $p_1 = 0.4$ with $\alpha = .01$ and a target power of .90, the following output results when the command `sampsi_fleming, a(.01) p(.90)` is used.

```
Sample size calculation for the Fleming design
-----------------------------------------------------
H0: p <= p0
H1: p > p0

p0 = .2 p1 = .4
With a sample size of 67
the null hypothesis is rejected if there are >= 22 respon-
ders
Type I error = 0.0093
Power        = 0.9082
```

Users of SAS Software may be interested in O'Brien and Castelloe (2007), which gives some illustrations of sample size analysis and power determination.

Although now outdated, Shih (1995) described the use of the software SIZE for determining sample size for clinical trials.

Software for sample size determination for clinical trials using Bayesian methods has not existed in the recent past and that is apparently still true.

7.14   SUMMARY

Although simple sample size formulas are desirable if hand calculations are necessary, "one size fits all" approaches should be avoided. Flaherty (2004) stated that 400 subjects is a reliable sample size for a study to have adequate statistical power. Fogel (2004) disputed this broad generalization, pointing out that of the first 40 abstracts of papers in the *Journal of the American Medical Association* that he looked at, 52% did not meet this requirement.

There is much to consider regarding sample size and power in clinical trials. Readers may be interested in the discussions in Proschan, Lan, and Wittes (2006), especially Chapter 3, which is entitled "Power: Conditional, Unconditional and Predictive," and Bacchetti (2010) is also recommended, as stated previously.

REFERENCES

A'Hern, R. P. (2001). Sample size tables for exact single-stage Phase II designs. *Statistics in Medicine*, **20**, 859–866.

Ahn, C. and S.-H. Jung (2005). Effect of dropouts on sample size estimates for test on trends across repeated measurements. *Journal of Biopharmaceutical Statistics*, **15**, 33–41.

Ahn, C., J. E. Overall, and S. Tonidandel (2001). Sample size and power calculations in repeated measurement analysis. *Computer Methods andPrograms in Biomedicine*, **64**(2), 121–124.

Allen, I. E. and C. A. Seaman (2009). Predicting success: Simulation can forecast probable success in clinical trials. *Quality Progress*, February, 60–63.

Bacchetti, P. (2002). Peer review of statistics in medical research: The other problem. *British Medical Journal*, **324**, 1271–1273.

Bacchetti, P. (2010). Current sample size conventions: Flaws, harms, and alternatives. *BMC Medicine*, **17** (electronic journal).

Bacchetti, P., C. E. McCulloch, and M. R. Segal (2008). Simple, defensible sample sizes based on cost efficiency. *Biometrics*, **64**, 577–585. Discussion: **64**, 586–594.

Bacchetti, P., L. E. Wolf, M. R. Segal, and C. E. McCulloch (2005). Ethics and sample size. *American Journal of Epidemiology*, **161**, 105–110.

Bamber, D. C. (1975). The area above the ordinal dominance graph and the area below the receiver operating characteristic curve graph. *Journal of Mathematical Psychology*, **12**, 387–415.

Bang, H., S.-H. Jung, and S. George (2005). Sample size calculation for simulation-based multiple-testing procedures. *Journal of Biopharmaceutical Statistics*, **15**, 957–967.

Barthel, F.M.-S., P. Royston, and A. Babiker (2005). A menu-driven facility for complex sample-size calculation in randomized control trials with a survival or a binary outcome: Update. *The Stata Journal*, **5**(1), 123–129.

Barthel, F.M.-S., P. Royston, and M. K. B. Parmar (2009). A menu-driven facility for sample-size calculation in novel multiarm, multistage, randomized controlled trials with a time-to-event outcome. *The Stata Journal*, **9**(4), 505–523.

Bartroff, J. and T. L. Lai (2008). Efficient adaptive designs with mid-course sample size adjustment in clinical trials. *Statistics in Medicine*, **27**, 1593–1611.

Baskerville, N. B., W. Hogg, and J. Lemelin (2001). The effect of cluster randomization on sample size in prevention research. *Journal of Family Practice*, **50**, 241–246.

Bassiakos, Y. and P. Katerelos (2006). Sample size calculation for the therapeutic equivalence problem. *Communications in Statistics: Simulation and Computation*, **35**, 1019–1026.

Bedard, P. L., M. K. Krzyzanowska, M. Pintillie, and I. F. Tannock (2007). Statistical power of negative randomized controlled trials presented at American Society for Clinical Oncology Annual Meetings. *Journal of Clinical Oncology*, **25**(23), 3482–3487.

Birkett, M. A. and S. J. Day (1994). Internal pilot studies for estimating sample size. *Statistics in Medicine*, **13**, 2455–2463.

Blackwelder, W. C. (1993). Sample size and power in prospective analysis of relative risk. *Statistics in Medicine*, **12**, 691–698.

Bloch, D. A. (1986). Sample size requirements and the cost of a randomized clinical trial with repeated measurements. *Statistics in Medicine*, **5**(6), 663–667.

Boyd, K. A., A. H. Briggs, E. Fenwick, J. Norrie, and S. Stock (2011). Power and sample size for cost-effectiveness analysis: fFN neonatal screening. *Contemporary Clinical Trials*, **32**(6), 893–901.

Bretz, F., F. Koenig, W. Brannath, E. Glimm, and M. Posch (2009). Adaptive designs for confirmatory clinical trials. *Statistics in Medicine*, **28**(8), 1181–1217.

Briggs, A. and A. Gray (1998). Power and sample size calculations for stochastic cost-effectiveness analysis. *Medical Decision Making*, **18**, Supplement, S81–S92.

Brutti, P. and F. De Santis (2008). Robust Bayesian sample size determination for avoiding the range of equivalence in clinical trials. *Journal of Statistical Planning and Inference*, **138**, 1577–1591.

Brutti, P., F. De Santis, and S. Gibbiotti (2008). Robust Bayesian sample size determination in clinical trials. *Statistics in Medicine*, **27**, 2290–2306.

Campbell, M., J. Grimshaw, and N. Steen (2000). Sample size calculations for cluster randomised trials. *Journal of Health Services Research Policy*, **15**, 12–16.

Chan, I. S. F. and N. Bohidar (1998). Exact power and sample size for vaccine efficacy studies. *Communications in Statistics—Theory and Methods*, **27**(6), 1305–1322.

Chan, I.-S. (2002). Power and sample size determination for noninferiority trials using an exact method. *Journal of Biopharmaceutical Statistics*, **12**(4), 457–469.

Chang, M. (2007). *Adaptive Design Theory and Implementation using SAS and R*. Boca Raton, FL. Chapman & Hall, CRC.

Chang, M. (2008). *Classical and Adaptive Clinical Trial Designs Using ExpDesign Studio*. Hoboken, NJ: Wiley.

Chang, M. N., J. J. Shuster, and J. L. Kepner (2004). Sample sizes based on exact unconditional tests for Phase II clinical trials with historical controls. *Journal of Biopharmaceutical Statistics*, **14**, 189–200.

Charles, P., B. Giraudeau, A. Dechartes, G. Bacon, and P. Ravaud (2009). Reporting of sample size calculations in randomised clinical trials: Review. *British Medical Journal*, **338**, 1732.

Chen, T. T. (1997). Optimal three-stage designs for Phase II cancer clinical trials. *Statistics in Medicine*, **16**, 2701–2711.

Chen, Y. H. J., D. L. DeMets, and K. K. G. Lan (2004). Increasing the sample size when the unblinded interim result is promising. *Statistics in Medicine*, **23**, 1023–1038.

Cheng, D., A. J. Branscum, and J. D. Stamey (2010). A Bayesian approach to sample size estimation for studies designed to evaluate continuous medical tests. *Computational Statistics and Data Analysis*, **54**(2), 298–307.

Cheng, Y., F. Su, and D. A. Berry (2003). Choosing sample size for a clinical trial using decision analysis. *Biometrika*, **90**, 923–926.

Chi, L., H. M. J. Hung, and S.-J. Wang (1999). Modification of sample size in group sequential trials. *Biometrics*, **55**, 853–857.

Chow, S. C. and M. Chang (2006). *Adaptive Design Methods in Clinical Trials*. New York: Chapman and Hall.

Chow, S.-C. and M. Chang (2008). Adaptive design methods in clinical trials—A review. *Orphanet Journal of Rare Diseases*, **3**(11), (electronic journal).

Chow, S.-C. and H. Wang (2001). On sample size calculation in bioequivalence trials. *Journal of Pharmacokinetics and Pharmacodynamics*, **28**, 155–169.

Chow, S.-C., J. Shao, and H. Wang (2008). *Sample Size Calculations in Clinical Research*, 2nd edition. Boca Raton, FL: Chapman & Hall/CRC.

Chuang-Stein, C. (2006). Sample size and the probability of a successful trial. *Pharmaceutical Statistics*, **5**(4), 305–309.

Chuang-Stein, C. and R. Yang (2010). A revisit of sample size decisions in confirmatory trials. *Statistics in Biopharmaceutical Research*, **2**(2), 239–248.

Chuang-Stein, C., K. Anderson, P. Gallo, and S. Collins (2006). Sample size reestimation: A review and recommendations. *Drug Information Journal*, **40**, 475–484.

Coffey, C. S. and J. A. Kairalla (2008). Adaptive clinical trials: Progress and challenges. *Drugs in R & D*, **9**(4), 229–242.

Dallow, N. and P. Fina (2011). The perils with the use of predictive power. *Pharmaceutical Statistics*, **10**(4), 311–317.

Dann, R. S. and G. G. Koch (2008). Methods for one-sided testing of the difference between two proportions and sample size considerations related to non-inferiority clinical trials. *Pharmaceutical Statistics*, **7**, 130–141.

Darken, P. F. and S.-Y. Ho (2004). A note in sample size savings with the use of a single well-controlled clinical trial to support the efficacy of a new drug. *Pharmaceutical Statistics*, **3**, 61–63.

Dawson, J. D. and S. W. Lagakos (1993). Size and power of two-sample tests of repeated measures data. *Biometrics*, **49**(4), 1022–1032.

De Martini, D. (2010). Adapting by calibration the sample size of a Phase III trial on the basis of Phase II data. *Pharmaceutical Statistics*, **10**(2), 89–95.

De Martini, D. (2011). Robustness and corrections for sample size adaptation strategies based on effect size estimation. *Communications in Statistics—Simulation and Computation*, **40**(9), 1263–1277.

DerSimonian, R. and N. Laird (1986). Meta-analysis in clinical trials. *Controlled Clinical Trials*, **7**, 177–188.

Dunnett, C. W. and M. Gent (1996). An alternative to the use of two-sided tests in clinical trials. *Statistics in Medicine*, **15**, 1729–1738.

Eng, J. (2003). Sample size estimation: How many individuals should be studied? *Radiology*, **227**, 309–313.

Eng, J. (2004). Sample size estimation: A glimpse beyond simple formulas. *Radiology*, **230**(3), 606–612.

Fang, H.-B., G.-L.Tian, W. Li, and M. Tang (2009). Design and sample size for evaluating combinations of drugs of linear and loglinear dose–response curves. *Journal of Biopharmaceutical Statistics*, **19**(4), 625–640.

Fayers, P. M. and D. Machin (1995). Sample size: How many patients are necessary? *British Journal of Cancer*, **72**, 1–9.

Fayers, K. W., A. Cushieri, J. Fielding, B. Uscinska, and L. S. Freedman (2000). Sample size calculation for clinical trials: The impact of clinician beliefs. *British Journal of Cancer*, **82**, 213–219.

Flaherty, R. (2004). A simple method for evaluating the clinical literature. *Family Practice Management*, **11**(5), 47–52 (May).

Fleming, T. R. (1982). One-sample multiple testing procedure for Phase II clinical trials. *Biometrics*, **38**, 143–151.

Fogel, J. (2004). Letter to the Editor. *Family Practice Management*, **11**(9), 14 (October).

Freedman, K. B., S. Back, and J. Bernstein (2001). Sample size and statistical power of randomised, controlled trials in orthopaedics. *The Journal of Bone and Joint Surgery*, **83-B**(3), 397–402.

Friede, T. and M. Kieser (2003). Blinded sample size reassessment with non-inferiority in non-inferiority and equivalence trials. *Statistics in Medicine*, **22**(6), 995–1007.

Friede, T. and M. Kieser (2011). Blinded sample size recalculation for clinical trials with normal data and baseline adjusted analysis. *Pharmaceutical Statistics*, **10**(1), 8–13.

Friede, T. and H. Schmidli (2010a). Blinded sample size reestimation with negative binomial counts in superiority and non-inferiority trials. *Methods of Information in Medicine*, **49**(6), 618–624.

Friede, T. and H. Schmidli (2010b). Blinded sample size reestimation with count data: Methods and applications in multiple sclerosis. *Statistics in Medicine*, **29**(10), 1145–1156.

Friede, T. and H. Stammer (2010). Blinded sample size recalculation in noninferiority trials: A case study in dermatology. *Drug Information Journal*, **44**(5), 599–607.

Frison, L. and S. J. Pocock (1992). Repeated measures in clinical trials: Analysis using mean summary statistics and its implications for design. *Statistics in Medicine*, **11**(13), 1685–1704.

Gajewski, B. J. and M. S. Mayo (2006). Bayesian sample size calculations in Phase II clinical trials using a mixture of informative priors. *Statistics in Medicine*, **25**, 2554–2566.

Galbraith, S. and I. C. Marschner (2002). Guidelines for the design of clinical trials with longitudinal outcomes. *Controlled Clinical Trials*, **23**(3), 257–273.

Gao, P., C. R. Mehta, and J. H. Ware (2008). Sample size re-estimation for adaptive sequential design in clinical trials. *Journal of Biopharmaceutical Statistics*, **18**, 1184–1196.

George, S. L. and M. M. Desu (1974). Planning the size and duration of a clinical trial studying the time to some critical event. *Journal of Chronic Diseases*, **27**(1/2), 15–24.

Gittins, J. C. and H. Pezeshk (2002). A decision theoretic approach to sample size determination in clinical trials. *Journal of Biopharmaceutical Statistics*, **12**, 535–551.

Gould, A. L. (1995). Planning and revising the sample size for a trial. *Statistics in Medicine*, **14**, 1039–1051.

Gould, A. L. (2001). Sample size re-estimation: Recent developments and practical considerations. *Statistics in Medicine*, **20**, 2625–2643.

Gould, A. L. and W. Shih (1992). Sample size re-estimation without unblinding for normally distributed outcomes with unknown variance. *Communications in Statistics—Theory and Methods*, **21**, 2833–2853.

Grouin, J.-M., M. Coste, P. Bunouf, and B. Lecoutre (2007). Bayesian sample size determination in non-sequential clinical trials: Statistical aspects and some regulatory considerations. *Statistics in Medicine*, **26**, 4914–4924.

Halvorsen, K.T. (1986). Combining results from independent investigations: Meta analysis in medical research. In *Medical Uses of Statistics* (J. C. Bailar III and F. Mosteller, eds.), pp. 392–418. Waltham, MA: NEJM Books.

Hauschke, D., V. W. Steinjans, E. Diletti, and M. Burke (1992). Sample size determination for bioequivalence assessment using a multiplicative model. *Journal of Pharmacokinetics and Biopharmaceutics*, **20**, 557–561.

He, Y., Z. Shun, and Y. Feng. (2010). Stopping boundaries of flexible sample size design with flexible trial monitoring. *Statistics in Biopharmaceutical Research*, **2**(3), 394–407.

Heo, M., Y. Kim, X. Xue, and M. Kim (2010). Sample size requirement to detect an intervention effect at the end of a follow-up in longitudinal cluster randomized trial. *Statistics in Medicine*, **29**, 382–390.

Herson, J. and J. Wittes (1993). The use of interim analysis for sample size adjustment. *Drug Information Journal*, **27**, 753–760.

Horrobin, D. F. (2003). Are large clinical trials in rapidly lethal diseases usually unethical? *Lancet*, **361**, 695–697.

Hosmane, B., C. Locke, and Y.-L. Chiu (2010). Sample size and power estimation in thorough QT/QTc studies with parallel group design. *Journal of Biopharmaceutical Statistics*, **20**(3), 595–603.

Huang, P., R. F. Woolson, and P. C. O'Brien (2008). A rank-based sample size method for multiple outcomes in clinical trials. *Statistics in Medicine*, **27**, 3084–3104.

Huang, P., B. C. Tilley, R. F. Woolson, and S. Lipsitz (2005). Adjusting O'Brien's test to control Type I error for the generalized nonparametric Behrens–Fisher problem. *Biometrics*, **61**(2), 532–538.

Ivanova, A., B. Qaqish, and D. A. Schoenfeld (2011). Optimality, sample size, and power calculations for the sequential parallel comparison design. *Statistics in Medicine*, **30**(23), 2793–2803.

Jackson, D., J. Bowden, and R. Baker (2010). How does the DerSimonian and Laird procedure for random effects meta-analysis compare with its more efficient but harder to compute counterparts? *Journal of Statistical Planning and Inference*, **140**(4), 961–970.

Jackson, D., I. R. White, and S. G. Thompson (2010). Extending DerSimonian and Laird's methodology to perform multivariate random effects meta-analyses. *Statistics in Medicine*, **29**, 1282–1297.

Jahn-Eimermacher, A. and G. Hommel (2007). Performance of adaptive sample size adjustment with respect to stopping criteria and time of interim analysis. *Statistics in Medicine*, **26**, 1450–1461.

Jennison, C. and B. W. Turnbull (2003). Mid-course sample size modification in clinical trials based on the observed treatment effect. *Statistics in Medicine*, **22**, 971–993.

Jennison, C. and B. W. Turnbull (2010). *Group Sequential and Adaptive Methods for Clinical Trials*, 2nd edition. New York: Chapman and Hall.

Jiang, K. (2011). Optimal sample sizes and go/no-go decisions for Phase II/III development programs based on probability of success. *Statistics in Biopharmaceutical Research*, **3**(3), 463–475.

Jiang, Q. and S. Snapinn (2009). Nonproportional hazards and the power of sequential trials. *Statistics in Biopharmaceutical Research*, **1**(1), 66–73.

Julious, S. A. (2004). Tutorial in biostatistics: Sample sizes for clinical trials with normal data. *Statistics in Medicine*, **23**, 1921–1986.

Julious, S. A. (2009). *Sample Sizes for Clinical Trials*. Boca Raton, FL: CRC Press.

Jung, S. H. and C. Ahn (2003). Sample size estimation for GEE method comparing slopes in repeated measurements data. *Statistics in Medicine*, **22**(8), 1305–1315.

Kenward, M. G. and B. Jones (2003). *Design and Analysis of Cross-Over Trials*. New York: Chapman and Hall.

Kikuchi, T. and J. Gittins (2009). A behavioral Bayes method to determine the sample size of a clinical trial considering efficacy and safety. *Statistics in Medicine*, **28**, 2307–2324.

Kikuchi, T., H. Pezeshk, and J. Gittins (2008). A Bayesian cost–benefit approach to the determination of sample size in clinical trials. *Statistics in Medicine*, **27**, 68–82.

Kim, K. and D. L. DeMets (1992). Sample size determination for group sequential clinical trials with immediate response. *Statistics in Medicine*, **11**, 1391–1399.

Kirby, A., V. Gebski, and A. C. Keech (2002). Determining the sample size in a clinical trial. *Medical Journal of Australia*, **177**(5), 256–257.

Kraemer, H. C., J. Mintz, A. Noda, J. Tinjlenberg, and J. A. Yesavage (2006). Caution regarding the use of pilot studies to guide power calculations for study proposals. *Archives of General Psychiatry*, **63**, 484–489.

Kwong, K. S., S. H. Cheung, and M.-J. Wen (2010). Sample size determination in step-up procedures for multiple comparisons with a control. *Statistics in Medicine*, **29**(26), 2743–2756.

Lachin, J. M. (2005). A review of methods for futility stopping based on conditional power. *Statistics in Medicine*, **24**(18), 2747–2764.

Lai, T. L. and M.-C. Shih (2004). Power, sample size and adaptation consideration in the design of group sequential clinical trials. *Biometrika*, **91**(3), 507–528.

Lakatos, E. (1986). Sample size determination in clinical trials with time-dependent rates of losses and noncompliance. *Controlled Clinical Trials*, **7**, 189–199.

Lan, K. K. G. and Z. Shun (2009). A short note on sample size estimation. *Statistics in Biopharmaceutical Research*, **1**(4), 356–361.

Lan, K. K. G. and J. T. Wittes (2012). Some thoughts on sample size: A Bayesian-frequentist approach. *Clinical Trials*, **9**(5), 561–569.

Lan, K. K. G., P. Hu, and M. A. Proschan (2009). A conditional power approach to the evaluation of predictive power. *Statistics in Biopharmaceutical Research*, **1**(2), 131–136.

Landau, S. and D. Stahl (2013). Sample size and power calculations for medical studies by simulation when closed form expressions are not available. *Statistical Methods in Medical Research*, (to appear).

Lehmacher, W. and G. Wassmer (1999). Adaptive sample-size calculations in group sequential trials. *Biometrics*, **55**, 1286–1290.

Lemeshow, S., D. W. Hosmer, J. Klar, and S. K. Lwanga (1990). *Adequacy of Sample Size in Health Studies*. Chichester, UK: Wiley.

Li, G., W. J. Shih, T. Xie, and J. Lu (2002). A sample size adjustment procedure for clinical trials based on conditional power. *Biostatistics*, **3**(2), 277–287.

Lin, X., D. C. Parks, J. Greshock, R. Wooster, and K. R. Lee (2011). Effect of predictive performance of a biomarker for the sample size of targeted designs for randomized clinical trials. *Statistics in Biopharmaceutical Research*, **3**(4), 536–548.

Liu, P-Y. and S. Dahlberg (1995). Design and analysis of multiarm clinical trials with survival endpoints. *Controlled Clinical Trials*, **16**(2), 119–130.

Lu, K., X. Luo, and P.-Y. Chen (2008). Sample size estimation for repeated measures analysis in randomized clinical trials with missing data. *The International Journal of Biostatistics*, **4**(1), 1–16.

Lu, Q., S-. C. Chow, S. K. Tse, Y. Chi, and L. Y. Tang (2009). Sample size estimation based on event data for a two-stage survival adaptive trial with different durations. *Journal of Biopharmaceutical Statistics*, **19**, 311–323.

Machin, D., M. J. Campbell, S.-B. Tan, and S.-H. Tan (2009). *Sample Size Tables for Clinical Studies*. London : BMJ Books.

Machin, D., M. Campbell, P. Fayers, and A. Pinol (1997). *Sample Size Tables for Clinical Studies*. New York: Wiley.

Maki, E. (2006). Power and sample size considerations in clinical trials with competing risk endpoints. *Pharmaceutical Statistics*, **5**, 159–171.

Makuch, R. W. and R. M. Simon (1980). Sample size comparisons for non-randomised comparative studies. *Journal of Chronic Diseases*, **33**, 175–181.

Makuch, R. W. and R. M. Simon (1982). Sample size requirements for comparing time-to-failure among *k* treatment groups. *Journal of Chronic Diseases*, **35**(11), 861–867.

Malhotra, R. K. and A. Indrayan (2010). A simple nomogram for sample size for estimating sensitivity and specificity of medical tests. *Research Methodology*, **58**(6), 519–522.

McMahon, R. P., M. Proschan, N. L. Geller, P. H. Stone, and G. Sopko (1994). Sample size calculations for clinical trials in which entry criteria and outcomes are counts of events. *Statistics in Medicine*, **13**(8), 859–870.

Mehta, C. R. (2011). Sample size reestimation for confirmatory clinical trials. In *Designs for Clinical Trials: Prospectives on Current Issues* (D. Harrington, ed.). New York: Springer.

Mehta, C. R. and N. R. Patel (2006). Adaptive, group, sequential and decision theoretic approaches to sample size determination. *Statistics in Medicine*, **25**, 3250–3269.

Mehta, C. R. and S. J. Pocock (2011). Adaptive increase in sample size when interim results are promising: A practical guide with examples. *Statistics in Medicine*, **30**(28), 3267–3284.

Mehta, C. R. and A. A. Tsiatis (2001). Flexible sample size considerations using information based interim monitoring. *Drug Information Journal*, **35**, 1095–1112.

Moher, D., C. S. Dulberg, and G. A. Wells (1994). Statistical power, sample size, and their reporting in randomized controlled trials. *Journal of the American Medical Association*, **272**(2), 122–124. (Available at http://www.ncbi.nlm.nih.gov/pubmed/8015121.)

Morgan, C. C. (2003). Sample size re-estimation in group sequential response-adaptive clinical trials. *Statistics in Medicine*, **22**, 3843–3857.

O'Brien, P. C. (1984). Procedures for comparing samples with multiple endpoints. *Biometrics*, **40**, 1079–1087.

O'Brien, R. G. and J. M. Castelloe (2007). Sample size analysis for traditional hypothesis testing: Concepts and issues. In *Pharmaceutical Statistics Using SAS: A Practical Guide* (A. Dmitrienko, C. Chuang-Stein, and R. D'Agostino, eds.), pp. 237–271, Chapter 10. Cary, NC: SAS.

Ogungbenro, K. and L. Aarons (2010a). Sample size/power calculations for population pharmacodynamic experiments involving repeated-count measurements. *Journal of Biopharmaceutical Statistics*, **20**(5), 1026–1042.

Ogungbenro, K. and L. Aarons (2010b). Sample-size calculations for multi-group comparison in population experiments. *Pharmaceutical Statistics*, **9**, 255–268.

Ogungbenro, K., L. Aarons, and G. Graham (2006). Sample size calculations based on generalized estimating equations for population pharmacokinetic experiments. *Journal of Biopharmaceutical Statistics*, **16**, 135–150.

O'Malley, A. J., S.-L. T. Norman, and R. E. Kuntz (2002). Sample size calculation for a historically controlled clinical trial with adjustment for covariates. *Journal of Biopharmaceutical Statistics*, **12**(2), 227–247.

Orloff, J., F. Douglas, J. Pinheiro, S. Levinson, M. Branson, P. Chaturvedi, E. Ette, P. Gatto, G. Hirsch, C. Mehta, N. Patel, S. Sabir, S. Springs, D. Stanski, M. R. Evers, E. Fleming, N. Singh, T. Tramontin, and H. Golub (2009). The future of drug development: Advancing clinical design. *Nature Reviews Drug Discovery*, **8**, 949–957.

Parker, R. A. and N. G. Berman (2003). Sample size: More than calculations. *The American Statistician*, **57**(3), 166–170.

Patel, N. R. and S. Ankolekar (2007). A Bayesian approach for incorporating economic factors in sample size design for clinical trials of individual drugs and portfolios of drugs. *Statistics in Medicine*, **26**, 4976–4988.

Peace, K. E. (2009). *Design and Analysis of Clinical Trials with Time-to-Event Endpoints*. Boca Raton, FL: Chapman and Hall, CRC.

Peters, S. A., M. K. Palmer, H. M. den Ruitjer, D. E. Grobbee, J. R. Crouse III, D. H. O'Leary, G. W. Evans, J. S. Raichlen, and M. L. Bots (2012). Sample size requirements in trials using repeated measurements and the impact of trial design. *Current Medical Research and Opinion*, **28**(5), 681–688.

Pezeshk, H. (2003). Bayesian techniques for sample size determination in clinical trials: A short review. *Statistical Methods in Medical Research*, **12**, 489–504.

Posch, M. and P. Bauer (2000). Interim analysis and sample size reassessment. *Biometrics*, **56**, 1170–1176.

Proschan, M. A. (2005). Two-stage sample size re-estimation based on a nuisance parameter— A review. *Journal of Biopharmaceutical Statistics*, **15**, 559–574.

Proschan, M.A. (2009). Sample size re-estimation in clinical trials. *Biometrical Journal*, **51**, 348–357.

Proschan, M. A. and S. A. Hunsbarger (1995). Designed extension of studies based on conditional power. *Biometrics*, **51**, 1315–1324.

Proschan, M., K. K. G. Lan, and J. T. Wittes (2006). *Statistical Monitoring of Clinical Trials: A Unified Approach*. New York: Springer.

Rahardja, D. and Y. D. Zhao (2009). Unified sample size computations using the competing probability. *Statistics in Biopharmaceutical Research*, **1**(3), 323–327.

Richardson, D. J. and S. Leurgans (1998). Sample size justification in Phase III/IV clinical trials. *Neuroepidemiology*, **17**(2), 63–66.

Royston, P. and A. Babiker (2002). A menu-driven facility for complex sample size calculation in randomized controlled trials with a survival or a binary outcome. *The Stata Journal*, **2**(2), 151–163.

Royston, P. and F. M.-S. Barthel (2005). Projection of power and events in clinical trials with a time-to-event outcome. *The Stata Journal*, **10**(3), 386–394.

Sahu, S. K. and T. M. F. Smith (2006). A Bayesian method of sample size determination with practical applications. *Journal of the Royal Statistical Society, Series A: Statistics in Society*, **169**, 235–253.

Sathian, B., J. Sreedharan, N. S. Baboo, K. Sharan, E. S. Abhilash, and E. Rajesh (2010). Relevance of sample size determination in medical research. *Nepal Journal of Epidemiology*, **1**(1), 4–10.

Schouten, H. J. A. (1999). Planning group sizes in clinical trials with a continuous outcome and repeated measures. *Statistics in Medicine*, **18**(3), 255–264.

Schulz, K. F. and D. A. Grimes (2005). Sample size calculations in randomised trials: Mandatory and mystical. *The Lancet*, **365**, 1348–1353.

Schwartz, T. A. and J. S. Denne (2006). A two-stage sample size recalculation procedure for placebo- and active-controlled non-inferiority trials. *Statistics in Medicine*, **25**(19), 3396–3406.

Senn, S. J. (2002). *Cross-over Trials in Clinical Research*, 2nd edition. New York: Wiley.

Senn, S. and F. Bretz (2007). Power and sample size when multiple endpoints are considered. *Pharmaceutical Statistics*, **6**, 161–170.

Sethuraman, V. S., S. Leonov, L. Squassante, T. R. Mitchell, and M. D. Hale (2007). Sample size calculation for the power model for dose proportionality studies. *Pharmaceutical Statistics*, **6**, 35–41.

Shen, Y. and J. Cai (2003). Sample size reestimation for clinical trials with censored survival data. *Journal of the American Statistical Association*, **98**(462), 418–426.

Shih, J. H. (1995). Sample size calculation for complex clinical trials with survival endpoints. *Controlled Clinical Trials*, **16**, 395–407.

Shih, W. J. (1993). Sample size re-estimation for triple blind clinical trials. *Drug Information Journal*, **27**, 761–764.

Shih, W. J. (2009). Two-stage sample size reassessment using perturbed unblinding. *Statistics in Biopharmaceutical Research*, **1**(1), 74–80.

Shih, W. J. and P. L. Zhao (1997). Design for sample size re-estimation with interim data for double blind clinical trials with binary outcomes. *Statistics in Medicine*, **16**, 1913–1923.

Shun, Z., Y. He, Y. Feng, and M. Roessner (2009). A unified approach to flexible sample size design with realistic constraints. *Statistics in Biopharmaceutical Research*, **1**(4), 388–398.

Shuster, J. J. (1992). *Practical Handbook of Sample Size Guidelines for Clinical Trials*. Boca Raton, FL: CRC Press.

Shuster, J. J. (2010). Empirical vs. natural weighting in random effects meta-analysis. *Statistics in Medicine*, **29**, 1259–1265. Discussion: **29**, 1266–1281.

Simon, R. (1989). Optimal two-stage designs for Phase II clinical trials. *Controlled Clinical Trials*, **10**, 1–10.

Siqueira, A. L., A. Whitehead, S. Todd, and M. M. Lucini (2005). Comparison of sample size formulae for 2 × 2 cross-over designs applied to bioequivalence studies. *Pharmaceutical Statistics*, **4**(4), 233–243. Discussion: **5**, 231–233.

Sjögren, P. and L. Hedström (2010). Sample size determination and statistical power in randomized controlled trials. Letter to the Editor. *Oral Surgery, Oral Medicine, Oral Pathology, Oral Radiology, and Endodontology*, **109**(5), 652–653.

Sozu, T., T. Sugimoto, and T. Hamasaki (2010). Sample size determination in clinical trials with multiple co-primary binary endpoints. *Statistics in Medicine*, **29**(21), 2169–2179.

Sozu, T., T. Sugimoto, and T. Hamasaki (2011). Sample size determination in superiority clinical trials with multiple co-primary correlated endpoints. *Journal of Biopharmaceutical Statistics*, **21**, 650–668.

Sozu, T., T. Sugimoto, and T. Hamasaki (2012). Sample size determination in clinical trials with multiple co-primary endpoints including mixed continuous and binary variables. *Biometrical Journal*, **54**(5), 716–729.

Spiegelhalter, D. J., L. S. Freedman, and P. R. Blackburn (1986). Monitoring clinical trials: Conditional or predictive power? *Controlled Clinical Trials*, **7**, 8–17.

Stalbovskaya, V., B. Hamadicharef, and E. Ifeachor (2007). Sample size determination using ROC analysis. *Proceedings of the 3rd International Conference on Computational Intelligence in Medicine and Healthcare*, July 25–27. Plymouth, U.K.

Stone, G. W. and S. J. Pocock (2010). Randomized trials, statistics, and clinical inference. *Journal of American College of Cardiology*, **55**, 428–431.

Su, G. (2005). Sample size and power analysis for endometrial safety studies. *Journal of Biopharmaceutical Statistics*, **15**, 491–499.

Tan, M. T., H.-B. Fang, and G.-L. Tian (2009). Dose and sample size determination for multidrug combination studies. *Statistics in Biopharmaceutical Research*, **1**(3), 301–316.

Tango, T. (2009). Sample size formula for randomized controlled trials with counts of recurrent events. *Statistics and Probability Letters*, **79**, 466–472.

Thabane, L., J. Ma, R. Chu, J. Cheng, A. Ismalia, L. P. Rios, R. Robson, M. Thabane, L. Giangregorio, and C. H. Goldsmith (2010). A tutorial on pilot studies: The what, why and how. *BMC Medical Research Methodology*, **10**(1), open access journal.

Tracy, M. (2009). *Methods of Sample Size Calculations for Clinical Trials*. Master of Science thesis, University of Glasgow, Glasgow, Scotland. (Available at `http://theses.gla.ac.uk/671`.)

Tseng, C.-H. and Y. Shao (2010). Sample size analysis for pharmacogenetic studies. *Statistics in Biopharmaceutical Research*, **2**(3), 319–328.

Vickers, A. J. (2003). Underpowering in randomized trials reporting a sample size calculation. *Journal of Clinical Epidemiology*, **56**, 717–720.

Waksman, J. A. (2007). Assessment of the Gould–Shih procedure for sample size reestimation. *Pharmaceutical Statistics*, **6**(1), 53–65.

Wang, H. and S.-C. Chow (2007). Sample size calculation for comparing time-to-event data. In *Wiley Encyclopedia of Clinical Trials*, pp. 1–7. Hoboken, NJ: Wiley.

Wang, H., S.-C. Chow, and M. Chen (2005). A Bayesian approach on sample size calculation for comparing means. *Journal of Biopharmaceutical Statistics*, **15**, 799–807.

Wang, H., S.-C. Chow, and G. Li (2002). On sample size calculations based on odds ratios in clinical trials. *Journal of Biopharmaceutical Statistics*, **12**, 471–483.

Wang, H., B. Chen, and S.-C. Chow (2003). Sample size determination based on rank tests in clinical trials. *Journal of Biopharmaceutical Statistics*, **13**(4), 735–751.

Wang, M.-D. (2007). Sample size reestimation by Bayesian prediction. *Biometrical Journal*, **49**(3), 365–377.

Wassmer, G. (2011). On sample determination in multi-armed confirmatory adaptive designs. *Journal of Biopharmaceutical Statistics*, **21**(4), 802–817.

Wernicke, J. F., Y. L. Pritchett, D. N. D'Souza, A. Waninger, P. Tran, S. Iyengar, and J. Raskin (2006). A randomized controlled trial of duloxetine in diabetic peripheral neuropathic pain. *Neurology*, **67**, 1411–1420.

Whitehead, J., E. Valdés-Márquez, P. Johnson, and G. Graham (2008). Bayesian sample size for exploratory clinical trials incorporating historical data. *Statistics in Medicine*, **27**, 2307–2327.

Whitley, E. and J. Bell (2002). Statistics review: Sample size calculations. *Critical Care*, **6**(4), 335–341.

Willan, A. R. (2008). Optimal sample size determinations from an industry perspective based on the expected value of information. *Clinical Trials*, **5**(6), 587–594.

Willan, A. and S. Eckerman (2010). Optimal clinical trial design using value of information methods with imperfect implementation. *Health Economics*, **19**(5), 549–561.

Willan, A. R. and M. E. Kowgier (2008). Determining optimal sample sizes for multi-stage randomized clinical trials using value of information methods. *Clinical Trials*, **5**, 289–300.

Willan, A. R. and E. M. Pinto (2005). The expected value of information and optimal clinical trial design. *Statistics in Medicine*, **24**(12), 1791–1806. (Correction: **25**, 720.)

Wittes, J. (2002). Sample size calculations for randomized controlled trials. *Epidemiologic Reviews*, **24**(1), 39–53.

Wittes, J. and E. Brittain (1990). The role of internal pilot studies in increasing the efficiency of clinical trials. *Statistics in Medicine*, **9**, 65–72.

Wolbers, M., D. Heemskerk, T. T. H. Chan, N. T. B. Yen, M. Caws, J. Farrar, and J. Day (2011). Sample size requirements for separating out the effects of combination treatments: Randomised controlled trials of combination therapy vs. standard treatment compared to factorial designs for patients with tuberculous meningitis. *Trials*, **12**, 26.

Wu, M., M. Fisher, and D. DeMets (1980). Sample sizes for long-term medical trials with time-dependent dropout and event rates. *Controlled Clinical Trials*, **9**, 119–136.

Wust, K. and M. Keiser (2003). Blinded sample size recalculation for normally distributed outcomes using long- and short-term data. *Biometrical Journal*, **45**(8), 915–930.

Xiong, C., K. Yu, Y. Yan, and Z. Zhang (2005). Power and sample size for clinical trials when efficacy is required in multiple endpoints: Application to an Alzheimer's treatment trial. *Clinical Trials*, **2**(5), 387–393.

Yan, X. and X. Su (2006). Sample size determination for clinical trials in patients with nonlinear disease progression. *Journal of Biopharmaceutical Statistics*, **16**, 91–105.

Yin, Y. (2002). Sample size calculation for a proof of concept study. *Journal of Biopharmaceutical Statistics*, **12**, 267–276.

You, Z., O. D. Williams, I. Aban, E. K. Kabagambe, H. K. Tiwari, and G. Cutter (2011). Relative efficiency and sample size for cluster randomized trials with variable cluster sizes. *Clinical Trials*, **8**(1), 27–36.

Zaslavsky, B. G. (2009). Bayes models of clinical trials with dichotomous outcomes and sample size determination. *Statistics in Biopharmaceutical Research*, **1**(2), 149–158.

Zaslavsky, B. G. (2012). Bayesian sample size estimates for one sample test in clinical trials with dichotomous and countable outcomes. *Statistics in Biopharmaceutical Research*, **4**(1), 76–85.

Zhang, S. and C. Ahn (2010). Effects of correlation and missing data on sample size estimation in longitudinal clinical trials. *Pharmaceutical Statistics*, **9**, 2–9.

Zhang, S. and C. Ahn (2011). Adding subjects or adding measurements in repeated measurement studies under financial constraints. *Statistics in Biopharmaceutical Research*, **3**(1), 54–64.

Zhang, S., J. Cao, and C. Ahn (2010). Calculating sample size in trials using historical controls. *Clinical Trials*, **7**, 343–353.

Zhang, W. and V. Sethuraman (2010). On power and sample size calculation in ethnic sensitivity studies. *Journal of Biopharmaceutical Statistics*, **21**(1), 18–23.

Zwarenstein (2002). Letter to the Editor and discussion. *British Medical Journal*, **325**, 491.

EXERCISES

7.1. Consider a single-stage Phase II clinical trial with desired power of .90 and $\alpha = .05$. The maximum response rate of a poor treatment is .10 and the minimum response rate of a good treatment is .25. Use PASS 11 or other software to determine the required sample size for the clinical trial. For what numbers of responses will the null hypothesis be rejected?

7.2. Why should there be concern over survey results of research articles that give the results of clinical trials?

7.3. What is one advantage that the method of competing probability has from the viewpoint of a patient over other methods for sample size determination that were discussed in the chapter?

CHAPTER 8

Quality Improvement

Statistical methods for quality improvement have been used extensively in the United States, for example, especially during the past 25 years. Unlike a t-test to compare two means or ANOVA used to analyze data from an experimental design, some of these statistical methods are used repeatedly. When this is the case, the concept of power, which applies to a single analysis, is not appropriate.

For example, control chart usage may involve a small sample of items being taken every 30 minutes, with the objective of maintaining tight control over a process. The properties of a single sample are almost irrelevant since many samples will be obtained in a given day. Hence, sample size determination is viewed in a different way and different statistics are used. This is discussed in Section 8.1.3, in particular.

8.1 CONTROL CHARTS

There are two phases of control chart usage: analysis of past data and real-time process monitoring, and charts are constructed using either individual observations or subgroups, which might be groups of 4 or 5 observations obtained every 30 minutes, say, from some process. (The analysis of past data and real-time process monitoring are herein termed Stage 1 and Stage 2, respectively; they have also been designated as Phase 1 and Phase 2 by some writers.) For Stage 1, there is a question of how much past data to use in computing the necessary parameter estimates. If an insufficient amount of data is used, control chart performance could have both unacceptable variability and unacceptable properties, on average.

Sample Size Determination and Power, First Edition. Thomas P. Ryan.
© 2013 John Wiley & Sons, Inc. Published 2013 by John Wiley & Sons, Inc.

Note that 3-sigma control chart limits are typically used. For a normal distribution, the tail areas outside $\mu \pm 3\sigma$ are each .000135. Since this is a very small value, we don't have a hypothesis testing situation with $\alpha = .05$ or .01. Rather, we can, loosely speaking, think of $\alpha = .000135$ for a one-sided test and $\alpha = 2(.00135) = .0027$ for a two-sided test. [There are dissimilarities between control chart usage and hypothesis testing, however; see Woodall (2000).]

8.1.1 Shewhart Measurement Control Charts

A measurement control chart is a chart for which a measured process characteristic is being monitored, such as a diameter. The standard 3-sigma control charts are often referred to as "Shewhart charts" since Dr. Walter A. Shewhart first sketched out the basic idea of a control chart in 1924, with the first chart proposed being a p-chart.

An attribute control chart, such as a p-chart, is one for which a unit is declared to be either conforming or nonconforming, or else the number of nonconformities of a certain type or all types are counted. (A p-chart is the former.) Sample size determination for attribute control charts is discussed in Section 8.1.2.

To illustrate the use of measurement charts, let's assume that the objective is to control the mean of some process characteristic, which we will assume has a normal distribution, and we will also assume that individual observations will be plotted on a (control) chart. The 3-sigma control limits will be at $\hat{\mu} \pm 3\hat{\sigma}$ and the chart is called an X-chart. The mean, μ, would logically be estimated by the average of the past data values, $\bar{X}$. The estimation of $\hat{\sigma}$ is not as simple, however. The usual approach in Stage 1 is to use $\hat{\sigma} = \overline{\text{MR}}/1.128$, with $\overline{\text{MR}}$ denoting the average of moving ranges of size two of the time-ordered past data and 1.128 being the constant that makes the estimator unbiased. For Stage 2, Cryer and Ryan (1990) showed that $\hat{\sigma} = S/c_4$ is the preferred estimator, as that estimator has a smaller variance than the estimator based on moving ranges, with s denoting the standard deviation of the Stage 1 (historical) data, and c_4 is the constant, which depends on the number of observations, that makes the estimator unbiased. Ideally, the moving range estimator should be used to help identify the data that have not come from the in-control distribution. These data would then be removed and the remaining data used to compute both $\bar{X}$ and S/c_4 for Stage 2. (The reason that the moving range estimator should be used in Stage 1 is that it is less sensitive to aberrant data than is the standard deviation, with the resultant control limits thus being better at helping the control chart user to identify data that is not from the in-control distribution.)

The control chart parameters should be estimated with sufficient data so that the point at which signals are received after a change in the process mean does not have high variability. That is, for example, we would not want to receive a signal on the 5th plotted point one time and on the 85th plotted point the next time. Control chart properties have high variability because of the small probability associated with 3σ limits, even when the parameters are assumed known; the problem should not be exacerbated by using a small amount of data to estimate the parameters.

The results given by Quesenberry (1993) are useful in determining the total number of observations to be used in Stage 1, which for subgroup data is the number of subgroups times the subgroup size and is the number of individual observations for a control chart of individual observations. As a rule-of-thumb, at least 100 observations should be used to compute trial control limits, with approximately 300 observations used for "permanent" limits. (Processes change over time, so parameters must eventually be reestimated.)

When data are in subgroups rather than as individual observations, subgroup averages can be plotted on a chart. When this is done, the chart is called an $\bar{X}$-chart. Then a decision must be made regarding the subgroup size as well as the number of subgroups of past data that will be used for parameter estimation. Historically, subgroups of 4 or 5 have been used, without any attention given to the power associated with each subgroup size for a given mean shift. Dockendorf (1992) made this point and provided two graphs that could be used as an aid in determining subgroup size. Unfortunately, however, an "allowable shift in standard deviation units" is on the horizontal scale of each of the graphs, with 1.5 in the middle of the scale. This greatly limits the value of the graphs as a shift of less than one standard deviation unit would typically be an acceptable shift, with CUSUM schemes, for example, typically designed with the focus of detecting (at least) a one standard deviation shift.

It should be noted that the sample size need not be constant, as it is reasonable to decrease the subgroup size or increase the sampling interval, or both, when a process seems to be running smoothly with a process disturbance creating an out-of-control situation being very unlikely. When that is the case, a variable sample size might be used. Such charts are discussed in Section 8.1.5.

Consider Table 8.1, which indicates how power changes with subgroup size changes for a given shift in the mean from μ to $\mu + \sigma$. Control chart users think in

Table 8.1   Power of Detecting a 1σ Upward Mean Shift with an $\bar{X}$-Chart with Subgroup Size n (μ and σ Assumed Known)

n	Power (ARL)
1	.02275 (43.96)
2	.05639 (17.73)
3	.10241 (9.76)
4	.15866 (6.30)
5	.22245 (4.50)
6	.29098 (3.44)
7	.36158 (2.77)

terms of average run lengths (ARLs), however, which is the expected number of points to be plotted after a change in the parameter(s) being monitored for a signal to be received from a point plotting outside the control limits. Although power is not typically mentioned when control charts are designed, the probability of a point plotting outside the control limits after the parameter that is being monitored (such as a mean) has changed can be termed the "power" of the control chart, loosely speaking. ARL is then equal to 1/power. Parameter changes for measurement charts are generally expressed in terms of the number of standard deviation units of what is being plotted, and ARLs are given for parameter changes expressed in this manner.

Thus, if subgroup averages are being plotted, which would be the case when an $\bar{X}$-chart is used, the change would be expressed in terms of a multiple of $\sigma_{\bar{x}}$. That won't work in trying to determine subgroup size, however, because the subgroup size is then "lost." Specifically, $Z = [\mu + 3\sigma_{\bar{x}} - (\mu + a\sigma)]/\sigma_{\bar{x}}$ is a function of n, whereas $Z = [\mu + 3\sigma_{\bar{x}} - (\mu + a\sigma_{\bar{x}})]/\sigma_{\bar{x}}$ is not a function of n, with $\mu + 3\sigma_{\bar{x}}$ denoting the upper control limit (UCL) of an $\bar{X}$-chart, and $(\mu + a\sigma)$ representing the new mean as a function of σ, and similarly for $\mu + a\sigma_{\bar{x}}$. Therefore, it is the first of these two forms for Z that was used in the power and ARL values that are shown in Table 8.1, which is based on the assumption of known μ and σ. (This assumption will later be relaxed.)

Note that none of the power values are even remotely close to .8 or .9, but that is of no consequence since, unlike a typical hypothesis testing problem, sampling is often done very frequently (such as every 15 minutes), and the ARL values show that the shift should be detected after just a few plotted points when the subgroup size is around five. Thus, power really isn't an issue when control charts are used, nor are very small differences in ARL values of any concern. Thus, the choice between, say, a subgroup size of 5 and a subgroup size of 6 should be based on factors other than those shown in Table 8.1.

Regarding the number of subgroups of past data to use, which is also a sample size determination problem of sorts, applying the Quesenberry (1993) results would lead to at least 20 subgroups of size 5 being used for Stage 1, or at least 25 subgroups of size 4 (i.e., at least 100 observations). This would be applied to measurement control charts such as $\bar{X}$-, R-, and X-charts, which are virtually the most frequently used control charts. Since individual observations are plotted on an X-chart, this means that at least 100 individual observations would be needed for Stage 1, and about 2 or 3 times that many when (semi-) permanent control limits are used in Stage 2 (the process monitoring stage). Sample size determination for other types of charts will be discussed later.

Regarding the choice of subgroup size, since we may view control chart usage as being similar to hypothesis testing since a decision of "in control" or "out of control" is made each time a point is plotted, a very large subgroup would be impractical and would likely result in changes being detected that are not of practical significance, for changes that are expressed as $\mu + a\sigma$ or $\mu - a\sigma$.

(Note that this is the same type of consideration that must be made when hypothesis testing is used, in general.) On the other hand, even small changes may be of significance in medical applications and the failure to detect such changes could have serious consequences.

We want the ARL to be large when the process is in control and to be small for changes that are deemed to be consequential, analogous to having both a small Type I error probability and a small Type II error probability for general hypothesis testing. The objective is to detect changes before they have serious consequences. There are many types of statistical process control charts and control procedures but the general objective should be the same with each one. That is, enough data should be used to estimate control chart parameters so that control chart performance does not have large variability, and the number of observations used at each time period when a point is plotted on the chart should be such that the control chart scheme has desirable ARL properties. That is, a control chart signal should be received very infrequently when the process is in statistical control (i.e., false signals should be rare), but a signal should be received very quickly when there is evidence of a process change that is of a magnitude that one wishes to detect quickly. Unfortunately, for decades ARLs were given based on the assumption of known parameter values, which is essentially analogous to acting as if an infinite sample size was used in estimating the parameters. Note, however, that the assumption of known parameters in determining ARLs is similar to assuming a known value of σ and determining a sample size, as was done in Chapters 2 and 3, for example. Recall from the discussion in Section 3.2, though, that it would be much better to utilize parameter estimation variability in such a way that a confidence interval on power is obtained. If very large numbers of observations are used in estimating parameters, confidence intervals on those parameters would be quite narrow and the parameter estimates would have very little sampling variability, which in turn would mean that power would have very little sampling variability and would render a confidence interval for power unnecessary. With control charts, there may be enough historical data available that a large amount of data could be used for parameter estimation, although it is important that such data be recent.

8.1.2 Using Software to Determine Subgroup Size

Release 11 of PASS can be used to determine subgroup size for various control charts, with PASS using simulation exclusively. Simulation wouldn't be necessary if the parameters were assumed to be known, as then the appropriate statistical theory would be used. Simulation *is* necessary when parameters are estimated, however. One very useful way in which PASS can be used is to vary the number of subgroups that are used for estimating the parameters and see how this directly affects the properties of the chart. This will essentially duplicate the work of Quesenberry (1993) but it can be a good learning tool.

8.1.2.1 $\bar{X}$-Chart

To illustrate, it is well known that the ARL for determining a $1\sigma_{\bar{x}}$ shift in the process mean when an $\bar{X}$-chart is used is 43.89 when the parameters are assumed to be known. Therefore, if an extremely large amount of historical data is used for parameter estimation, the ARL for such a shift obtained by simulation should be approximately 43.89 if a very large number of simulations are performed. Setting the number of observations for parameter estimation at 1000 in PASS and performing 50,000 simulations produces an ARL of 44.2 and a median run length of 30.0. (The difference between the last two numbers illustrates why ARL values are often supplemented with other information from the run length distribution, such as the median and various percentiles, because the run length distribution is very skewed and with highly skewed distributions the average is not a very good measure.) Here the ARL of 44.2 is slightly different from the theoretical value of 43.9 even though two large numbers were used: 1000 observations for parameter estimation and 50,000 simulations. Such differences can be explained as follows. Since 3-sigma limits on an $\bar{X}$-chart are being used and there are very small tail areas (.00135 on each end) when normality is assumed, even very small errors in parameter estimation can result in probabilities that differ more than slightly from .00135. When this occurs, run lengths can be more than slightly affected. Furthermore, the standard deviation of the run lengths will be of the same order of magnitude as the average run length, so run lengths exhibit considerable variability and some large run lengths invariably result when simulations are performed.

Thus, there are factors at work that will cause the simulated average run length to differ slightly from the theoretical value.

The in-control (i.e., no parameter change) ARL for the chart is known to be 370.37 in the parameters-known case. The run length standard deviation is, at 369.87, almost the same as the ARL, so some very large and some very small run lengths will be generated when simulations are performed, and for this reason the simulated ARL should not be expected to be very close to the theoretical ARL. The simulations will take some time since almost all of the in-control run lengths will be large. Using PASS, the simulated in-control ARL was 372.6 and the median run length was 258.0 when 20,000 simulations were performed and the parameters were estimated from 1000 observations. The simulations took 10.69 minutes.

The simulated in-control ARL, which was obtained in PASS by letting the out-of-control distribution be the same as the in-control distribution, is thus very close to the theoretical value.

All of this is fine for gaining an understanding of the importance of using a large amount of historical data in Stage 1 and obtaining a good idea of just how much data to use, but what if we are interested in determining the subgroup size? Let's again assume that there is a shift from $N(\mu, \sigma) = N(0, 2)$ to $N(1, 2)$, with N signifying a normal distribution with mean μ and standard deviation σ. It was stated earlier in this section that the simulated ARL was 44.2. Now let's assume that we want the ARL for detecting this change to have a target value of 20. How large should the subgroup size be? PASS gave $n = 8$ as the desired subgroup size, as this produced an ARL value of 17.8, not far from the target ARL of 20. This was obtained using 50,000 simulations (Monte Carlo samples in the PASS vernacular), with the chart parameters assumed known [i.e., $N(0, 2)$]. This result is almost identical when the parameters are estimated from the simulated data, but then the simulations take a very long time to run (1.17 hours when 20,000 simulations were run and for each simulated sample the parameters were estimated from 1000 observations).

The necessary sample size is easy to compute analytically for an $\bar{X}$-chart, under the assumption of normality and known parameter values. The mechanics involve computing the appropriate Z-statistic and computing the probability using the normal distribution. Specifically,

$$Z = \frac{\mu + 3\sigma_{\bar{x}} - \mu^*}{\sigma_{\bar{x}}} \tag{8.1}$$

with μ denoting the mean that was used in computing the control limits, and μ^* denoting the mean after the mean shift. Here those two means are 0 and 1, respectively. We want the value of the Z-statistic to be such that $P(Z > Z_0) = .05$ since $1/.05 = 20$, the desired ARL for this mean shift. We can usually generally ignore the other tail of the standard normal distribution (i.e., the tail that is on the opposite side of the shift), as is being done here, because that will usually have no effect on the solution. Substituting the two mean values and $\sigma = 2$ into Eq. (8.1), we obtain

$$Z = \frac{0 + 3(2/\sqrt{n}) - 1}{2/\sqrt{n}}$$

$$= 3 - \frac{\sqrt{n}}{2}$$

Since we want $P(Z > Z_0) = .05$, it follows that $Z_0 = 1.645$. Thus, $1.645 = 3 - \sqrt{n/2}$, so that $\sqrt{n} = 2.710$ and $n = 7.34$. If we require that the in-control ARL be *at most* 20, we would round up to $n = 8$, which would give an ARL of 17.73, whereas $n = 7$ gives an ARL of 21.39. PASS follows this rule, which is quite reasonable and is in the same spirit as solving for a sample size such that the power is at least equal to the target value. That is, here the ARL is at least as desirable as the target value since the smaller a parameter-change ARL, the better.

8.1.2.2 S-Chart and S²-Chart

Now let's assume that a process standard deviation is being monitored, still assuming a normal distribution, and the objective is to detect an increase from 0.1 to 0.2 within 20 samples, so the target ARL is 20. When a two-sided S-chart with .00135 probability limits is specified, using PASS with 20,000 simulations results in $n = 2$ being selected, under the assumption of normality for the individual observations. [Note that it is much better to use an S-chart with probability limits than an S-chart with 3-sigma limits because there will be no lower control limit (LCL) when the subgroup size is less than 6.]

We could try to obtain an analytical solution as was done with an $\bar{X}$-chart, but we encounter problems immediately. To illustrate, when the individual observations have a normal distribution, $W = (n-1)s^2/\sigma^2$ has a χ^2 distribution with $(n-1)$ degrees of freedom, so that $\sqrt{W}$ has a chi distribution. The upper control limit for the S-chart using .00135 probability limits is

$$\text{UCL} = \sigma \sqrt{\frac{\chi^2_{.00135,n-1}}{n-1}}$$

Since the numerator is a function of n, it can't be specified without knowing n, which is what we are trying to solve for! (Of course, we encounter the same problem when the t-distribution is involved in sample size determination.) The necessary solution can be obtained numerically, but that won't be pursued here. If a numerical solution must be obtained, which might be difficult for many control chart users without experience in obtaining numerical solutions, then one might as well use software such as PASS and use its capability to solve for n using simulation.

Since the control chart capabilities in PASS are only in the latest release (PASS 11), it seems reasonable to assume that not very many control chart users have used PASS for determining control chart subgroup sizes. Therefore, it is of interest to see how well the sample size approximation for an S^2-chart given by Bonett and Al-Sunduqchi (1994) works, and especially how it works relative to PASS, which can be regarded as the gold standard provided that a very large number of simulations is used, which of course would be the case for any software that uses simulations.

The approximation that Bonett and Al-Sunduqchi (1994) stated as being the best is the average of n_1 and n_2, with n_1 given by

$$n_1 = \left(\frac{k^{1/2} Z_{\alpha/2} + \sigma Z_\beta}{Z_{p1}} \right)^2$$

with $Z_{p1} = 2^{1/2}|k^{1/2} - \sigma|$ and $\sigma^2 = k$ is the hypothesized value of σ^2, which for an S^2-chart or S-chart would be the in-control value of σ^2. As indicated by Bonett and Al-Sunduqchi (1994), this sample size expression results from a simple approximation given by Duncan (1986, p. 601). They stated that Duncan's approximation is very accurate when $\alpha = \beta$, but only when $\alpha = \beta$. This condition almost certainly will not be met when an S^2-chart or S-chart is used, however, because we want α to be very small, such as .0027 as when probability limits are used, and if $\beta = .0027$, then the power would be .9973—a much larger value than a practitioner would want to use as, in particular, an extremely large sample size would often be required. Furthermore, as Table 8.1 indicates, we don't need a large power value in order to have a very small and desirable ARL.

The expression for n_2 is

$$n_2 = \left(\frac{Z_{\alpha/2} + Z_\beta}{Z_{p2}} \right)^2$$

with $Z_{p2} = (|\ln(\sigma^2) - \ln(k)|)/2^{1/2}$. (It should be noted that although the title of their paper was on control charts, the methodology is presented as if the focus was on hypothesis testing. In particular, there is no mention of ARLs.)

■ **EXAMPLE 8.1**

Assume that the in-control value of σ^2 is 9, $\alpha = .0027$ (i.e., .00135 probability limits), we want to detect $\sigma^2 = 4$, as that would indicate significant improvement, and the desired power is .90. The value of n_1 is then

$$n_1 = \left[\frac{9^{1/2}3 + (2)(1.28)}{2^{1/2}} \right]^2$$
$$= 66.8$$

It can be shown that the value of $n_2 = 86.0$. Of course, no one is going to use subgroup sizes this large in practice. Since we know that n_1 should not be a good approximation to the necessary sample size, what should the ARL be if we use a sample size of 86? Not surprisingly, PASS gives the ARL and median run length as 1.0, using 20,000 simulations. Thus, these sample size formulas are actually for a one-sample hypothesis test of σ^2, not for an S^2-chart, despite the way that the material is presented by Bonett and Al-Sunduqchi (1994). That is, the sample size is being determined for immediate rejection of $\sigma^2 = 9$ when $\sigma^2 = 4$. That is not of any particular interest in quality control work because immediate detection of a change in any parameter is not necessary. Apparently Bonett and Al-Sunduqchi (1994) were not aware of the fact that control chart procedures are evaluated using ARL properties.

Castagliola, Celano, and Chen (2009) considered the properties of an S^2-chart when the in-control process variance is estimated and concluded that at least 200

Stage 1 samples are needed so that the S^2-chart will have properties similar to the properties in the known variance case. They also derived new control limits when a small number of Stage 1 samples are used.   ■

8.1.3   Attribute Control Charts

The situation with attribute charts is much different from the use of charts for measurement data (which are also called variables charts), because, for example, a large number of units of production might form a sample when nonconforming units are being charted, so the sample size may be in the hundreds, or even in the thousands.

The standard deviation of a sample proportion is a function of the sample size, so it would be preferable to think about detecting a specified change in the true (population) proportion, p, rather than thinking about detecting a change that is a function of $\sigma_{\hat{p}}$, the standard deviation of the sample proportion.

For example, since a p-chart should be used, in particular, to detect an improvement in product quality, we might want to detect a reduction in nonconforming (i.e., defective) items from, say, 2% to 1%. Of course, a control chart user might also be concerned about the possibility of p increasing to, say, .3, but the primary use of an attribute control chart should be to see if improvement is occurring, assuming that the quality has not already reached an acceptable level. Attribute charts simply provide a picture of quality over time; they can't be used to help identify problems that are causing quality to be less than desired.

A decision must be made regarding the form of the control limits. When p is approximately .01, the regression-based control limits of Ryan and Schwertman (1997) are superior to the customary use of 3-sigma limits since the use of the latter implies that the distribution of nonconforming units is approximately symmetric, which won't be the case when p is that small, regardless of the value of n. Those control limits for a p-chart are

$$\text{UCL} = 0.6195/n + 1.00523p + 2.983\sqrt{p/n}$$

$$\text{LCL} = 2.9529/n + 1.0195p - 3.2729\sqrt{p/n}$$

When p is assumed to be .02, for example, LCL $= 2.9529/n + 1.0195(.02) - 3.2729\sqrt{.02/n}$. Considering only the LCL for the moment, and assuming the desired power is .80, simply for illustration, we want

$$P(\hat{p} < 2.9529/n + 0.0204 - 0.4629/\sqrt{n} \mid p = .01) = .80 \qquad (8.2)$$

Note that Eq. (8.2) does not lend itself to an algebraic solution for n, which would have to be obtained iteratively.

Since the binomial distribution must be used directly, it would be preferable to convert Eq. (8.2) to a form corresponding to the number of nonconforming units being plotted rather than the proportion. That form, which is obtained by multiplying the inequality terms by n, is

$$P(\,X < 2.9529 + 0.0204n - 0.4629\sqrt{n}\,|\,p = .01) = .80 \qquad (8.3)$$

with $X \sim \text{Binomial}(n, .01)$ denoting the number of nonconforming units in a sample of size n. The iterative task can be simplified by starting with the solution obtained using available software, none of which uses the Ryan–Schwertman limits, but the solution should be a good starting point. The solution obtained using PASS is $n = 2460$ if we let $\alpha = .00135$. Substituting $n = 2460$ into Eq. (8.2) and solving for X produces $X = 30.18$. Since $P\,(X \le 30|\,n = 2460$ and $p = .01) = .8819$, this is not the solution for n that satisfies Eq. (8.2), although it is at least in the ballpark, as expected. [It should also be noted that $P(X \le 29|\,n = 2460$ and $p = .01) = .8401$, with 29 being the largest value of X that corresponds to a power of at least .80, so Eq. (8.2) misses the value of X by one unit for this example.]

Since there is apparently no software that uses the Ryan–Schwertman control limits, there is thus no software that can be used to solve for n given an initial starting value. It is not difficult to solve iteratively for n, however, such that Eq. (8.2) is satisfied. Using guided trial and error, if $n = 2165$, the LCL $= 25.58$ (giving a lower tail area of .00169), and $P(X \le 25|\,n = 2165$ and $p = .01) = .800469$. Thus, with the Ryan–Schwertman approach, a sample size of $n = 2165$ could be used and it can be noted that this time the use of Eq. (8.2) to solve for X does give the correct value as the solution is $X = 25.58$, so that the LCL expressed in terms of X is $X = 26$. Note also that this gives the *actual* power here, conditioned on the assumed value of p, because the power is computed using the binomial distribution. (It should be noted that the Ryan–Schwertman approach was not intended to be used to determine sample size, however.)

This might seem like a very large sample size, but if p is small, a large sample would have to be used in order to observe any nonconforming units. This is not built into any sample size determination algorithm in software, but it is an important consideration when the control chart is used. For example, if $p = .001$, many samples of $n = 1000$ would not have any nonconforming units.

There is not much chance that a sample of size $n = 2165$ would be devoid of nonconforming units if $p = .01$, however, since the expected number of nonconforming units is 21.65. Therefore, it isn't necessary to use this large a sample in order to virtually ensure that some nonconforming units will be present. Furthermore, we don't need power as large as .80, since that would produce ARL $= 1/.80 = 1.25$. Although it would certainly be desirable to detect a 50% reduction in the true proportion this quickly, quality practitioners would almost certainly prefer slower detection and a smaller sample size.

It should be noted that samples are obtained repeatedly when control charts are used, so sample size considerations that are made when a single hypothesis test is to be performed do not apply to control charts.

Therefore, let's now assume that power of .20 would be acceptable, which would produce an ARL of 5. Unfortunately, using "Tests for One Proportion (Proportions)" in PASS won't work because when a power is less than .50, PASS uses 1 minus the specified power, and the same thing happens with the other PASS routines for proportions. MINITAB cannot be used to determine sample size for a p-chart in quality improvement work using the binomial distribution because it uses a normal approximation in its hypothesis testing for proportions, but that won't work when p is small. The use of nQuery, which uses the exact binomial test, shows a power of .2008 for $n = 905$, this apparently being as close as one can come to .20 and still be at least .20, this result being obtained through trial and error because in nQuery it is not possible to solve for the sample size for a stated value of the power in testing a proportion. Since the expected number of nonconforming units is 9.05 for a sample of this size, the sample size should be adequate.

Thus, if we lower the power substantially so as to produce a slightly larger ARL value, the sample size can be reduced considerably.

This approach can be compared with the methods discussed by Morris and Riddle (2008), although they gave only a lower bound on sample size for each of the methods that they presented and they did not consider hypothesis testing or changes in the value of p. Instead, they concentrated on the sample size necessary to make the probability of zero nonconforming units in a sample correspond to the probability that $Z \leq -3$, with $Z \sim N(0, 1)$. In other words, they appropriately focused on the use of a p-chart to detect quality improvement, with the latter detectable by having a LCL with the lower tail area being approximately what it would be for a chart with 3σ limits under the assumption of normality.

Morris and Riddle (2008) presented four methods, the first of which was based on the normal approximation to the binomial distribution, and they gave a lower bound for n, which was $n \geq 9(1-p)/p$. That isn't quite right, however, because it can easily be shown that the LCL on both a p-chart and an np-chart with 3σ limits will be zero when $n = 9(1-p)/p$. Zero cannot be a LCL because the definition of a LCL is that it is a value below which a plotted point can fall. So the lower bound on n in order for the LCL to exist is $n > 9(1-p)/p$.

The normal approximation won't work well at all when p is quite small, however, as was demonstrated by Ryan (2011, Chapter 8). (Of course, in quality improvement applications we hope that p is indeed very small!) Recognizing this shortcoming, Morris and Riddle (2008) presented the minimum sample size for the modified p-chart given by Winterbottom (1993), although they again erred slightly in giving the minimum sample size such that the LCL could be zero. Another approach that they gave was to determine the minimum sample size by working directly with the binomial distribution, which leads to the well-known result $n > \log(.00135)/\log(1-p)$, which results from setting $P(X=0)$ to .00135, which is reasonable when p is very small. The other method that they gave was a rule-of-thumb based on the Poisson approximation to the binomial distribution, which was $n \geq 6.608/p$. They stated that it is better to use $n \geq 6.6/p$ when $p \geq 0025$. That rule-of-thumb won't work for a chart with 3σ limits, however, because the requirement that $n > 9(1-p)/p$ is not met when $p = .01$, for example, so there would not be a LCL.

Of the four methods that they presented, the authors indicated their preference for determining the minimum sample size directly from the binomial distribution.

Yang, Xie, Kuralmani, and Tsui (2002) considered the determination of sample size for a geometric chart, which is an alternative to a p-chart when p is extremely small (such as .001), as then no method of determining the LCL for a p-chart will result in the chart having satisfactory properties.

Nomograms are also available for determining sample sizes, but these of course are for a specific form of a hypothesis test statistic and, more specifically, standard forms. Many such nomograms are given by Brush (1988).

8.1.4 CUSUM and EWMA Charts

CUSUM and EWMA charts are alternatives to the use of Shewhart charts and differ from those charts in the sense that data are accumulated over time and used in computing the value of each statistic at each point in time, whereas with a Shewhart chart only the data at each point in time are used when a chart is constructed. The name "CUSUM" reflects the nature of the chart, as the acronym stands for "cumulative sum" chart, whereas "EWMA" stands for "exponentially weighted moving average" chart.

Both types of charts use recent data in addition to the current data, but they do so in different ways. A basic CUSUM scheme employs two cumulative sums

$$S_{H_i} = \max[0, (Z_i - k) + S_{H_{i-1}}] \qquad S_{Li} = \min[0, (Z_i + k) + S_{Li-1}]$$

with i denoting the current subgroup or individual observation and Z_i is the "Z-score" as used in introductory statistics courses (i.e., it is the number of standard deviation units that the subgroup mean or individual observation is from the assumed mean), and as used in Section 2.1. The first cumulative sum is for detecting mean increases and the second is for detecting mean decreases. The value of k is chosen to be one-half the mean shift, in standard deviation units, that one wishes to quickly detect. Thus, if the focus is on quickly detecting a one-sigma shift, then k would be set to 0.5. There are variations of the basic CUSUM, but those will not be discussed here. See Ryan (2011, Chapter 8).

An exponentially weighted moving average (EWMA) chart weights data based on their proximity to the current point in time. The weighting, when subgroup averages are used, is done as

$$w_t = \lambda \bar{x}_t + (1 - \lambda) w_{t-1} \tag{8.4}$$

with λ the weight applied to the current subgroup average (i.e., at time "t"), with w_{t-1} denoting the value of the EWMA statistic at the previous time period.

Both types of charts can be used either with individual observations or with subgroups, as indicated previously.

8.1.4.1 Subgroup Size Considerations for CUSUM Charts

When used with subgroups, the CUSUM user can determine a reasonable subgroup size by looking at the ARLs for various subgroup sizes. These are given in Table 8.2 for a basic CUSUM for the same range of possible subgroup sizes as was used in Table 8.1.

The ARL values in parentheses are the ones obtained using the getarl .exe program of Professsor Doug Hawkins, which can be accessed at ftp://ftp.stat.umn.edu/pub/cusum. Those ARL values are computed analytically and note the almost exact agreement between the simulated values using PASS and the analytical values, as would be expected when 50,000 simulations are used. (PASS can be used to solve for either the subgroup size or the run length distribution. The former is illustrated in Table 8.4 in Section 8.1.4.3.) It should also be noted that these are "zero start" ARLs; that is, the CUSUM values for S_H and S_L are assumed to equal zero at the time that the shift occurs. Of course, the values won't necessarily be zero and Hawkins's applet additionally shows the

Table 8.2 ARL for Detecting a 1σ Upward Mean Shift with a Basic CUSUM Chart with Subgroup Size n ($k = 0.5, h = 5$), Using PASS with 50,000 Simulations

n	ARL	Median RL	Value of a in $a\,\sigma_{\bar{x}}$ Mean Change
1	10.39 (10.38)	9.00	1.00
2	6.23 (6.22)	6.00	1.41
3	4.79 (4.78)	4.00	1.73
4	4.01 (4.01)	4.00	2.00
5	3.52 (3.52)	3.00	2.24
6	3.18 (3.18)	3.00	2.45
7	2.93 (2.93)	3.00	2.65
8	2.73 (2.73)	3.00	2.83
9	2.57 (2.57)	2.00	3.00
10	2.45 (2.44)	2.00	3.16

"steady state ARL," which is obtained after the CUSUM has been running and reached a "steady state" and is lower than the zero start ARL. Although PASS has some CUSUM options, it does not give steady state ARLs, so a comparison with the results of Hawkins's applet thus cannot be made for steady state ARLs.

The purpose of the last column is to show the magnitude of the mean shift in units of multiples of $\sigma_{\bar{x}}$ such that the upward mean shift equals $\mu + \sigma_x$, as stated. because this is how the shift is customarily given in research papers on CUSUM procedures and SPC books. In particular, this facilitates comparison with tabular values for the integer values of $a = 1, 2$, and 3 that are given in such sources and there is agreement for those values. The numbers in that column show that most of the mean shifts in the table are large ones in terms of $\sigma_{\bar{x}}$, so the corresponding ARL values are small.

Comparing Table 8.2 with Table 8.1, note that an $\bar{X}$-chart is more powerful than the Basic CUSUM once the sample size reaches 5. It is well-known that the $\bar{X}$-chart is more powerful than the Basic CUSUM at detecting large shifts, and by fixing the shift at σ, as is done here, rather than in terms of $\sigma_{\bar{x}}$ as is usually done, the shift relative to $\sigma_{\bar{x}}$ is thus increasing relative to the latter as n increases since $\sigma_{\bar{x}}$ decreases as n increases. So, viewed in this way, the shift is becoming "larger." For example, for a $3\sigma_{\bar{x}}$ upward shift in the mean, the ARL for the $\bar{X}$-chart is 2.0 since the probability of a point plotting above the UCL is .5, since the distribution with the new mean is centered at the UCL. This is less than the ARL for a Basic CUSUM for that shift, which is 2.57.

8.1.4.2 CUSUM and EWMA Variations

There are variations of Basic CUSUM and EWMA charts that, for example, try to capture the value of an $\bar{X}$-chart for detecting large mean shifts. This is accomplished by adding Shewhart-type limits, with the resultant charts being called Shewhart–CUSUM and Shewhart–EWMA charts, respectively. PASS will determine sample size for Shewhart–CUSUM and Shewhart–EWMA charts, as well as a fast initial response (FIR) CUSUM, which is protection against all of the assignable causes possibly not removed after a process is stopped and the search for assignable causes initiated. The sample size for each type of chart is determined using simulation.

8.1.4.3 Subgroup Size Determination for CUSUM and EWMA Charts and Their Variations

For an EWMA chart, the tables of Lucas and Saccucci (1990) can be used to select the subgroup size, the value of λ [in Eq. (8.4)], and the value of L for L-sigma control limits. Alternatively, PASS could be used to determine subgroup size and in general to design an EWMA chart. This can be illustrated and discussed relative to the Lucas and Saccucci (1990) tables, as follows. A small value of λ is often recommended and expanded tables beyond those given in Lucas and Saccucci (1990) suggest that a reasonable combination is $L = 3.00$ and $\lambda = .25$.

**Table 8.3   ARL for Detecting a 1σ Upward Mean Shift with a
Basic EWMA Chart with Subgroup size n ($L = 3.00$, $\lambda = .25$),
Using PASS with 200,000 Simulations**

n	ARL	Median RL	Value of a in $a\,\sigma_{\bar{x}}$ Mean Change
1	10.40	8.00	1.00
2	5.31	5.00	1.41
3	3.71	3.00	1.73
4	2.94	3.00	2.00
5	2.47	2.00	2.24
6	2.15	2.00	2.45
7	1.92	2.00	2.65
8	1.75	2.00	2.83
9	1.61	1.00	3.00
10	1.51	1.00	3.16

As in Table 8.2, we will assume a 1σ increase in the population mean and will look at ARLs for the same values of n (see Table 8.3).

It is of interest to run PASS and see what sample size it selects for each of these charts. Following Ryan (2011, p. 275), we will assume Shewhart limits of 3.7σ for the Shewhart–CUSUM chart (and also for the Shewhart–EWMA chart), with $h = 5.2$ and the headstart value for FIR CUSUM then $5.2/2 = 2.6$. The results are given in Table 8.4.

Jones, Champ, and Rigdon (2001) examined the properties of an EWMA chart with estimated parameters. One of their conclusions was that the effect of estimating σ was most pronounced when λ was small. In particular, they stated that when $\lambda = .1$, 400 samples of size 5 in Stage 1 are needed to achieve the same in-control performance as in the parameter known case. Jones et al. (2001) obtained their results analytically but we can, of course, also obtain the results by simulations in PASS. For example, when the mean and variance are estimated using 250 samples of size 5 and the EWMA chart parameters are $L = 3$ and

**Table 8.4   Subgroup Sizes and ARLs for Basic CUSUM and EWMA
Charts and Their Variations, Using PASS with 50,000 Simulations
and a Target ARL of 3.0 for Detecting a 1σ Mean Shift**

Chart Type	Sample Size	ARL
CUSUM	8	2.815
Shewhart–CUSUM	7	2.786
FIR CUSUM	3	2.873
EWMA	4	2.916
Shewhart–EWMA	4	2.939

$\lambda = .1$, the ARL for detecting a 1σ mean shift is 2.448 using 20,000 simulations. When the parameters are assumed to be known, the ARL is 2.446. Thus, the ARLs are essentially the same, as expected because of the number of samples that were used. (The results should be virtually the same with a larger number of simulations.) When only 40 preliminary samples are used, however, the ARL is 2.46 for the 20,000 simulations, thus showing a 0.57% ARL inflation. It is much worse when only 20 preliminary samples are used, as then the ARL is 2.513, which is a 2.7% inflation, and the ARL is 2.576 when only 10 preliminary samples of size 5 are used, again when 20,000 simulations are used (and 2.595 using 100,000 simulations). Practitioners may not be overly concerned about these differences, however.

8.1.4.4 EWMA Applied to Autocorrelated Data
Autocorrelated data frequently occur in practice and Lu and Reynolds (1999) briefly considered the number of observations that are needed for parameter estimation. They concluded that values of 100 or less that are typically used in applications are much too small and that the number "should be larger by an order of magnitude." Köksal, Kantar, Ula, and Testik (2008) also considered EWMA and other types of charts applied to autocorrelated data and addressed the question of how large the Stage 1 sample size should be for effective process monitoring in Stage 2.

8.1.5 Adaptive Control Charts

It was stated in Chapter 7 that adaptive clinical trials have become popular. The same general concept can be applied to control charts. That is, the sample size and sampling interval can be variable rather than fixed and be determined by recent control chart results. For example, if a process has stabilized and out-of-control conditions are very rare, there is no point in collecting data as frequently as data were collected when the process was not doing very well. There has been a moderate amount of research on designing control charts with variable sample size and variable sampling interval. Included in this category are papers by Wu and Luo (2004), Wu, Zhang, and Wang (2007), Tseng, Tang, and Lin (2007), Jensen, Bryce, and Reynolds (2008), and Zhou, Wang, and Li (2009). Jensen et al. (2008) recommended that adaptive control charts be used for "mature processes." Certainly, that is good advice as processes should be stable and have a recent history of stability so that their performance is fairly predictable.

8.1.6 Regression and Cause-Selecting Control Charts

A regression control chart was proposed by Mandel (1969) and is used for testing a process or product characteristic that naturally changes over time, but might change at an unexpectedly fast rate and thus be out of control. An example would be tool wear. Tools wear out but the wear at any point in time should be within expected limits.

The concept is similar to a prediction interval in simple linear regression, whose width depends partly on the sample size. Specifically, the centerline on the chart is at $\hat{Y} = \hat{\beta}_0 + \hat{\beta}_1 X$ and the control limits are given by $\hat{Y} \pm 2s$, rather than from

$$\hat{Y} + 2s \sqrt{1 + \frac{1}{n} + \frac{(X_0 - \bar{X})^2}{\sum (X - \bar{X})^2}}$$

which would seem to be the natural choice for obtaining the control limits. The argument given by Mandel (1969) is that the use of control limits obtained from $\hat{Y} \pm 2s$ will provide tighter control for extreme values of X_0, which is where tight control is generally desired. Thus, Y is controlled through $\hat{Y}$. Since the control limits are not a direct function of n, general guidelines, such as the 10:1 rough rule-of-thumb proposed by Draper and Smith (1998), could be employed to determine the sample size.

A cause-selecting control chart is similar to a regression control chart, with the former used to distinguish between quality problems that occur in one stage of a process from quality problems that occur at a previous stage. Letting Y denote the output from the "current" stage and X denote the output from the previous stage, Zhang (1984, 1985) termed a plot of the standardized residuals of Y on X a cause-selecting control chart. Since a residual that is outside the control limits could signify that either Y or X is out of control, or both, a control chart on X would be maintained to check on the control of X. As recommended by Ryan (2011, p. 420), the control limits for X should be constructed as $\bar{x} \pm 3s_x/c_4$ for Stage 2. Although c_4 is a function of n, the values of c_4 are almost constant in the neighborhood of sample sizes that are likely to be used. Therefore, sample sizes that are used should be determined by rules-of-thumb such as the one given at the beginning of this section.

Kim, Mahmoud, and Woodall (2003) proposed a method for monitoring a linear regression equation in Stage 2 (Phase 2, in their terminology) that utilized three separate EWMA charts: one for the Y-intercept, one for the slope, and one for the error variance. They did not address the sample size that should be used, however. Although an EWMA chart applied to data in subgroups would generally have the same subgroup size as an $\bar{X}$-chart, that won't work for monitoring a linear profile because it would be undesirable to try to estimate three parameters—β_0, β_1, and σ_ϵ^2 (the variance error) using only 4 or 5 observations. Therefore, even though subgroups would be obtained with the same frequency as when an $\bar{X}$-chart is used, it would be desirable to use a subgroup size of approximately 10 so that the estimates of the three parameters would not have a large sampling variability.

Although the control limits recommended by Kim et al. (2003) for monitoring β_0 and σ_ϵ^2 are a function of the subgroup size, this is not the case for the EWMA chart for monitoring β_1 since the variance of $\hat{\beta}_1$ is not a function of the sample size. Whether the control limits reflect the sample size or not, it is desirable to use enough observations to estimate the parameters so that the sampling variability will not be excessive and the performance of the chart will not have unacceptable variability.

This issue has apparently not been addressed in the quality improvement literature and the problem is bypassed by selecting a value for L with L-sigma limits such that the in-control ARL is acceptable.

8.1.7 Multivariate Control Charts

Multivariate analogues to the univariate control charts that have been presented in this chapter have been given in the literature, but unfortunately there is apparently no software that can be used to determine subgroup size for a multivariate chart for subgroup averages, or to solve for sample size for a multivariate attributes chart. Therefore, guidance must come from the literature.

Champ, Jones-Farmer, and Rigdon (2005) studied the properties of a T^2 control chart and gave their recommendations for the amount of historical data to use for parameter estimation in Stage 1, in addition to the subgroup size for Stage 2. One of their recommendations is that the subgroup size should move in the opposite direction as the number of variables used in a T^2 control chart, so that the subgroup size needed to achieve desired performance decreases as the number of variables increases.

They also pointed out that when parameters are estimated (which of course will almost always be the case), the T^2 control chart, which has only a UCL, will not have an in-control ARL of $1/\alpha$ when the mean vector and covariance matrix are estimated, with the UCL given as

$$\text{UCL} = \frac{p\,(m+1)\,(n-1)}{m\,(n-1)+1-p} F_{1-\alpha,\,p,\,mn-m-p+1}$$

with p denoting the number of variables, m the number of subgroups, and n the subgroup size, and $F_{1-\alpha,\,p,\,mn-m-p+1}$ is the $(1-\alpha)$ percentile of the F-distribution with p and $(mn-m-p+1)$ degrees of freedom.

In particular, their Table 1 gave in-control ARL values when the parameters were estimated using $m = 50$ subgroups of size $n = 5$. The ARLs ranged from 11% higher than the in-control ARL assuming known parameter values when $p = 10$ to 17% higher when $p = 2$. A somewhat nonintuitive result from their research was their statement that the out-of-control performance of the T^2-chart depends only on the "statistical distance between the in-control and out-of-control mean vectors" and thus does not depend on their parameter values or their estimates, and thus must also not depend on the sample size. This is true provided that the control limit is adjusted so that the in-control ARL with the adjusted limit matches the in-control ARL for the standard limit based on the assumption of known parameter values.

Therefore, they focused attention on the number of subgroups and subgroup size that should be used for a given number of variables so that the in-control ARL differs from the theoretical in-control ARL by a specified percentage and provided graphs that users could utilize in designing a T^2 control chart. For example, let p = the number of variables, m = number of subgroups, and n = subgroup size. For $p = 10$, they recommended $mn > 550$, if the goal is to have the in-control ARL no more than 5% higher than the desired ARL of 200. As they stated, this might consist of 110 subgroups of size 5. Their recommendations for other numbers of variables monitored by the chart were given in their Table 3. Specifically, they recommended sample sizes greater than 900, 700, 650, and 600 for $p = 2, 4, 6$, and 8, respectively.

Champ et al. (2005) stated that their sample size recommendations call for the use of a larger amount of data than do the recommendations of Lowry and Montgomery (1995) and Nedumaran and Pignatiello (1999), and they explain that is due to goals being different.

8.2 MEDICAL APPLICATIONS

Certain applications, such as medical applications, present special challenges and problems that do not exist in manufacturing applications. For example, whereas a decision could be made to chart the average diameter of five ball bearings every 15 minutes when thousands are rolling off an assembly line every hour, it certainly would not be possible to chart the average of some characteristic relating to coronary bypass operations every 15 minutes, as the operations almost certainly would not be performed at virtually the same time. Therefore, as Shahian, Williamson, Svensson, Restuccia, and D'Agostino (1996) discussed, it is more convenient to analyze the patients on a time interval, such as a week, month, or quarter. This will invariably result in a varying sample size and the term "subgroup" is not particularly applicable since the measurements are not being made close together in time, although the authors did use that term, while recognizing that measurements should be made close enough together in time so that conditions are uniform. The authors stated: "In the instance of cardiac surgical morbidity and mortality, which ranges from 2% to 5% for most adverse outcomes, a subgroup size of 50 to 100 patients would be desirable." This led them to choose quarterly reporting of data.

The authors also stated that for subgroup sizes greater than nine, an S-chart (a chart of subgroup standard deviations) should be used instead of an R-chart (a chart of subgroup ranges). So here a decision is being made as to what chart to use or recommend based on the subgroup size. This illustrates some "suboptimal thinking" because an S-chart should be used for any subgroup size, with the two charts being equivalent when the subgroup size is two. When the subgroup size is greater than two, all of the data are not being used in calculating the range since the range is the largest value minus the smallest value. Efficiency is lost—with any statistical procedure—when data that have been recorded are not used. There is also a problem with the acceptable minimum number of subgroups that they mention, as they state the minimum as being 10. The minimum should depend on the subgroup size, as the total number of observations should be at least 100. In their case, they used 17 consecutive quarters, so more than enough data were used in determining control limits. Of course, many changes in conditions could occur over such a long period of time. They obviously recognized this possibility in stating that any changes in the patient population, staff, procedures, or equipment should be noted.

It is not clear from their article whether they are distinguishing between Stage 1 and Stage 2, however, and this is true of many articles on control charts in the applied literature.

Unfortunately, there have been many applications of control charts in which the number of observations used to determine the control limits is far less than desirable. For example, Mohammed, Worthington, and Woodall (2008) cited Carey (2003) as stating that at least 20–25 observations are needed to compute the control limits for an X-MR chart, which is a combined chart of individual observations and moving ranges. As indicated in Section 8.1.1, that is far less than the number of observations that should be used.

8.3 PROCESS CAPABILITY INDICES

Process capability indices are used to determine how well a process performs relative to engineering tolerances. Many such indices have been proposed during the past 25 years and no attempt will be made to review them here, other than to state that improved indices appeared starting in the mid-1980s and on through the 1990s. These indices were superior to the most frequently used index during the early 1980s, which was $C_p = (\text{USL} - \text{LSL})/6\sigma$, with USL and LSL denoting the upper specification limit and the lower specification limit, respectively. This index was of limited value because it was not a function of the process mean. A better capability index is C_{pk}, which is defined as $C_{pk} = \frac{1}{3}Z_{\min}$, with $Z_{\min}$ defined as the minimum of $Z_1 = (\text{USL} - \mu)/\sigma$ and $Z_2 = (\mu - \text{LSL})/\sigma$. C_{pk} is thus a function of a z-score, and if USL and LSL are a large distance from μ, relative to σ, so as to make Z_1 and Z_2 large, estimating C_{pk} is then almost like estimating an extreme percentile of a distribution, which generally requires thousands of observations. Here μ and σ are being estimated, however, not a percentile, but the effect is similar since, for example, if $(USL - \mu)$ is large, misestimation of σ by a large percentage amount could have a sizable effect on the Z-score.

The reader interested in a detailed presentation of process capability indices is referred to Pearn and Kotz (2006), Kotz and Lovelace (1998), and Kotz and Johnson (1993).

Process capability indices must be estimated, so the necessary sample size for such estimation must be addressed. The following statements are made at `http://www.itl.nist.gov/div898/handbook/pmc/section1/pmc16.htm`: "Most capability indices estimates are valid only if the sample size used is 'large enough.' Large enough is generally thought to be about 50 independent data values." Most capability indices assume a normal distribution and the indices are sensitive to that assumption. It would be preferable to have somewhat more than 50 observations to test the normality assumption. Of course, "power" is not relevant here, because nothing is changing (presumably), so it is not a matter of having a large enough sample size to detect a change quickly. Instead, the objective should be to use a large enough sample so that a good picture of the present can be obtained. Sample size determination for one of the process capability indices, C_{pm}, has been considered by Zimmer, Hubele, and Zimmer (2001). See also Pearn and Shu (2003) and Shu and Wang (2006), as the latter reviewed existing formulas for the lower confidence bounds of certain process capability indices and proposed a new approach for sample size determination for C_p and C_{pm}.

8.4 TOLERANCE INTERVALS

The most commonly used type of tolerance interval is an interval on population values that a user can state, with a specified degree of confidence, will contain at least a certain proportion of population values. A lesser-known type of tolerance interval is one that contains at least a certain proportion of the center of the population with a specified degree of confidence, which is usually referred to as an equal-tailed tolerance interval (Krishnamoorthy and Mathew, 2009, p. 4).

Tolerance intervals are used in engineering statistics and in quality improvement work. Interest in determining sample size for tolerance intervals dates at least from the work of Wilks (1941), who presented both a nonparametric approach and a method based on the assumption of a normal distribution. With the former it was a matter of determining how large a sample should be so that the largest and smallest sample values can form the tolerance interval.

Of course, there has been much research work on tolerance intervals since 1941 and, for example, Chapter 9 of Hahn and Meeker (1991) is a 37-page chapter entitled "Sample Size Requirements for Tolerance Intervals, Tolerance Bounds, and Demonstration Tests," although the chapter consists almost entirely of nomograms.

The term "tolerance interval" has been used in a potentially confusing way in some places. For example, the Power and Precision software gives a "Tolerance Interval for the 95%, 1-tailed Confidence Interval" for the *t*-test option where the parameters are being estimated. First, there is no such thing as a one-tailed confidence interval, as one of the endpoints is either plus infinity or minus infinity, so we cannot have a finite confidence *interval*. The appropriate term is "confidence bound" or perhaps "confidence limit." This is a somewhat common error, however.

Second, the terms "tolerance interval" and "confidence interval" should not be used in the same expression, as they are totally different. The Power and Precision software is simply indicating a range for the confidence intervals that would occur with repeated sampling. Although that is certainly of some interest as an aid in understanding confidence interval variability, only one sample is generally taken.

What the two types of intervals do have in common is that their width is a direct function of the variability of the estimator of σ, as *s* is used in constructing a tolerance interval just as it is used in constructing a confidence interval for the mean of a normal distribution. Specifically, the tolerance interval is $\bar{x} \pm ks$ if the interval is to be symmetric about $\bar{x}$, with *k* chosen from a table to give the desired coverage probability with the desired degree of confidence. Thus, since the expression for the endpoints of the interval is not a function of *n*, we can't use the expression to solve for *n*.

The situation is different for a nonparametric tolerance interval, as there the objective is to take a large enough sample so that, for example, the largest and smallest observations in the sample can form the tolerance interval. Algorithms for determining sample size for this purpose date from at least Brooker and Shelby (1975), although the latter does not guarantee approximately equal tail probabilities, whereas the approach of Neave (1978) does so, as well as the tolerance interval approach given by Chou and Mee (1984). See also Chou and Johnson (1987), who gave tables of minimum sample sizes. See also the tables of sample sizes for normality-based and nonparametric tolerance intervals given by Kirkpatrick (1977). Another excellent source is Odeh and Owen (1980) but that book has been out of print for many years.

Although tolerance intervals are generally either based on the assumption of normality or else are nonparametric tolerance intervals, Chen and Yang (1999) gave Monte Carlo algorithms for estimating the sample size and coverage for tolerance intervals for nonnormal distributions.

A two-sided β-expectation tolerance interval is defined (see, e.g., Mee, 1984) in the following way for a normally distributed random variable, *X*: $E_{\hat{\mu}\hat{\sigma}}\{P_x[\hat{\mu} - k\hat{\sigma} < X < \hat{\mu} + k\hat{\sigma}|\hat{\mu}, \hat{\sigma}]\} = \beta$. In words, the expectation of the tolerance interval with endpoints $\hat{\mu} - k\hat{\sigma}$ and $\hat{\mu} + k\hat{\sigma}$ is β, so on average the coverage is β. There is no guarantee about the coverage in each tail of the distribution but Chou (1984) went a step further and determined sample sizes for β-expectation tolerance intervals that control the proportion in each tail of a normal distribution. Odeh, Chou, and Owen (1989) explained the difference between a β-expectation tolerance interval and a β-content tolerance interval, with the latter constructed to contain at least $100\beta\%$ of the population with a stated degree of confidence. This is the most frequently used of the two types.

Fountain and Chou (1991) determined minimum sample sizes for two-sided β-content tolerance intervals. This type of tolerance interval differs from a β-expectation tolerance interval in that it is defined as $P_{\hat{\mu}\hat{\sigma}}\{P_x[\hat{\mu} - k\hat{\sigma} < X < \hat{\mu} + k\hat{\sigma} \mid \hat{\mu}, \hat{\sigma}]\} \geq \beta$ for some confidence coefficient γ.

Early work on sample size determination for tolerance limits includes Faulkenberry and Weeks (1968) and Faulkenberry and Daly (1970). See also Sa and Razaila (2004), who proposed an algorithm for constructing one-sided tolerance limits continuously over time for any distribution. They showed that the sample size required by their method is reduced over time. Wang and Tsung (2009) considered tolerance intervals for binomial and Poisson random variables and proposed procedures for calculating the minimum and average coverage probabilities.

8.5 MEASUREMENT SYSTEM APPRAISAL

Measurement variability consists of variability due to materials and people, such as parts and operators. Variance components are estimated (such as σ_{parts}^2) and enough observations must be used in order to obtain good estimates of those components. When used in measurement system appraisal this is called a Gauge R and R study, with the two Rs representing "reproducibility" and "repeatability," respectively.

Confidence intervals are often constructed for variance components and a desired maximum width of such intervals might be specified, which would lead to sample size determination. Readers interested in more information about confidence intervals for variance components are referred to Burdick and Larsen (1997). Their general recommendation is that it is important to obtain enough samples and operators, these being more important than replicates. Specifically, they stated that 10 samples, 3 operators, and 3 replicates is typical in published Gauge R and R studies.

8.6 ACCEPTANCE SAMPLING

Sample size determination is covered briefly here (and deliberately placed at the end of the chapter) because some practitioners still use it, not because it has any particular value relative to the current quality objectives of most organizations. As the prominent industrial statistician Harold F. Dodge (1893–1976) stated decades ago: "You can't inspect quality into a product."

Although tables have long been used to determine how many items to inspect and the criteria used to determine when to accept or reject a lot (such as the charts in Hahn, 1974), software can of course also be used for this purpose. STATGRAPHICS is one such software package, as it can be used for acceptance sampling with measurement data and for attribute data. These methods have historically been referred to as acceptance sampling for variables and acceptance sampling for attributes, respectively.

MINITAB can also be used to determine a sample size and sampling plan. To illustrate sample size determination for Acceptance Sampling by Variables, assume that the lot size is 25,000 units, the producer's risk (α) is to be .05; the consumer's risk (β) is set at .10; the acceptable quality level (AQL) in terms of nonconforming units per million is 10 and the rejectable quality level (RQL) is 50 nonconforming units per million. The USL is 100 and the LSL is 50. The necessary sample size given by MINITAB is 564. MINITAB could also be used to determine a sample size and sampling plan for Acceptance Sampling by Attributes.

Hauck and Shaikh (2001) stated that one approach employed in the pharmaceutical industry is to use a two-sided tolerance interval and accept a given batch if the tolerance interval falls entirely within an acceptance interval. They addressed the problem of determining power and sample size for such an approach.

8.7   RELIABILITY AND LIFE TESTING

Product reliability is also an important part of quality and quality improvement. Moura (1991) is a compact source of information on sample size determination for accelerated life testing, and Chapter 9 of Mathews (2010) contains some information on sample size determination for reliability. The Weibull probability distribution has historically played a key role in reliability analysis. Jeng (2003) gave a sample size determination approach that was based on a combination of simulation and asymptotic theory for a Weibull test plan when there is complete data or time censored data.

Since reliability is the industrial counterpart to survival analysis, reliability is also discussed briefly in Section 9.2.

8.8   SOFTWARE

Unfortunately, software developers in general have not focused attention on sample size determination for the tools that were presented in this chapter, with PASS being the most useful software and MINITAB having value in designing acceptance sampling schemes.

8.9 SUMMARY

Although control chart users have not concentrated on subgroup (sample) size determination, that doesn't mean that it shouldn't be done. Certainly, determining the amount of data to use for parameter estimation in Stage 1 is extremely important. The need for sample size determination in Stage 2 is lessened somewhat, however, by the fact that control chart usage is a continuous process, whereas hypothesis testing in general is not. Sample size determination has always been important in acceptance sampling, however, and in tolerance interval construction.

REFERENCES

Bonett, D. G. an M. S. Al-Sunduqchi (1994). Approximating sample size requirements for s^2 charts. *Journal of Applied Statistics*, **21**(5), 425–429.

Brooker, P. and M. J. P. Shelby (1975). Algorithm AS 92: The sample size for a distribution free tolerance interval. *Applied Statistics*, **24**, 388–390.

Brush, G. G. (1988). *How to Choose the Proper Sample Size*. Milwaukee, WI: American Society for Quality Control.

Burdick, R. K. and G. A. Larsen (1997). Confidence intervals on measures of variability in *R&R* studies. *Journal of Quality Technology*, **29**(3), 261–273.

Carey, R. G. (2003). *Improving Health Care with Control Charts: Basic and Advanced SPC Methods and Case Studies*. Milwaukee, WI: Quality Press.

Castagliola, P., G. Celano, and G. Chen (2009). The exact run length distribution and design of the S^2 chart when the in-control variance is estimated. *International Journal of Reliability, Quality, and Safety Engineering*, **16**(1), 23–28.

Champ, C. W., L. A. Jones-Farmer, and S. E. Rigdon (2005). Properties of the T^2 control chart when parameters are estimated. *Technometrics*, **47**(4), 437–445.

Chen, H. and T.-K. Yang (1999). Computation of the sample size and coverage for guaranteed-coverage nonnormal tolerance intervals. *Journal of Statistical Computation and Simulation*, **63**, 299–320.

Chou, Y. M. (1984). Sample sizes for β-expectation tolerance limits which control both tails of the normal distribution. *Naval Research Logistics Quarterly*, **31**(4), 601–607.

Chou, Y.-M. and G. M. Johnson (1987). Sample sizes for strong two-sided distribution-free tolerance intervals. *Statistical Papers*, **28**, 117–131.

Chou, Y.-M. and R. W. Mee (1984). Determination of sample sizes for setting β-content tolerance intervals controlling both tails of the normal distributions. *Statistics and Probability Letters*, **2**, 311–314.

Cryer, J. D. and T. P. Ryan (1990). Estimation of sigma for an X chart: $\overline{MR}/d_2$ or S/c_4? *Journal of Quality Technology*, **22**, 187–192.

Dockendorf, L. (1992). Choosing appropriate sample subgroup sizes for control charts. *Quality Progress*, October, 160.

Draper, N. R. and H. Smith (1998). *Applied Regression Analysis*, 3rd edition. New York: Wiley.

Duncan, A. J. (1986). *Quality Control and Industrial Statistics*, 5th edition. Homewood, IL: Irwin.

Faulkenberry, G. D. and J. C. Daly (1970). Sample size for tolerance limits on a normal distribution. *Technometrics*, **12**(4), 813–821.

Faulkenberry, G. D. and D. L. Weeks (1968). Sample size determination for tolerance limits. *Technometrics*, **10**(2), 343–348.

Fountain, R. L. and Y.-M. Chou (1991). Minimum sample sizes for two-sided tolerance intervals for finite populations. *Journal of Quality Technology*, **23**(2), 90–95.

Hahn, G. J. (1974). Minimum size sampling plans. *Journal of Quality Technology*, **6**(3), 121–127.

Hahn, G. J. and W. O. Meeker (1991). *Statistical Intervals: A Guide for Practitioners*. New York: Wiley.

Hauck, W. W. and R. Shaikh (2001). Sample sizes for batch acceptance from single- and multistage designs using two-sided normal tolerance intervals with specified content. *Journal of Biopharmaceutical Statistics*, **11**, 335–346.

Jeng, S. L. (2003). Exact sample size determination for a Weibull test plan when there is time censoring. *Journal of Statistical Computation and Simulation*, **73**, 389–408.

Jensen, W. A., G. R. Bryce, and M. R. Reynolds, Jr. (2008). Design issues for adaptive control charts. *Quality and Reliability Engineering International*, **24**, 429–445.

Jones, L. A., C. W. Champ, and S. E. Rigdon (2001). The performance of exponentially weighted moving average charts with estimated parameters. *Technometrics*, **43**(2), 156–167.

Kim, K., M. A. Mahmoud, and W. H. Woodall (2003). On the monitoring of linear profiles. *Journal of Quality Technology*, **35**, 317–328.

Kirkpatrick, R. L. (1977). Sample sizes to set tolerance limits. *Journal of Quality Technology*, **9**(1), 6–12.

Köksal, G., B. Kantar, T. Ali Ula, and C. Testik (2008). The effect of Phase I sample size on the run length performance of control charts for autocorrelated data. *Journal of Applied Statistics*, **35**, 67–87.

Kotz, S. and N. L. Johnson (1993). *Process Capability Indices*. New York: Chapman and Hall.

Kotz, S. and C. R. Lovelace (1998). *Process Capability Indices in Theory and Practice*. London: Hodder Arnold.

Krishnamoorthy, K. and T. Mathew (2009). *Statistical Tolerance Regions: Theory, Applications, and Computation*. Hoboken, NJ: Wiley.

Lowry, C. A. and D. C. Montgomery (1995). A review of multivariate control charts. *IIE Transactions*, **27**, 800–810.

Lu, C. W. and M. R. Reynolds (1999). EWMA control charts for monitoring the mean of autocorrelated processes. *Journal of Quality Technology*, **31**, 166–188.

Lucas, J. M. and M. S. Saccucci (1990). Exponentially weighted moving average control schemes: Properties and enhancements (with discussion). *Technometrics*, **32**, 1–29.

Mandel, B. J. (1969). The regression control chart. *Journal of Quality Technology*, **1**(1), 1–9.

Mathews, P. (2010). *Sample Size Calculations: Practical Methods for Scientists and Engineers*. Fairport Harbor, OH: Mathews, Malnar, and Bailey, Inc.

Mee, R. W. (1984). β-expectation and β-content tolerance limits for balanced one-way ANOVA random model. *Technometrics*, **26**(3), 251–254.

Mohammed, M. A., P. Worthington, and W. H. Woodall (2008). Plotting basic control charts: Tutorial notes for health care practitioners. *Quality and Safety in Health Care*, **17**, 137–145.

Morris, R. L. and E. J. Riddle (2008). Determination of sample size to detect quality improvement in *p*-charts. *Quality Engineering*, **20**(3), 281–286.

Moura, E. C. (1991). *How to Determine Sample Size and Estimate Failure Rate in Life Testing*. Milwaukee, WI: ASQC Quality Press.

Neave, H. (1978). Algorithm AS 124: Sample sizes for one-sided and strong two-sided distribution-free tolerance intervals. *Applied Statistics*, **27**, 188–190.

Nedumaran, G. and J. J. Pignatiello, Jr. (1999). On constructing T^2 control charts for on-line process monitoring. *IIE Transactions*, **31**, 529–536.

Odeh, R. E. and D. B. Owen (1980). *Tables for Normal Tolerance Limits, Sampling Plans, and Screening*. New York: Marcel Dekker.

Odeh, R. E., Y. M. Chou, and D. B. Owen (1989). Sample size-determination for two-sided β-expectation tolerance intervals for a normal distribution. *Technometrics*, **31**(4), 461–468.

Pearn, W. L. and S. Kotz (2006). *Encyclopedia and Handbook of Process Capability Indices: A Comprehensive Exposition of Quality Control Measures*. Series on Quality, Reliability, and Engineering Statistics, Vol. 12. Hackensack, NJ: World Scientific Publishing.

Pearn, W. L. and M.-H. Shu (2003). Lower confidence bounds with sample size information for C_{pm} applied to production yield assurance. *International Journal of Production Research*, **41**(15), 3581–3599.

Quesenberry, C. P. (1993). The effect of sample size on estimated limits for $\bar{X}$ and X control charts. *Journal of Quality Technology*, **25**, 237–247.

Ryan, T. P. (2011). *Statistical Methods for Quality Improvement*, 3rd edition. Hoboken, NJ: Wiley.

Ryan, T. P. and N. C. Sohwertman (1997). Optimal limits for attribute control charts. *Journal of Quality Technology*, **29**, 86–98.

Sa, P. and L. Razaila (2004). One-sided continuous tolerance limits and their accompanying sample size problem. *Journal of Applied Statistics*, **31**, 419–434.

Shahian, D. M., W. A. Williamson, L. G. Svensson, J. D. Restuccia, and R. S. D'Agostino (1996). Applications of statistical quality control to cardiac surgery. *Annals of Thoracic Surgery*, **62**, 1351–1358.

Shu, M. H. and C. H. Wang (2006). A review and extensions of sample size determination for estimating process precision and loss with a designated accuracy ratio. *The International Journal of Advanced Manufacturing Technology*, **27**(9/10), 1038–1046.

Tseng, S.-T., J. Tang, and C.-H. Lin (2007). Sample size determination for achieving stability of double multivariate exponentially weighted moving average controller. *Technometrics*, **49**(4), 409–419. Technical Note: *Technometrics*, **51**, 335–338.

Wang, H. and F. Tsung (2009). Tolerance intervals with improved coverage probabilities for binomial and Poisson variables. *Technometrics*, **51**, 25–33.

Wilks, S. S. (1941). Determination of sample sizes for setting tolerance limits. *The Annals of Mathematical Statistics*, **12**(1), 91–96.

Winterbottom, A. (1993). Simple adjustments to improve control limits on attribute charts. *Quality and Reliability Engineering International*, **9**, 105–109.

Woodall, W. H. (2000). Controversies and contradictions in statistical process control (with discussion). *Journal of Quality Technology*, **32**(4), 341–350.

Wu, Z. and H. Luo (2004). Optimal design of the adaptive sample size and sampling interval *np* control chart. *Quality and Reliability Engineering International*, **20**, 553–570.

Wu, Z., S. Zhang, and P. Wang (2007). A CUSUM scheme with variable sample sizes and sampling intervals for monitoring the process mean and variance. *Quality and Reliability Engineering International*, **23**, 157–170.

Yang, Z., M. Xie, V. Kuralmani, and K.-L. Tsui (2002). On the performance of geometric control charts with estimated control limits. *Journal of Quality Technology*, **34**(4), 448–458.

Zhang, G. X. (1984). A new type of control charts and a theory of diagnosis with control charts. In *ASQC Annual Quality Congress Transactions*, pp. 175–185. Milwaukee, WI. American Society for Quality Control.

Zhang, G. X. (1985). Cause-selecting control charts—A new type of quality control charts. *The QR Journal*, **12**, 221–225.

Zhou, M.-Y., X.-L. Wang, and X.-Y. Li (2009). The Effects of VSSI $\bar{X}$ chart when control limits are estimated. *Journal of Data Analysis*, **4**, 1–14 (in Chinese).

Zimmer, L. S., N. F. Hubele, and W. J. Zimmer (2001). Confidence intervals and sample determination of C_{pm}. *Quality and Reliability Engineering International*, **17**, 51–68.

EXERCISES

8.1. Derive the values for $n = 2$ that were given in Table 8.1 for power and ARL.

8.2. Control chart properties that are given in textbooks and in journal articles are based on the assumption that the observations have come from a common distribution, such as a normal distribution, or that the Central Limit Theorem can be invoked to assume approximate normality for subgroup means. The Central Limit Theorem does not apply, even approximately, for subgroup sizes that are typically used for variables control charts, such as an $\bar{X}$-chart. Assume that a Shewhart $\bar{X}$-chart with 3-sigma limits and a subgroup size of 5 is in operation. Use appropriate software to determine the ARL for detecting a mean increase of $1.5\sigma_{\bar{x}}$ when the individual observations are from a logistic distribution. Based on your answer, what would you suggest be done before control chart limits be constructed? Explain.

CHAPTER 9

Survival Analysis and Reliability

9.1 SURVIVAL ANALYSIS

The term "survival analysis" is obviously self-explanatory. The objectives are to determine the proportion of a population that will survive past a particular point in time, as well as determining the rate at which death or "failure," in general, is occurring at some point in time, and what the factors are that can cause a change in the survival rate. Two-group survival studies are often used, with survival examined for each group over a specified length of time and sample size determined to detect a specified difference in the survival proportions at the conclusion of a study for a selected power value.

Industrial reliability analysis, on the other hand, is concerned with the functionality of manufactured items rather than people. More specifically, in that context, reliability is the probability that the unit will function adequately for the intended length of time. That type of reliability should be distinguished from other types of reliability. For example, interobserver reliability studies are conducted to investigate the reproducibility and level of agreement among people, as in rating products such as food items. Sample size can be determined for these other types of reliability studies, and this has been discussed in the literature, but in this chapter we will consider only industrial-type reliability studies since this parallels survival analysis since a unit of production will eventually die (or be discarded), just as a person will die.

The emphasis in this chapter, however, is on determining sample size for survival studies, as comparatively little attention has been given to determining sample size for reliability analyses. In general, sample size computations for survival studies are based on either (1) an estimate of surviving proportions for one or two groups at a fixed point in time, or (2) a model for an entire survival curve.

Sample Size Determination and Power, First Edition. Thomas P. Ryan.

Determining sample size for a survival analysis can be very challenging. Quoting from Simon (2004), "sample size is a tricky problem, and it is especially tricky for survival data models." The author pointed out that it is the number of deaths (or events, in general, not the number of patients) that is most important. This same point has been emphasized by other authors, including Collett (2003, p. 300). Simon (2004) also stated: "You can make some simplifying assumptions, but generally, power calculations for a survival data model are a mess." This is partly due to the nonconstant nature of the number of people who are part of the study at a given point in time, with some people entering, some dropping out, and some dying along the way. Consequently, some software that has sample size capability for survival analysis make some simplifying assumptions that serve to make sample size determination less complicated, although obviously also less precise. There is one well-known software package that allows the user to provide information regarding accrual periods, dropout rate, hazard rate, and sample size for each period and computes power using simulations. It cannot be used to directly determine sample size for survival studies, however. Another well-known software package permits the same type of information to be entered but determines sample size rather than computing power. Freeware for survival analysis falls into both categories.

Noncompliance is one of the complications as participants can discontinue use of study medication. Almost all existing sample size methods assume that when patients do discontinue, they do so independently of their risk of an endpoint, so that noncompliance is noninformative. Jiang, Snapinn, and Iglewicz (2004) pointed out that this is not always the case, however, and introduced a modified version of the sample size method proposed by Lakatos (1988) in the presence of informative noncompliance.

A detailed comparison of software and freeware for survival analysis is provided in Section 9.4. Since there is so much to chose from, a user needs to be careful in selecting software or freeware that will correspond to input that the user can provide and will give output in the form(s) that is needed.

9.1.1 Logrank Test

The logrank test is the most commonly used method in clinical trial work for comparing the total survival of two or more groups of individuals (Lakatos and Lan, 1992). The test can be used in clinical trial work to compare two types of treatments, such as two types of drugs. This might consist of a standard drug recommended for a certain physical condition, and a new drug that shows promise as possibly being superior to the standard drug.

There are several versions of a logrank test, depending on what is assumed. One version is the simplest logrank test because it is actually a nonparametric type of test as no assumption is made about the shape of the survival curve for any of the groups, nor is there an assumption about the distribution of survival times. This is the method of analysis advocated by Bland and Altman (2004) and can be illustrated as follows. We will assume an example with two groups. The null hypothesis is that there is no difference between the two populations in the probability that an event (such as death) occurs at any point in time. Computations are performed each time there is an event and are based on the times of those events. For example, assume that there are 50 people in group #1 and 40 people in group #2, and that the first death occurs in week #4, and the person was in group #1. The probability of a person dying in week #4 is 1/90 since there were 90 people alive at the start of the week. Under the null hypothesis, the expected number of deaths in group #1 is $50/90 = 5/9$ and $40/90 = 4/9$ for group #2. Assume that the second death occurs in week #10 and the person is in group #2. There were 89 people alive at the start of that week, so the risk of dying was 1/89. The expected number of deaths were $49/89 = .55$ for group #1 and $40/89 = .44$ for group #2, respectively.

These calculations continue each time a death occurs and the deaths and expected number are summed for each group. The analysis that is then performed is just a simple chi-square test using the observed and expected figures for each group. For example, assume that the number of deaths in group #1 is 16 and the expected number is 13.82, with the number of deaths in group #2 being 18 and the expected number is 20.18. The usual χ^2 goodness-of-fit statistic is then computed as $\sum_g \left(O_g - E_g\right)^2 / E_g$, with g denoting the group, O representing the observed value, and E denoting the expected value. For this example, $\chi^2 = (16 - 13.82)^2/13.82 + (18 - 20.18)^2/20.18 = 0.58$. The number of degrees of freedom is the number of groups minus 1. The calculated value of χ^2 is quite small, for any number of degrees of freedom and for any significance level, and since $\chi^2_{.05,1} = 3.84$, the null hypothesis would not be rejected.

This is a simple test that has both advantages and disadvantages. The primary advantage is that it avoids the specification of a survival distribution for each population, which is likely to be skewed since there can be many events that occur early and much fewer that occur later. Specifying a specific skewed distribution could be difficult, however, and the assumption would not be possible to test with any reasonable amount of power in the absence of a considerable amount of data. The disadvantages of the test are that it is strictly a significance test and as such cannot provide an estimate of the size of the difference between the groups or a confidence interval on the mean difference.

Some readers may be interested in the short tutorial on the logrank test given by Bland and Altman (2004). Yateman and Skene (1992) may also be of interest because they approximated survival and loss distributions with piecewise exponential distributions and patient entry with a piecewise linear distribution, which they claimed significantly reduces the required computation and enables the expected number of deaths to be routinely evaluated.

As discussed in Section 9.1, power is based on the number of events (deaths), not the sample size, so it is desirable to determine the required number of deaths, although obviously this cannot be fixed as one fixes a sample size. Nevertheless, it is important to know how may deaths are needed. Collett (2003, p. 300) gave the formula for the required number of deaths for the logrank test, while pointing out that the formula also applies to the Cox proportional hazards model (see Section 9.1.5). The formula is

$$d = \frac{4(Z_{\alpha/2} + Z_\beta)^2}{\theta_R^2} \tag{9.1}$$

with θ_R denoting the true log-hazard ratio and $Z_{\alpha/2}$ and Z_β as defined and used in earlier chapters. The log-hazard ratio is defined as $\log(S_2)/\log(S_1)$, with S_1 and S_2 denoting the proportion surviving in the first and second groups, respectively. The designation of first and second group doesn't matter for Eq. (9.1) because the log of the hazard ratio if the latter had been defined as $\log(S_1)/\log(S_2)$ would just be the negative of the log of the hazard ratio as originally defined here, and since that number is squared in Eq. (9.1), the manner in which the hazard ratio is defined relative to the subscripts is immaterial.

Equation (9.1) is based on the assumption that there are equal proportions of individuals assigned to each treatment group. If the proportions differ, so that the proportions are π and $(1 - \pi)$ for the two groups, the appropriate formula is then

$$d = \frac{(Z_{\alpha/2} + Z_\beta)^2}{\pi(1 - \pi)\theta_R^2}$$

Since $\pi(1 - \pi)$ has its maximum value when $\pi = 0.5$, the required number of deaths is inflated by the disparity in the proportions, although that inflation will be slight unless the respective proportions differ greatly.

The derivation of this formula is given by Collett (2003) and is based on the assumption that the logrank statistic has approximately a normal distribution. Thus, the formula is an approximation since the Z-variates in the formulas for equal and unequal proportions are based on the assumption of a normal distribution.

Hsieh (1987) gave a simple method for determining sample size for the logrank test (or t-test) for designs with unequal sample sizes, with simulation used to compare the performance of that method with other methods. Hsieh (1992) compared that method with several others and found that no method was uniformly best.

Zhang and Quan (2009) pointed out that the proportional hazards model won't always hold when the logrank test is used and derived formulas for calculating the asymptotic power of the logrank test under a nonproportional hazards alternative. In general, a modified approach will often be necessary when the logrank test is used since the assumptions for its use won't necessarily be met. This was also addressed by Song, Kosorok, and Cai (2008), who proposed modified logrank tests that are robust with respect to different data-generating processes and gave the accompanying sample size formulas. Jung, Kang, McCall, and Blumenstein (2005) proposed modification of the logrank test for noninferiority trials with a survival endpoint and developed an accompanying sample size formula. Lu and Pajak (2000) considered sample size and power for a logrank test when change point(s) in treatment effect are given. Jung and Hui (2002) considered rank tests in general for comparing more than two survival distributions and gave both an asymptotic and approximate sample size formula. Jung (2008) introduced a sample size formula for weighted rank test statistics used with paired two-sample survival data. Gail (1985) compared a logrank test with a test of two proportions relative to sample size and power and found that each test has comparative advantages and disadvantages under certain conditions.

9.1.1.1 Freedman Method

Lakatos and Lan (1992) compared several methods of determining sample size for the logrank test. One of these is due to Freedman (1982), whose sample size formula is based on the expected value and variance of the logrank test. With that method, sample size is determined as follows. Let θ denote the hazard ratio, which can be expressed in several ways, one of which is $\theta = \log(S_1)/\log(S_2)$, with S_1 denoting the proportion of subjects in group #1 who are surviving at the end of the clinical trial, and S_2 defined the same way for group #2. The hazard ratio is assumed to remain constant throughout the trial and time periods are not stated, nor is accrual considered.

Assume that in a particular clinical trial those proportions are $S_1 = .3$ and $S_2 = .4$ and that there are an equal number of subjects who begin. Then if θ is defined as $\theta = \log(S_1)/\log(S_2)$, we obtain $\theta = \log(.3)/\log(.4) = 1.314$. Assume further that the power is to be .80 and $\alpha = .05$ and that a two-sided test is to be used with equal group sizes. The sample size, n, is then determined as

$$n = \left[\frac{\theta + 1}{\theta - 1}\right]^2 (z_{\alpha/2} + z_\beta)^2 / (2 - S_1 - S_2)$$

$$= \left[\frac{1.314 + 1}{1.314 - 1}\right]^2 (1.96 + 0.8416)^2 / (2 - .3 - .4)$$

$$= 327.96$$

so $n = 328$ would be used and this would be the sample size used in each of the two groups. [Note that if θ had been defined as $\theta = \log(S_2)/\log(S_1)$, the bracketed expression would have been $(1 + 1.314)/(1 - 1.314)$ and that would have produced the same sample size since $(1.314 - 1)^2 = (1 - 1.314)^2$.]

This solution can also be produced by several software. Specifically, PASS would be used for this example by first selecting "Survival" from the menu, and then selecting "Logrank Tests (Freedman)," then entering the values for α, power, S_1, and S_2, and specifying that a two-sided test is to be used. PASS shows the power to be .8001—virtually identical to the target value—with $n_1 = n_2 = 328$ given as the solution, in accordance with the hand computation. The output also shows the total number of events (i.e., deaths) that must be observed for the two groups combined (427, in this case) in order for the stated power to be attained.

The user of nQuery would first select "Survival (Time to Event)" and then select "Logrank test for equality of survival curves." That output also shows $n_1 = n_2 = 328$ but shows 421 for the total number of events, in disagreement with the result given by PASS. [Although not listed in the menu, the reference for the procedure is Freedman (1982), suggesting that sample size is being determined using the Freedman approach.]

Similarly, the Freedman method is the default for the logrank test in Stata, which gives the same sample size for each, $n = 328$, but gives 428 as the "estimated number of events," thus differing slightly from the 427 given by PASS and more than slightly from the 421 events given by nQuery. This discrepancy may be due to different assumptions or different methods of estimation, but that isn't clear. The expected number of events, E, is given by $4(z_{\alpha/2} + z_\beta)^2/\log^2(1/\theta)$. This computation yields $E = 420.8$, which supports the solution given by nQuery.

If a one-sided test is desired, $z_{\alpha/2}$ in the formula for n would be replaced by z_α, so 1.645 would be used in place of 1.96. For this example, the sample size would then be computed as $n = 258.36$, so $n = 259$ would be used. This is the sample size given by PASS and nQuery, with the former indicating that the power is .8002 and nQuery showing that 332 events for the two groups combined are required to reach that power. Stata also gives $n = 259$ but gives 336 as the necessary number of events, again disagreeing with nQuery. Hand computation gives $E = 331.45$, which again supports the solution of nQuery.

9.1.1.2   Other Methods

A parametric test can be justified if there is faith in the distributional assumption that must be made. For example, survival might be considered to be exponential over time. The software nQuery has the capability for sample size determination for a test of equal exponential survival for two groups. For example, if $\alpha = .05$, a two-sided test is used, power $= .90$, the exponential parameter (mean) is 2 for one group and 3 for the other group, the total number of required events is 256.

Cantor (1992), however, explained that the assumption of an exponential distribution is inappropriate when a nonzero proportion of the population is expected to have indefinite survival. A Gompertz model was stated as being a reasonable alternative for such a scenario. A method was given for calculating the required accrual time for a clinical trial in which the treatments have Gompertz survival distributions that satisfy the proportional hazards assumption. A computer program that performs the necessary computations was also provided.

For the case when stratification is present, Ahnn and Anderson (1995) derived the sample size formula for the stratified logrank test, extending the result of Palta and Amini (1985). See also Ahnn and Anderson (1998).

9.1.2 Wilcoxon–Breslow–Gehan Test

A variation of the logrank test is used if a person considers events at different times to be of different importance, such as deaths early in a survival curve being of more importance than later deaths if a new treatment that is purported to be beneficial in avoiding early mortality is part of a comparison study. Thus, early deaths would have a high weight (i.e., penalty). In general, different times would be weighted unequally and the chi-square statistic would be

$$\chi^2 = \sum_{gt} \frac{R_t(O_{gt} - E_{gt})^2}{R_t^2 E_{gt}}$$

with R_t denoting the weight that is assigned at time t. This test has various names, one of which is the Wilcoxon–Breslow–Gehan test in recognition of the fact that it is a modification of the Wilcoxon test and has been proposed by both Breslow and Gehan.

This test can be performed in Stata, in addition to the logrank test and other variations of the logrank test. More specifically, the `stpower logrank` command in Stata estimates required sample size, power, and effect size for survival analysis comparing survivor functions in two groups using the logrank test. It provides options for unequal allocation of subjects to the two groups, possible withdrawal of subjects from the study, plus uniform accrual of subjects into the study.

It does not, however, provide the capability of determining sample size for the Wilcoxon–Breslow–Gehan test, nor does other sample size determination software.

9.1.3 Tarone–Ware Test

This is another weighted logrank test and it was proposed by Tarone and Ware (1977), who claimed that it may be more powerful against a range of alternatives than the logrank test and Wilcoxon–Breslow–Gehan test. Ahnn and Anderson (1998) gave a sample size formula for testing the equality of at least two survival distributions using the Tarone–Ware class of test statistics in the case of nonproportional hazards, time-dependent losses, noncompliance, and drop-in. Chow, Shao, and Wang (2008) described the Tarone–Ware test in their Section 7.4.1, which included the formula for sample size, and they gave an example of its use in Section 7.4.2.

9.1.4 Other Tests

Schumacher (1981) proposed distribution-free tests for use with censored data, with one test based on McNemar's (1947) test.

9.1.5 Cox Proportional Hazards Model

The Cox proportional hazards model (Cox, 1972) is also known as Cox regression, which was the topic of Section 5.3, where it was presented in some detail and will be presented in less detail here, with an emphasis on applications in survival analysis. It is covered in this chapter because the model is used in the comparison of survival curves for treatment groups and is often used to adjust for covariates such as patient age and disease stage.

As such, an understanding of the term "proportional hazards" is needed. As defined in Section 5.3, a hazard function is the probability of failure (i.e., death in survival analysis) at time t divided by the probability of survival until time t. As such, a hazard function is a function of time and a set of covariates, which might vary over time. The proportional hazards model separates these two effects, so that the model is written

$$h(t; \mathbf{x}) = \lambda(t) \exp[G(\mathbf{x}; \beta)]$$

using the notation of McCullagh and Nelder (1989), with $\lambda(t)$ denoting the baseline hazard and $G(\mathbf{x}; \beta)$ the model that contains the parameters and the set of covariates.

As explained by McCullagh and Nelder (1989), it is conventional, but not necessary, to assume that the covariates have a multiplicative effect on the hazard. If so, the model could then be written

$$h(t; \mathbf{x}) = \lambda(t) \exp(\beta_1 X_1 + \beta_2 X_2 + \cdots + \beta_m X_m) \tag{9.2}$$

where $X_1, X_2, \ldots, X_m$ denote the covariates, and $\lambda(t)$ is the baseline hazard, with $X_1, X_2, \ldots, X_m$ the covariates. The word "proportional" comes from the $\lambda(t)$ term and the fact that there is no other term on the right side of the model that is a function of the time, t. The term $\lambda(t)$ might seemingly be a continuous, smooth function of time, but for the proportional hazards model it is defined only at times that events occur and, as stated by McCullagh and Nelder (1989), plays the role of a blocking factor in a blocked experimental design (see Section 6.2.5).

The model can be written in the form of a linear model by dividing each side of Eq. (9.2) by $\lambda(t)$ and then taking the logarithm of each side, producing

$$\log \left(\frac{h\{(t), (X_1, X_2, \ldots, X_m)\}}{\lambda(t)} \right) = \beta_1 X_1 + \beta_2 X_2 + \cdots + \beta_m X_m \tag{9.3}$$

Notice that this is similar to the way that the alternative form of the logistic regression model was produced at the beginning of Section 5.2.

The development of sample size formulas for comparing survival curves for the proportional hazards model dates at least from Schoenfeld (1983) and includes Schoenfeld and Borenstein (2005). Schoenfeld's sample size formula for the logrank test for two-sample censored data is well known and widely used according to Eng and Kosorok (2005), who derived a sample size formula based on the limiting distribution of the two-sided supremum-weighted logrank statistic. Gangnon and Kosorok (2004) gave a simple formula for weighted logrank statistics applied to clustered survival data with variable cluster sizes and arbitrary treatment assignment within clusters that reduces to the Schoenfeld's (1983) formula when there is either no clusters or else independence within clusters. Xie and Waksman (2003) also derived a sample size formula for clustered survival data.

Schoenfeld (1983) illustrated how adjusting for covariates permits a reduction in sample size for the same power, giving an example in which the necessary sample size for 80% power was reduced from 272 to 212 when there was an adjustment for covariates.

Despite the popularity of the proportional hazards model in survival analysis work, adequacy of model fit should be assessed whenever it is applied, as with any other model. In particular, if the proportional hazards assumption is not met, the relative risk for variables in the model can be either overestimated or underestimated, with the result that the power for testing the corresponding parameters is reduced. Stablein, Carter, and Novak (1981) discussed how the appropriateness of the proportional hazards model in a particular setting can be tested.

What if the proportional hazards assumption is not met and there is a time dependency? There are two schools of thought on this: (1) use weighted estimation in Cox regression and (2) model the time-dependent effects.

As noted in Section 5.3, maximum likelihood won't always be the best estimation method for the Cox proportional hazards model (see also Heinze and Schemper, 2001), which presents a problem relative to sample size determination because the sample size determination methods that have been proposed, such as Hsieh and Lavori (2000), have been presented assuming that maximum likelihood is the method of estimation. Heinze and Dunkler (2008) presented a solution to the monotone likelihood problem that can occur with Cox regression and extended Firth's (1993) procedure to Cox regression with time-dependent effects.

9.1.6 Joint Modeling of Longitudinal and Survival Data

Although joint modeling of longitudinal and survival data has become popular in recent years, not much attention has been devoted to design aspects. Chen,

Ibrahim, and Chu (2011) derived a sample size formula for estimating the effect of the longitudinal process in joint modeling and extended Schoenfeld's (1983) sample size formula for estimating the overall treatment effect in the joint modeling setting.

9.1.7 Multistage Designs

Desseaux and Porcher (2007) presented a flexible design with sample size reevaluation for survival trials in the context of a two-stage design.

9.1.8 Comparison of Software and Freeware

Since survival analysis is such a commonly used statistical tool, it is not surprising that there is adequate software and freeware from which to choose. The capabilities and input requirements vary considerably, however, and this is potentially confusing to users who might use multiple software packages.

nQuery has two options for its logrank test with the difference between the two being the components of the total input information. Specifically, the user specifies the significance level and indicates whether the test is one-sided or two-sided.

PASS has several options, one of which determines sample size using the method of Freedman (1982). The way that this routine differs from the other logrank routines in PASS is indicated by the following statement from the PASS online help system: "Time periods are not stated. Rather, it is assumed that enough time elapses to allow for a reasonable proportion of responses to occur. If you want to study the impact of accrual and follow-up time, you should use one of the other logrank modules also contained in *PASS*." Thus, it is possible to account for accrual and follow-up time with PASS, but not with the Freedman logrank routine.

Power and Precision also has the capability for sample size determination for comparing two survival curves and provides several options, not in terms of test selection but relative to how a study is performed. Specifically, the user can choose between a hazard rate that is either constant or varies; either no attrition, constant attrition, or attrition that varies; and either subjects entering prior to the first study interval, entering during that study at a constant rate, or entering at a rate that varies.

Stata will perform sample size calculations for survival studies, including the logrank test, through its `stpower` command. Specifically, `stpower logrank` is used for determining sample size and power when the logrank test is used. Options that are provided include being able to account for unequal allocation of subjects between the two groups, withdrawal of subjects from the study, and uniform accrual of subjects into the study.

The `stpower cox` command in Stata estimates the required sample size, power, and effect size using Cox proportional hazard models with one or more covariates. Its options include accounting for possible correlation between the covariate of interest and other predictors, and for withdrawal of subjects from the study. The other Stata command for sample size determination and power in survival analysis is `stpower exponential`, which can be used for estimating sample size and power for comparing two exponential survivor functions.

In addition to the built-in capabilities, some menu driven programs have been contributed that add to Stata's sample size determination capability for survival analysis. This includes the programs of Royston and Babiker (2002) and Barthel, Royston, and Babiker (2005), with the latter updating the former. Barthel, Babiker, Royston, and Parmar (2006) contributed a Stata program, ART, that utilized a general framework for sample size calculation in survival studies for comparing two or more survival distributions using any one of a class of tests that includes the logrank test. The program has considerable flexibility and allows for the possible presence of nonuniform patient entry, nonproportional hazards, loss to follow-up, and treatment changes including crossover between treatments. Of course, power can be determined using simulation and Feiverson (2002) showed how to write programs that estimate the power of virtually any test that Stata can perform.

The overall survival analysis capabilities in Stata, including sample size determination, are described in Cleves, Gould, Gutierrez, and Marchenko (2008).

There is other software that have been available during the past few decades. For example, Dupont and Plummer (1990) described freeware that they contributed that can be used for studies with a survival response measure as well as dichotomous and continuous outcomes, with the software downloadable from `http://biostat.mc.vanderbilt.edu/twiki/bin/view/Main/PowerS ampleSize`.

An applet for determining sample size when a survival curve is to be compared against a historical control is available at `http://www.cct.cuhk.edu .hk/stat/survival/Dixon1988.htm`.

Although software can render tables and nomograms unnecessary, they are still undoubtedly in use by many people. Chapter 8 of Machin, Campbell, Tan, and Tan (2009), which was cited in Chapter 7, contains three sample size tables for comparing survival rates and Schoenfeld and Richter (1982) provided nomograms for calculating the number of patients needed for a clinical trial that has survival as an endpoint.

9.2 RELIABILITY ANALYSIS

It should be noted that there are different types of reliability, as the reliability of a test instrument used in education is another type of reliability, and the term "reliability" is used often in that literature. Although sample sizes can, of course, also be determined for nonindustrial reliability, as in Shoukri, Asyali, and Donner (2004), that will not be the focus of this section.

Meeker, Hahn, and Doganaksoy (2004) discussed the planning, including sample size determination, of life tests to demonstrate reliability. They gave an example for which the requirement was for a newly designed bearing for a washing machine to run flawlessly on 99% of all units for 4000 cycles. That is, the reliability was to be $R = .99$ and the objective was to demonstrate that with $100(1 - \alpha)\% = 90\%$ confidence. Thus, $\alpha = .10$. Meeker et al. (2004) gave the required sample size as $n = \log(\alpha)/\log(R)$, with this formula having been given previously by Hahn (1974). Thus, $n = \log(.10)/\log(.99) = 229.105$, so $n = 230$ bearings would be used.

They stated that the requisite number of test units can be reduced by running each unit beyond the specified lifetime, provided that some assumptions can be made about the distribution of time to failure based on experience and knowledge of the failure mechanism. Meeker and Escobar (1998) showed that under the assumption of a Weibull distribution as the life distribution, a zero failure demonstration test run for k multiples of the specified lifetime requires that

$$n = \frac{1}{k^\beta} \left[\frac{\log(\alpha)}{\log(R)} \right]$$

units be tested, with β the shape parameter of the Weibull distribution, α the significance level for the test, and R the reliability. As the title of their paper indicates, McKane, Escobar, and Meeker (2005) addressed sample size and number of failure requirements for demonstration tests when location-scale and log-location-scale distributions are involved and there is failure censoring. That is, a test is run until a specified number of failures occurs. They addressed sample size determination using graphs, estimating the necessary sample size from a graph. Unfortunately, whereas software for sample size determination in survival analysis is plentiful, software for determining sample size in various types of (industrial) reliability tests seems to be virtually nonexistent.

9.3 SUMMARY

Much has been written about sample size determination for tests used in survival analysis. In particular, several different methods of sample size determination have been proposed for the logrank test. Software developers have responded to this level of activity, with the result that PASS, in particular, has 15 procedures for determining sample size. There has not been a similar interest in software for reliability testing, however. Consequently, users need to rely on sample size formulas given in research papers and in books such as Mathews (2010), which covers more reliability tests than were given in this chapter.

REFERENCES

Ahnn, S. and S. J. Anderson (1995). Sample size determination for comparing more than two survival distributions. *Statistics in Medicine*, **14**, 2273–2282.

Ahnn, S. and S. J. Anderson (1998). Sample size determination in complex clinical trials using the log-rank test. *Statistics in Medicine*, **17**, 2525–2534.

Barthel, F. M.-S., P. Royston, and A. Babiker (2005). A menu-driven facility for complex sample size calculations in randomized controlled trials with a survival or a binary outcome. *Stata Journal*, **5**, 123–129.

Barthel, F. M.-S., A. Babiker, P. Royston, and M. K. B. Parmar (2006). Evaluation of sample size and power for multi-arm survival trials allowing for non-uniform accrual, non-proportional hazards, and loss to follow-up and cross-over. *Statistics in Medicine*, **25**, 2521–2542.

Bland, J. M. and D. G. Altman (2004). The logrank test. *British Medical Journal*, **328** (Number 7447, May 1), 1073. (Available online with free subscription at http://www.bmj.com/cgi/content/full/328/7447/1073.)

Cantor, A. B. (1992). Sample size calculations for the log rank test: A Gompertz model approach. *Journal of Clinical Epidemiology*, **45**(10), 1131–1136.

Chen, L. M., J. G. Ibrahim, and H. Chu (2011). Sample size and power determination in joint modeling of longitudinal and survival data. *Statistics in Medicine*, **30**(18), 2295–2309.

Chow, S.-C., J. Shao, and H. Wang (2008). *Sample Size Calculations in Clinical Research*, 2nd edition. Boca Raton, FL: Chapman and Hall/CRC.

Cleves, M. A., W. W. Gould, R. G. Gutierrez, and Y. Marchenko (2008). *An Introduction to Survival Analysis Using Stata*, 2nd edition. College Station, TX: Stata Press.

Collett, D. (2003). *Modeling Survival Data in Medical Research*, 2nd edition. London: Chapman and Hall.

Cox, D. R. (1972). Regression models and life tables. *Journal of the Royal Statistical Society, Series B*, **34**, 187–220.

Desseaux, K. and R. Porcher (2007). Flexible two-stage design with sample size reassessment for survival trials. *Statistics in Medicine*, **26**, 5002–5013.

Dupont, W. D. and W. D. Plummer (1990). Power and sample size calculations: A review and computer program. *Controlled Clinical Trials*, **11**, 116–128.

Eng, K. H. and M. R. Kosorok (2005). A sample size formula for the supremum log-rank statistic. *Biometrics*, **61**, 86–91.

Feiverson, A. H. (2002). Power by simulation. *Stata Journal*, **2**, 107–124.

Firth, D. (1993). Bias reduction of maximum likelihood estimates. *Biometrika*, **80**, 27–38.

Freedman, L. S. (1982). Tables of the number of patients required in clinical trials using the logrank test. *Statistics in Medicine*, **1**, 121–129.

Gail, M. H. (1985). Applicability of sample size calculations based on a comparison of proportions for use with the log rank test. *Controlled Clinical Trials*, **6**, 112–119.

Gangnon, R. E. and M. R. Kosorok (2004). Sample-size formula for clustered survival data using weighted log rank statistics. *Biometrika*, **91**, 263–275.

Hahn, G. J. (1974). Minimum size sampling plans. *Journal of Quality Technology*, **6**(3), 121–127.

Heinze, G. and D. Dunkler (2008). Avoiding infinite estimates of time-dependent effects in small-sample survival studies. *Statistics in Medicine*, **27**(30), 6455–6469.

Heinze, G. and M. Schemper (2001). A solution to the problem of monotone likelihood in Cox regression. *Biometrics*, **57**(1), 114–119.

Hsieh, F. Y. (1987). A simple method of sample size calculation for unequal-sample-size designs that use the logrank or *t*-test. *Statistics in Medicine*, **6**(5), 577–581.

Hsieh, F. Y. (1992). Comparing sample size formulas for trials with unbalanced allocation using the logrank test. *Statistics in Medicine*, **11**, 1091–1098.

Hsieh, F. Y. and P. W. Lavori (2000). Sample size calculations for the Cox proportional hazards model with nonbinary covariates. *Controlled Clinical Trials*, **21**(6), 552–560.

Jiang, Q., S. Snapinn, and B. Iglewicz (2004). Calculation of sample size in survival trials: The impact of informative noncompliance. *Biometrics*, **60**, 800–806.

Jung, S.-H. (2008). Sample size calculation for the weighted rank statistics with paired survival data. *Statistics in Medicine*, **27**, 3350–3365.

Jung, S.-H. and S. Hui (2002). Sample size calculation for rank tests comparing k survival populations. *Lifetime Data Analysis*, **8**, 361–373.

Jung, S.-H., S. Kang, L. McCall, and B. Blumenstein (2005). Sample size computation for two-sample noninferiority log-rank test. *Journal of Biopharmaceutical Statistics*, **15**, 969–979.

Lakatos, E. (1988). Sample sizes based on the logrank test in complex clinical trials. *Biometrics*, **44**, 229–241.

Lakatos, E. and K. K. G. Lan (1992). A comparison of sample size methods for the logrank test. *Statistics in Medicine*, **11**(2), 179–191.

Lu, J. and T. F. Pajak (2000). Statistical power for a long-term survival trial with a time-dependent treatment effect. *Controlled Clinical Trials*, **21**(6), 561–573.

Machin, D., M. J. Campbell, S.-B. Tan, and S.-H. Tan (2009). *Sample Size Tables for Clinical Studies*. London: BMJ Books.

Mathews, P. (2010). *Sample Size Calculations: Practical Methods for Engineers and Scientists*. Fairport Harbor, OH: Mathews Malnar and Bailey, Inc.

McCullagh, P. and J. A. Nelder (1989). *Generalized Linear Models*, 2nd edition. London: Chapman and Hall.

McKane, S. W., L. A. Escobar, and W. Q. Meeker (2005). Sample size and number of failure requirements for demonstration tests with log-location-scale distributions and failure censoring. *Technometrics*, **47**, 182–190.

McNemar, Q. (1947). Note on the sampling error of the differences between correlated proportions or percentages. *Psychometrika*, **12**, 153–157.

Meeker, W. Q. and L. A. Escobar (1998). *Statistical Methods for Reliability Data*. New York: Wiley.

Meeker, W. Q., G. J. Hahn, and N. Doganaksoy (2004). Planning life tests for reliability demonstration. *Quality Progress*, August, 80–82.

Palta, M. and S. B. Amini (1985). Consideration of covariates and stratification in sample size determination for survival studies. *Journal of Chronic Diseases*, **38**, 801–809.

Royston, P. and A. Babiker (2002). A menu-driven facility for complex sample size calculation in randomized controlled trials with a survival or binary outcome. *Stata Journal*, **2**, 151–163.

Schoenfeld, D. (1983). Sample-size formula for the proportional-hazards regression model. *Biometrics*, **39**, 499–503.

Schoenfeld, D. and M. Borenstein (2005). Calculating the power or sample size for the logistic and proportional hazards models. *Journal of Statistical Computation and Simulation*, **75**, 771–785.

Schoenfeld, D. and J. Richter (1982). Nomograms for calculating the number of patients needed for a clinical trial with survival as an endoint. *Biometrics*, **38**, 163–170.

Schumacher, M. (1981). Power and sample size determination for survival time studies with special regard to the censoring mechanism. *Methods of Information in Medicine*, **20**, 110–115.

Shoukri, M. M., M. H. Asyali, and A. Donner (2004). Sample size requirements for the design of reliability study: Review and new results. *Statistical Methods in Medical Research*, **13**, 251–271.

Simon, S. (2004). Sample size for a survival data model. (Electronic resource at `www.pmean.com/o4/survival.html`.)

Song, R., M. R. Kosorok, and J. Cai (2008). Robust covariate-adjusted log-rank statistics and corresponding sample size formula for recurrent events data. *Biometrics*, **64**, 741–750.

Stablein, D. M., W. H. Carter, Jr., and J. W. Novak (1981). Analysis of survival data with nonproportional hazard functions. *Controlled Clinical Trials*, **2**, 149–159.

Tarone, R. E. and J. H. Ware (1977). On distribution-free tests for equality of survival distributions. *Biometrika*, **64**, 156–160.

Williamson, J. M., H.-M Lin, and H.-Y. Kim (2009). Power and sample size calculations for current status survival analysis. *Statistics in Medicine*, **28**, 1999–2011.

Xie, T. and J. Waksman (2003). Design and sample size estimation in clinical trials with clustered survival times as the primary endpoint. *Statistics in Medicine*, **22**(18), 2835–2846.

Yateman, N. A. and A. M. Skene (1992). Sample sizes for proportional hazards survival studies with arbitrary patient entry and loss to follow-up distributions. *Statistics in Medicine*, **11**, 1103–1113.

Zhang, D. and H. Quan (2009). Power and sample size calculation for logrank test with a time lag in treatment effect. *Statistics in Medicine*, **28**, 2617–2638.

EXERCISE

9.1. Use PASS or other software to verify the sample size of 328 that was given in Section 9.1.1.1. If you use PASS, you will notice that the output includes the number of events for each group.

CHAPTER 10

Nonparametric Methods

Nonparametric methods are frequently used with small sample sizes as large sample properties of parametric tests then do not apply. Nonparametric methods have less power than their corresponding parametric methods when the assumptions for the parametric methods are met. This is well known, but computing power for nonparametric tests when the assumption of a specific distribution is not met poses special problems. This is because a specified distribution is used in computing probabilities for parametric methods (as seen in previous chapters), with such probabilities being the power values. For these reasons, it is best to use parametric methods if it appears, for a given set of data, that the parametric distribution assumptions are not seriously violated. But when we are at the point of trying to determine sample size for use with a nonparametric method, we don't yet have any data! Therefore, we can't test for any distribution assumption.

In general, we would use a nonparametric approach if we seriously doubt that the distribution assumption for a parametric test is likely to not even be approximately met, such as more than slight nonnormality. We need to consider the type of test being used, however, as some tests are robust to violations of the test assumptions and some are not. Robustness of various statistical methods is discussed by Rasch and Guirard (2004).

We need not be concerned with the actual distribution when the test is performed, but, somewhat paradoxically, a distribution must be assumed when sample size is determined for a specified power because power depends on the actual distribution! Of course, if we knew the actual distribution, we wouldn't use a nonparametric (distribution-free) approach in the first place! Because of these difficulties, one conservative approach would be to inflate the sample size for the corresponding parametric approach. This is discussed in Section 10.2. Certainly any such simple rule-of-thumb would avoid the complexities involved in sample size determination for nonparametric methods, in general.

Sample Size Determination and Power, First Edition. Thomas P. Ryan.
© 2013 John Wiley & Sons, Inc. Published 2013 by John Wiley & Sons, Inc.

Although the focus in this chapter is on determining sample size when a nonparametric test is used, Walker (2003) considered a Bayesian nonparametric decision theoretic approach to sample size calculations, independent of any specific test. Mumby (2002) pointed out that the power of nonparametric tests has not been discussed to any extent in the literature and advocated the use of simulation for power and sample size determination.

10.1 WILCOXON ONE-SAMPLE TEST

The Wilcoxon (1945) one-sample test, which is often called the Wilcoxon signed rank test, is used to test whether the median of a symmetric distribution is equal to a specified number. (With a normal distribution, the median and mean are the same.) For observations x_i, the test entails computing $|x_i - \text{median}|$ for $i = 1, 2, \ldots, n$, and ranking the absolute values from smallest to largest, while keeping track of which values of $(x_i - \text{median})$ are positive and which are negative. Let T_+ denote the total of the ranks for the positive deviations and let T_- denote the total of the ranks for the negative deviations. Typically, the smaller of the two totals is used as the test statistic, but that doesn't really matter.

If the sample data support the hypothesized median, the two totals should be about the same. If, however, the data do not support the hypothesized median, we would expect the totals to differ considerably.

In general, if a parametric test assumption is normality and a nonparametric test is to be used but normality is specified for the purpose of comparing the sample size with the required sample size for the parametric procedure, the sample sizes will of course differ. For example, it was shown in Example 2.1 that $n = 56$ when $H_0: \mu = 100$ is tested against the alternative $H_a: \mu > 100$, using $\alpha = .05$ and the desired power being .80 for detecting $\mu = 101$ under the assumption $\sigma = 3$. If the nonparametric counterpart, the one-sample Wilcoxon test, is used to test that the median is equal to a specified value (such as 100 in this case), the sample size will be greater than 56 if normality is assumed because the ranks of the data are used relative to the median, rather than the distance from the median being used. Since information from a sample is less when ranks are used rather than the actual observations, the necessary sample size must be greater than when the latter are used.

The term *asymptotic relative efficiency* (A.R.E.) is used in comparing nonparametric tests to the corresponding parametric test in terms of power, computed assuming that the assumptions of the parametric test are met. The A.R.E. is defined as $100 \lim_{n \to \infty}(n_a/n_b)$, with $n_a = $ sample size for the parametric test and $n_b = $ sample size for the nonparametric test, using of course the same null hypothesis and assumed true parameter value, α, and power.

For the Wilcoxon test, the A.R.E. is $3/\pi = 95.5\%$. The term *relative efficiency* is $100 n_a/n_b$. PASS can be used to show that $n = 59$ for this example. The relative efficiency is then $100(56/59) = 94.9\%$, slightly less than the A.R.E. If the power is increased to .99, the sample sizes are 149 and 142, respectively, with $100(142/149) = 95.3\%$—very close to the asymptotic result and expectedly closer to 95.5% than with sample sizes of 59 and 56, respectively, since the sample sizes are much larger.

As explained by Conover (1980, p. 291) and Lehmann (2006, p. 80), the A.R.E. of the Wilcoxon test relative to the t-test has a lower bound of 0.864, so a conservative approach would be to compute the sample size for the t-test and multiply it by $(1/0.864) = 1.1574$, and use that as the sample size for the Wilcoxon test. That would be a more defensible approach than what is done when sample size determination software is used because the user must specify a distribution, but if the distribution were known, a test could be performed using the appropriate theory for that distribution and it wouldn't be necessary to use the Wilcoxon test!

Noether (1987) gave the sample size expression for a one-sided test as

$$n = \frac{(z_\alpha + z_\beta)^2}{3(p' - 1/2)^2} \tag{10.1}$$

with α being the significance level of the test, z_α and z_β being as defined in previous chapters, and $p' = P(X + X' > \text{median})$, with X and X' denoting two independent observations. Equation (10.1) results from an approximation that is stated "for sufficiently large n." The existence of z_α and z_β in Eq. (10.1) implies that a normal approximation (i.e., asymptotic approach) is being used. Such approaches can be used when n is large, but whether or not n is large won't be known until it is calculated. How well Eq. (10.1) works for small n, which is an important question since nonparametric procedures are most often applied to small samples, is apparently unknown. It might not work very well, however, because the presence of z_α and z_β in the numerator means that there is the assumption of approximate normality of the test statistic.

The median in Noether's article is assumed to be zero, without loss of generality, but of course this isn't necessary, in general. This requires that the user have some prior knowledge regarding the actual distribution. Note that if symmetry does exist and the median is that specified by the null hypothesis, this would cause Eq. (10.1) to be undefined as the probability for a positive deviation would be .5, as would the probability of a negative deviation. This is essentially irrelevant, however, because sample size in general is for detecting a state that differs from what is specified in the null hypothesis. It wouldn't make any sense to speak of power if the null hypothesis were true. [See Noether (1987, p. 646) for the derivation of Eq. (10.1), which is an approximate large sample result.]

For the current example and the assumed mean of 101, $X + X'$ has a normal distribution with a mean of 202 (μ^*, say) and a standard deviation, $\sigma^* = \sqrt{18} =$

4.24, with the mean under the null hypothesis equal to 200. Then, $P(X + X' > 200 | \mu^* = 202$ and $\sigma^* = 4.24) = .6813$. Then

$$n = \frac{(z_\alpha + z_\beta)^2}{3(p' - 1/2)^2}$$

$$= \frac{(1.645 + 0.84)^2}{3(0.681324 - 1/2)^2}$$

$$= 62.61$$

so $n = 63$ would be used. This differs from the $n = 59$ obtained, as indicated previously, using PASS, but PASS computes the sample size in a different way. Specifically, PASS uses an adjustment from the sample size that would be required for a t-test, following the recommendation of Al-Sunduqchi (1990), who suggested multiplying the sample size required for the t-test (or z-test) by a factor that depends on the assumed distribution. For a normal distribution, as assumed in this example, the multiplier is $\pi/3 = 3.14159/3 = 1.0472$. So PASS obtains $n = 59$ as $56(1.0472) = 58.64$, so $n = 59$ would be used. This is an asymptotic adjustment that is based on the asymptotic relative efficiency of $3/\pi$ that was given previously. Of course, this adjustment should work well when the t-test sample size is large, but perhaps not so well when the t-test sample size is small. This is apparently unknown, however, and needs to be investigated, as does the Noether approximation. Although not specifically addressing this issue, Kolassa (1995) did examine the accuracy of some approximations to sample size and power and concluded that "in some cases one must exercise much care in using the simpler approximations."

Of course, the real value of nonparametric tests is when normality does *not* exist, but we would want to think twice about using a nonparametric test that was very inferior to the corresponding parametric test in terms of power when approximate normality *did* exist.

Note that determining the sample size to be used for a Wilcoxon one-sample test places considerable demands on the user. Unlike a parametric test of a single mean, which requires the user to state a value for the mean that the user wished to detect with the specified power, the user of the Wilcoxon test must not only specify a value for the median of the distribution (or the mean if PASS is used), but must also specify the *name* of the distribution. In reality, this could be anything; in PASS the options are normal, uniform, double exponential, and logistic. To see how the choice of distribution affects the sample size using PASS, the sample sizes produced under the assumption of a uniform, double exponential, and logistic distribution are 56, 38, and 52, respectively, so choice of distribution does have a sizable effect on the sample size when the choice is the double exponential distribution.

G*Power also has the capability for the Wilcoxon one-sample test. Its options for the assumed distribution are normal, Laplace, and logistic. The sample sizes that it produces for each of these are 60, 39, and 52, respectively. Thus, there is agreement between G*Power and PASS for the logistic distribution and a difference of 1 for a normal distribution. MINITAB, Power and Precision, and nQuery all do not have sample size determination capability for nonparametric tests.

If prior information suggests that the actual distribution probably cannot be adequately represented by any of these four distributions, the user might want to estimate p' using whatever distribution seems appropriate (or using prior knowledge, if it exists), and then use the formula given by Noether (1987). Even if one of these four distributions seemed appropriate in a given application, it might be a good idea to determine the sample size using both approaches and compare the results, especially since the work of Al-Sunduqchi was apparently never published.

Sample size expressions for the one-sample signed rank test were considered by Shieh, Jan, and Randles (2007); Wang, Chen, and Chow (2003) looked at sample size determination for both the one-sample test and the two-sample rank test (Section 10.2).

10.1.1 Wilcoxon Test for Paired Data

The Wilcoxon one-sample test can also be applied to paired data and be the nonparametric counterpart to a paired-t test when normality is assumed. That is, the one sample can be a sample of differences, computed by subtracting each of the second set of observations from each of the corresponding observations in the first sample. Then the null hypothesis is the same as when the starting point is just a single sample. This is probably the most common use of the Wilcoxon test.

The set of differences might be correlated, however, so Rosner, Glynn, and Lee (2003, 2006) proposed a modified Wilcoxon test for paired comparisons of clustered data and Rosner and Glynn (2011) proposed sample size determination methods for the test by extending their methods for the regular Wilcoxon test that were given in Rosner and Glynn (2009).

10.2 WILCOXON TWO–SAMPLE TEST (MANN–WHITNEY TEST)

The Wilcoxon two-sample test is more commonly referred to as the Mann–Whitney (1947) test and is sometimes called the Wilcoxon–Mann–Whitney test [as in Rahardja, Zhao, and Qu (2009) and Shieh, Jan, and Randles (2006)]. It is used for two independent samples to test whether the corresponding two populations have the same distribution when it is not reasonable to assume a normal distribution. As such, it is the most commonly used nonparametric test for comparing two populations. Okeh (2009) surveyed five biomedical journals and concluded that the Mann–Whitney two-sample test and the Wilcoxon one-sample test should be used more frequently in medical research, in which nonnormal data are widespread, with much data being ordinal (Rabbee, Coull, Mehta, Patel, and Senchaudhuri, 2003). Posten (1982) studied the power of the test relative to the independent sample t-test for various nonnormal distributions and concluded that the former is superior to the latter, although not for U- and J-shaped distributions. Wang, Chen, and Chow (2003) considered sample size determination for the two Wilcoxon tests and found that the methods work well under various alternative hypotheses for moderate sample sizes.

The two independent samples are merged when the Mann–Whitney test is used for the purpose of ranking the numbers from smallest to largest and the sum of the ranks is computed for each sample. The test statistic is then either the smaller or the larger of the two sums, as it doesn't make any difference which one is used.

As with nonparametric tests in general, there is both an exact test and an asymptotic form of the test. As discussed by Rahardja et al. (2009), the asymptotic version is the one that is most commonly used. One problem with exact tests is that they are generally computationally intensive, with the computations prohibitive for more than small-to-moderate sample sizes. Another problem is that they are generally conservative. For example, for the tests that they considered for a test of association in a small sample, unordered $r \times c$ tables, Lydersen, Pradhan, Senchaudhuri, and Laake (2007) found that "in general, we observe that the significance levels of the exact tests can be substantially lower than α, which demonstrates that exact tests are conservative." Thus, even though the term "*exact* tests" may have a good ring to it, such tests should not automatically be chosen over asymptotic tests. If a large sample size is used, the asymptotic test may be quite satisfactory.

Tied data points and thus tied ranks will often occur, necessitating the use of a method of handling ties. Zhao, Rahardja, and Qu (2008a) proposed such a method, which is incorporated in the R package `samplesize` (see `http://cran.r-project.org/web/packages/samplesize/index.html`).

Most sample size determination software do not have Mann–Whitney test capability, and that is also true for nonparametric tests in general, as noted previously. PASS 11 does have that capability, more or less, but that isn't readily apparent as the routine is not a menu item. This is because it is included as a variation of the parametric t-test, with the sample size computed by adjusting the sample size that would be used for the independent-sample t-test, with the adjustment factor being one of those given by Al-Sunduqchi (1990). Specifically, the appropriate sample size for the independent sample t-test is multiplied by 1 for a uniform distribution; 2/3 for a double exponential distribution; $9/\pi^2$ for logistic distribution; and $\pi/3$ for a normal distribution. It should be kept in mind that those adjustment factors are based on asymptotic theory so they could be off considerably for sample sizes that are not large. The efficacy of these adjustment factors has apparently not been investigated, and similarly, Al-Sunduqchi's (1990) work was apparently never published. Furthermore, since there is no stand-alone Mann–Whitney procedure, there is no adjustment in the case of ties, as in Zhao et al. (2008a).

The need to specify a distribution to determine the sample size for a nonparametric test is disturbing because if the distribution were known, at least approximately, then there wouldn't be a need to use a nonparametric test! To avoid this complication, one recommendation is if the corresponding parametric test is a t-test, one should add 15% to what the sample size should be if the t-test could be used. This is a commonly offered suggestion, provided that the sample sizes are reasonably large. This rule-of-thumb might be motivated by the fact that the A.R.E. of the Mann–Whitney test relative to the t-test cannot be less than 0.864, regardless of the actual distribution (see, e.g., Conover, 1980, p. 291). Since $1/0.864 = 1.157$, this would suggest an adjustment of 15% or 16% as the largest adjustment that should be needed.

Consider the example in Section 3.2 for which the required common sample size for a two-tailed test was given as 16. If we use a Mann–Whitney test with normality assumed for the purpose of determining the relative efficiency, we obtain $n = 17$ using PASS. A slight increase in the sample size would be expected since $n = 16$ is a small sample. We may note that $16/17 = .94$—essentially in line with what we would expect. This would suggest that the proxy for a true Mann–Whitney procedure that is available in PASS may produce reasonable results.

By comparison, nQuery can also be used for the Mann–Whitney test, but the inputs are quite different, as the user must specify $P(X < Y)$, with X and Y being the random variables corresponding to the two groups. A user may have difficulty deciding what value to input since a probability will generally be harder to estimate than a mean or standard deviation. The suggestion given by nQuery is to use the "Assistants" pull-down menu and select "Compute Effect Size." The user then enters each of the two population means and the common standard deviation, and the software computes $P(X < Y)$. For example, if the user enters 50 and 55 for the two population means and 2 for the common standard deviation, the software gives $P(X < Y) = .961$. This is based on the assumption of normality for each distribution as simple hand calculation gives this result since the variance of $(X - Y) = 8$ and $P[(X - Y) = 0 | \mu_1 - \mu_2 = -5]$ leads to $Z = 5/\sqrt{8} = 1.76777$ and $P(Z < 1.76777) = .96145$. Then for a two-sided test with $\alpha = .05$, power $= .90$, and $P(X < Y) = .961$, nQuery gives $n = 9$. Of course, this is a somewhat crude approach to sample size determination because if there was normality and a common standard deviation, a Mann–Whitney test wouldn't be used in the first place! By comparison, G*Power gives a sample size of $n = 10$, using the same inputs, although the user can select a normal distribution as one of the options and doesn't have to specify $P(X < Y)$.

Chakraborti, Hong, and van de Wiel (2006) gave the sample size expression, attributed to Noether (1987), for the Mann–Whitney test for continuous data and equal sample sizes as

$$n = \frac{[z_{\alpha/2} + z_\beta]^2}{6(p - 0.5)^2}$$

and briefly explained how it is derived, with p denoting $P(Y > X)$. See also how it is used in Walters (2004). To illustrate, again assume $\alpha = .05$, power $= .90$, and $P(X < Y) = .961$. This produces

$$n = \frac{[1.96 + 1.28]^2}{6(.961 - 0.5)^2}$$
$$= 8.23$$

so that $n = 9$ would be used, in agreement with the nQuery output. If the desired power had been .80, then $n = 7$ would be used. Although these are very small sample sizes, the inputs used to obtain the .961 probability corresponded to a difference in assumed population means of 1.77 times the standard deviation of $(X - Y)$ and 1.77 is not a small Z-value.

Chakraborti et al. (2006) also gave the sample size that results from solving for sample size from the power expression given by Lehmann (1975) for the Mann–Whitney test, pointing out that it should be more accurate than the expression given by Noether (1987) but it is also more demanding of the user in terms of inputs. Consequently, Chakraborti et al. (2006) proposed two new methods, both of which rely on pilot samples and one method involves bootstrapping.

It should be apparent that a rigorous approach to sample size determination for this test, as well as nonparametric tests in general, will be impossible without (sufficient) data from at least one pilot study. Rahardja et al. (2009) recommended the following:

> For a particular application, we recommend that readers study the plot data carefully and understand the underlying distribution. Then, readers can apply the method most suitable to their data. If possible, we also recommend that readers try various sample size formulas under different assumptions.

Although this is generally sound advice, a considerable amount of data is needed to gain insight into the underlying distribution.

It is well known that a t-test applied to the ranks of the data has the same power and Type I error probability as the Mann–Whitney test. Zimmerman (2011) showed that the power and Type I error probability remain about the same if the number of ranks is reduced from a very large number to a much smaller number by replacing sequences of ranks with a single number.

Divine, Kapke, Havstand, and Joseph (2010) examined the various methods that have been proposed for determining sample size for the Mann–Whitney test and found that under certain conditions the formula given by Zhao et al. (2008a) works just as well as the methods incorporated in nQuery Advisor and SAS 9.2 PROC POWER, although the latter two can be more accurate for certain allocation ratios.

Although exact tests, such as Fisher's exact test, are often computationally prohibitive, some research has been performed on determining sample size for exact tests, such as Hilton and Mehta (1993).

10.2.1 van Elteren Test—A Stratified Mann–Whitney Test

van Elteren (1960) proposed a test that is a form of the Mann–Whitney test and is applicable when the data are stratified and stratified factors are to be accounted for in the analysis. As discussed by Zhao, Rahardja, and Mei (2008b), it has been used in various fields of application, including ecological studies, epidemiological studies, and clinical trials. Qu, Zhao, and Rahardja (2008) compared the Mann–Whitney test when strata are used with the van Elteren test and found that the latter is preferable when the stratum effects are large and the Mann–Whitney test should be used when the effects are small.

Zhao (2006) considered the asymptotic version of the van Elteren test and presented three large-sample size estimation methods, in addition to presenting sample size estimation when the stratum fractions are unknown. Zhao, Qu, and Rahardja (2006) approximated the power of the test when the response data from a new treatment is limited to summary statistics.

10.3 KRUSKAL–WALLIS ONE-WAY ANOVA

This is the counterpart to one-factor ANOVA with normality assumed. The data are converted to ranks, which are used in the computations. PASS uses simulation to arrive at the common sample size and gives suggestions regarding the number of simulations to use, as it does for its many other procedures that use simulation.

Fan, Zhang, and Zhang (2011) used a bootstrap approach to determining sample size. Specifically, they adapted a particular bootstrap power calculation technique, the extended average X and Y method of Mahoney and Magel (1996), and then generalized the sample size calculation method for the Wilcoxon test given by Hamilton and Collings (1991) to the Kruskal–Wallis test. Sample size determination for this test was also considered by Rasch and Šimečková (2007).

10.4 SIGN TEST

Any test that uses only the sign of the number, relative to some criterion, is certainly going to have less power than tests that use the ranks of the numbers, such as the Wilcoxon one-sample test. Thus, the A.R.E. for the sign test will be less than the A.R.E. for the Wilcoxon one-sample test, and it is therefore presented herein after the sign test.

For a two-sided test of H_0: median$_0 = c$, the hypothesis would be rejected if there was a disproportionate number of plus signs (values above c) or minus signs (values below c). The objective would be to solve for n such that a rejection region of size approximately α and the desired power results for a specified value of median $\neq c$. For example, if $n = 17$, we can apply the binomial distribution and observe that below 5 and above 12 gives a significance level of $2(.02452) = .04904$, assuming that median $= c$ and there is a symmetric distribution. (Of course, "above 12" and "below 5" each imply the other when there are no values equal to c.) Let median$_0 = 0$ and median $= 1$, with $\sigma = 1$. Now what is the probability that the number of plus signs exceeds 12 when $\mu = 1$? That probability should be equal to the specified power, which for this example was given as .80.

PASS uses simulation to arrive at the necessary sample size, but that really isn't necessary because the appropriate formula was given by Noether (1987), as well as the development of it. The latter is similar to the development of Eq. (2.3) for the one-sided, one-sample mean test. That equation was given as

$$Z_\alpha + \frac{\mu_0 - \mu}{\sigma/\sqrt{n}} - Z_\beta \tag{10.2}$$

which can be rewritten

$$\frac{\mu - \mu_0}{\sigma/\sqrt{n}} = Z_\alpha + Z_\beta \tag{10.3}$$

Noether (1987) defines

$$Q(T) = \left(\frac{\mu(T) - \mu_0(T)}{\sigma_0(T)} \right)^2$$

as the noncentrality factor for the test T, with the sample size determined by setting $Q(T) = (Z_\alpha + Z_\beta)^2$ and solving for n. Note that this result has the same general form as would be obtained by squaring Eq. (10.3) and solving for n and also note that there is an implied assumption that $\sqrt{Q(T)}$ has a normal distribution, at least approximately.

For the sign test, let $S =$ the number of observations that exceed the hypothesized median [following Noether's (1987) notation]. Then $\mu(S) = np$ and $\sigma^2(S) = np(1 - p)$, with $p = P(X > \text{median}_0)$ and the mean and variance being those of the binomial distribution. With $p = 1/2$, by assumption, it follows that $\sigma_0^2(S) = n(1/2)(1 - 1/2) = n/4$. Then

$$Q(S) = \left(\frac{np - n(1/2)}{n/4}\right)^2 = 4n(p - 1/2)^2$$

Setting $Q(S) = (Z_\alpha + Z_\beta)^2$ and solving for n then produces

$$n = \frac{(z_\alpha + z_\beta)^2}{4(p - 1/2)^2} \tag{10.4}$$

Note that the p in Eq. (10.4) is the "true p." That is, it is the probability that an observation exceeds the hypothesized median, given the actual median. As with Noether's sample size expression for the one-sample Wilcoxon test, this expression depends on the assumption of normality of the test statistic.

To illustrate the use of Eq. (10.4), assume that the standard normal distribution, median = mean = 0, is hypothesized, but the mean and median = 1 instead of zero. Then $P(X > 0| \mu = 1) = .8413$.

Equation (10.2) applies whether the test is upper-tailed or lower-tailed, but if a two-sided test is to be used, z_α would be replaced by $z_{\alpha/2}$.

Assume a two-sided test. Since $P(X > 0| \mu = 1) = .8413$ when normality is assumed with $\sigma = 1$, it follows that

$$n = \frac{(1.96 + 0.84)^2}{4(.8413 - 1/2)^2}$$

$$= 16.955$$

PASS uses simulation to arrive at the same answer. [If the results differed more than slightly, this would suggest that the normal approximation that is inherent in the expression given by Noether (1987) is probably inadequate.] PASS similarly uses simulation to estimate the power and the documentation contains a table giving the degree of error to be expected in estimating the power for various numbers of simulations. When 100,000 simulations are specified, PASS does that many simulations for various sample sizes and converges to $n = 17$ for this example. The value of α is given as .049, which is correct because, as stated previously, $\alpha = .04904$. (This does not depend on the adequacy of a normal approximation because the value of α is, as indicated previously, the sum of two tail areas of the appropriate binomial distribution.) The value for the power is off slightly, however, because PASS gives .882, whereas the correct value, using the binomial distribution, is .88086. PASS does indicate, though, that the true value is between .880 and .884 for the particular set of simulations that I ran, although it is unnecessary to use simulations to compute power because a true distribution with specified parameter values must be assumed in order to compute power, and the power would be computed directly using that distribution.

Ahn, Hu, and Schucany (2011) extended Noether's formula to binary observations that are dependent within a cluster and a sign test is to be used to test a proportion. Specifically, they gave the sample size expression for each of three standardized test statistics, with those test statistics resulting from the use of equal weights to observations, equal weights to clusters, and optimal weights, respectively, while stating that all three standardized test statistics are the same if cluster sizes are constant.

10.5 McNEMAR'S TEST

McNemar's test is a test for significant changes. Lachenbruch (1992) considered the determination of sample size for that test under certain conditions and compared the results with sample sizes given previously in the literature. Lu and Bean (1995) considered the problem of testing the one-sided equivalence in the sensitivities of two medical diagnostic tests under a matched-pair design and derived conditional and unconditional sample size formulas. They claimed that their approach was superior to that of Lachenbruch (1992). Lachin (1992) compared various methods for determining sample size. PASS utilizes the approach given by Schork and Williams (1980).

10.6 CONTINGENCY TABLES

The simplest type of contingency table is a 2×2 table of counts, with the hypothesis that is tested being that the two classification factors are independent. Fisher's exact test is often used as the method of analysis, although it usually will be inapplicable as all four marginal totals would have to be fixed for the test to be applicable.

Very little research has been performed on determining sample size when a contingency table analysis is to be performed. Lydersen, Fagerland, and Laake (2009) give their recommended tests for testing for association in 2×2 tables and very briefly discussed power and sample size calculations for those tests. Some research has been performed for determining sample size for such tables. Dai, Li, Kim, Kimball, Jazwinski, and Arnold (2007) determined sample size for $2 \times 2 \times 2$ tables that are to be analyzed using Fisher's exact test, despite the fact that only two of the marginal totals were known.

10.7 QUASI-LIKELIHOOD METHOD

Mahnken (2009) showed that quasi-likelihood methods can be used for sample size determination when the response variable distribution is unknown but the relationship between the mean and variance is known, or assumed, as only knowledge of the variance as a function proportional to the mean is needed.

Sample size determination, which is done iteratively, is performed using an approach that is based on asymptotic arguments.

Numerical results showed that the results were more conservative than results obtained using Monte Carlo (MC) simulation, and that when the actual distribution was either a normal distribution or a mixture distribution, power estimates are different from the MC power estimates by less than .03 in the vast majority of cases.

10.8 RANK CORRELATION COEFFICIENTS

The Pearson correlation coefficient (see Section 5.7) is based on the assumption that the two random variables have a joint bivariate normal distribution, which implies that they have a linear relationship. As pointed out in Section 5.7, the bivariate normal distribution assumption will hardly ever be met and the relationship may not be linear, so it is then a question of how much of a departure there is from these assumptions.

As an alternative, there are various nonparametric correlation coefficients that are well known and have been used extensively. One of these is the Spearman correlation coefficient, which is the Pearson correlation computed using the ranks of the data. Specifically, the data in each sample are ranked from smallest to largest and the Pearson correlation is computed using those ranks.

Another correlation coefficient is Kendall's tau (τ), which is also a measure of agreement between ranks. As an example, assume that four student essays are ranked by each of two judges. There are multiple ways to compute the value of τ but the simplest way is as follows. List the ranks assigned by the first judge in ascending order and list the ranks of the second judge in juxtaposition and before the ranks of the first judge. Assume that the corresponding ranks of the second judge are, in order, 2 3 1 4. Let Q equal the total number of times that a smaller rank is to the right of each rank. That number is obviously 2 if the second judge's ranks are listed first. Kendall's τ is then computed as $\tau = 1 - 4Q/[n(n-1)]$, with n in this example denoting the number of student essays. Thus, $\tau = 1 - 4(2)/[4(4-1)] = .33$.

Bonett and Wright (2000) stated: "Testing the null hypothesis that a population correlation is equal to zero is not always interesting" and instead they considered sample size requirements for Spearman, Kendall, and Pearson correlation coefficients such that a Fisher confidence interval on the population correlation is of a desired width.

10.9 SOFTWARE

Software for sample size determination with nonparametric procedures is, unfortunately, far from plentiful. Chakraborti et al. (2006) noted that none of the most popular statistical packages provide any options for sample size calculations for the Mann–Whitney test, which motivated them to provide a routine in *Mathematica* that implements the methods that they proposed. As indicated in Section 10.2, however, PASS, nQuery, and G*Power all have Mann–Whitney sample size determination capability, and nQuery has a Mann–Whitney routine for ordered categories in addition to its routine for continuous data. Whereas both PASS and G*Power have capability for the Wilcoxon one-sample test, nQuery does not have that capability.

It should be noted that although PASS has considerable nonparametric capability, its procedures are not menu items and consequently may be difficult to find. For example, PASS can determine sample size for the McNemar test, as stated in Section 10.5, but the test is listed under "Proportions" rather than under "Nonparametric" in the main menu.

10.10   SUMMARY

Users of software for nonparametric procedures may be frustrated and confused when they discover that it is necessary to specify a distribution when a nonparametric test is considered, since nonparametric procedures are also referred to as distribution-free procedures. Power cannot be determined without specifying a distribution, however. All things considered, a simple rule-of-thumb that inflates the sample size for the corresponding parametric test by 10% or 15% to arrive at the sample size for each nonparametric test would undoubtedly have considerable practical appeal.

REFERENCES

Ahn, C., F. Hu, and W. R. Schucany (2011). Sample size calculation for clustered binary data with sign tests using different weighting schemes. *Statistics in Biopharmaceutical Research*, **3**(1), 65–72.

Al-Sunduqchi, M. S. (1990). *Determining the Appropriate Sample Size for Inferences Based on the Wilcoxon Statistics*. Unpublished Ph.D. dissertation. Department of Statistics, University of Wyoming, Laramie, Wyoming.

Bonett, D. G. and T. A. Wright (2000). Sample size requirements for estimating Pearson, Kendall, and Spearman correlations. *Psychometrika*, **65**(1), 23–25.

Chakraborti, S., B. Hong, and M. A. van de Wiel (2006). A note on sample size determination for a nonparametric test of location. *Technometrics*, **48**, 88–94.

Conover, W. J. (1980). *Practical Nonparametric Statistics*, 2nd edition. New York: Wiley.

Dai, J., L. Li, S. Kim, B. Kimball, S. M. Jazwinski, and J. Arnold (2007). Exact sample size needed to detect dependence in $2 \times 2 \times 2$ tables. *Biometrics*, **63**, 1245–1252.

Divine, G., A. Kapke, S. Havstad, and C. L. M. Joseph (2010). Exemplary data set sample size calculation for Wilcoxon–Mann–Whitney tests. *Statistics in Medicine*, **29**, 108–115.

Fan, C., D. Zhang, and C.-H. Zhang (2011). On sample size of the Kruskal–Wallis test with application to a mouse peritoneal cavity study. *Biometrics*, **67**, 213–224.

Hamilton, M. A. and B. J. Collings (1991). Determining the appropriate sample size for nonparametric tests for location shift. *Technometrics*, **33**, 327–337.

Hilton, J. F. and C. R. Mehta (1993). Power and sample size calculations for exact conditional tests with ordered categorical data. *Biometrics*, **49**, 609–616.

Kolassa, J. (1995). A comparison of size and power calculations for the Wilcoxon statistics for ordered categorical data. *Statistics in Medicine*, **14**, 1577–1581.

Lachenbruch, P. A. (1992). On the sample size for studies based upon McNemar's test. *Statistics in Medicine*, **11**, 1521–1525.

Lachin, J. M. (1992). Power and sample size evaluation for the McNemar test with application to case–control studies. *Statistics in Medicine*, **11**, 1239–1251.

Lehmann, E. L. (1975, 2006). *Nonparametrics: Statistical Methods Based on Ranks*, first edition and revised edition. New York: Springer.

Lu, Y. and J. A. Bean (1995). On the sample size for one-sided equivalence of sensitivities based upon McNemar's test. *Statistics in Medicine*, **14**, 1831–1839.

Lydersen, S., M. W. Fagerland, and P. Laake (2009). Recommended tests for association in 2 × 2 tables. *Statistics in Medicine*, **28**, 1159–1175.

Lydersen, S., V. Pradhan, P. Senchaudhuri, and P. Laake (2007). Choice of test for association in sample unordered $r \times c$ tables. *Statistics in Medicine*, **26**, 4328–4343.

Mahnken, J. D. (2009). Power and sample size calculations for models from unknown distributions. *Statistics in Biopharmaceutical Research*, **1**(3), 328–336.

Mahoney, M. and R. Magel (1996). Estimation of the power of the Kruskal–Wallis test. *Biometrical Journal*, **38**, 613–630.

Mann, H. B. and D. R. Whitney (1947). On a test of whether one or two random variables is stochastically larger than the other. *Annals of Mathematical Statistics*, **18**, 50–60.

Mumby, P. J. (2002). Statistical power of nonparametric tests: A quick guide for designing sampling strategies. *Marine Pollution Bulletin*, **44**(1), 85–87.

Noether, G. E. (1987). Sample size determination for some common nonparametric tests. *Journal of the American Statistical Association*, **82**, 645– 647.

Okeh, U. M. (2009). Statistical analysis of the application of Wilcoxon and Mann–Whitney U test in medical research studies. *Biotechnology and Molecular Biology Reviews*, **4**(6), 128–131.

Posten, H. O. (1982). Two-sample Wilcoxon power over the Pearson system and comparison with the *t*-test. *Journal of Statistical Computation and Simulation*, **16**(1), 1–18.

Qu, Y., Y. D. Zhao, and D. Rahardja (2008). Wilcoxon–Mann–Whitney test: Stratify or not? *Journal of Biopharmaceutical Statistics*, **18**(6), 1103–1111.

Rabbee, N., B. A. Coull, C. Mehta, N. Patel, and P. Senchaudhuri (2003). Power and sample size for ordered categorical data. *Statistical Methods in Medical Research*, **12**(1), 73–84.

Rahardja, D., Y. D. Zhao, and Y. Qu (2009). Sample size determinations for the Wilcoxon–Mann–Whitney test: A comprehensive review. *Statistics in Biopharmaceutical Research*, **1**(3), 317–322.

Rasch, D. and V. Guiard (2004). The robustness of parametric statistical methods. *Psychology Science*, **46**(2), 175–208.

Rasch, D. and M. Šimečková (2007). The size of experiments for the one-way ANOVA for ordered categorical data. MODA 8, June 4-8.

Rosner, B. and R. J. Glynn (2009). Power and sample size estimation for the Wilcoxon rank sum test with application to comparisons of C statistics from alternative prediction models. *Biometrics*, **65**, 188–197.

Rosner, B. and R. J. Glynn (2011). Power and sample size estimation for the clustered Wilcoxon test. *Biometrics*, **67**(2), 646–653.

Rosner, B., R. J. Glynn, and M.-L. T. Lee (2003). Incorporation of clustering effects for the Wilcoxon rank sum test: A large sample approach. *Biometrics*, **59**, 1089–1098.

Rosner, B., R. J. Glynn, and M.-L. T. Lee (2006). The Wilcoxon signed rank test for paired comparisons of clustered data. *Biometrics*, **62**, 185–192.

Schork, M. and G. Williams (1980). Number of observations required for the comparison of two correlated proportions. *Communications in Statistics—Simulation and Computation*, **B9**(4), 349–357.

Shieh, G., S.-L. Jan, and R. H. Randles (2006). On power and sample size determinations for the Wilcoxon–Mann–Whitney test. *Journal of Nonparametric Statistics*, **18**, 33–43.

Shieh, G., S.-L. Jan, and R. H. Randles (2007). Power and sample size determinations for the Wilcoxon signed-rank test. *Journal of Statistical Computation and Simulation*, **77**(8), 717–724.

van Elteren, P. H. (1960). On the combination of independent two sample tests of Wilcoxon. *Bulletin of the Institute of International Statistics*, **37**, 351–361.

Walker, S. G. (2003). How many samples? A Bayesian nonparametric approach. *The Statistician*, **52**(4), 475–482.

Walters, S. J. (2004). Sample size and power estimation for studies with health related quality of life outcomes: A comparison of four methods using the SF-36. *Health and Quality of Life Outcomes*, **2**, 26.

Wang, H., B. Chen and S.-C. Chow (2003). Sample size determination based on rank tests in clinical trials. *Journal of Biopharmaceutical Statistics*, **13**, 735–751.

Wilcoxon, F. (1945). Individual comparisons by ranking methods. *Biometrics*, **1**, 80–83.

Zhao, Y. D. (2006). Sample size estimation for the van Elteren test—A stratified Wilcoxon–Mann–Whitney test. *Statistics in Medicine*, **25**, 2675–2687.

Zhao, Y. D., D. Rahardja, and Y. Qu (2008a). Sample size calculation for the Wilcoxon–Mann–Whitney test, adjusting for ties. *Statistics in Medicine*, **27**(3), 462–468.

Zhao, Y. D., D. Rahardja, and Y. Mei (2008b). Sample size estimation for the van Elteren test adjusting for ties. *Journal of Biopharmaceutical Statistics*, **18**(6), 1112–1119.

Zhao, Y., Y. Qu, and D. Rahardja (2006). Power approximation for the van Elteren test based on location-scale family of distributions. *Journal of Biopharmaceutical Statistics*, **16**, 803–815.

Zimmerman, D. W. (2011). Power comparisons of significance tests of location, using scores, ranks, and modular ranks. *British Journal of Mathematical and Statistical Psychology*, **64**(2), 233–243.

EXERCISES

10.1. Justify the use of the 15% rule-of-thumb discussed in Section 10.1.

10.2. What is a major problem when sample size software is used to determine sample size for nonparametric tests?

CHAPTER 11

Miscellaneous Topics

In this chapter we briefly cover several topics that have not been covered to any extent, if at all, in previous chapters.

11.1 CASE–CONTROL STUDIES

A case–control study is an analytical study in which a group of people with a certain disease are compared with a group that does not have the disease, with the comparison made on one or more characteristics. These are retrospective, non-randomized studies and because of this they do not have the value of clinical trials and are generally rated as low quality. See Ury (1975) for a discussion of the efficiency of case–control designs. One option for determining sample size for a matched case–control study is the user-written command `sampsi_mcc` for Stata, which implements the approach described in Dupont (1988).

Satten and Kupper (1990) presented the calculation of sample sizes for unmatched case–control (or cohort) studies in which the objective is interval estimation of the odds ratio. Taylor (1986) discussed determining the number of controls to use in a case–control study. Many other papers have been written on determining sample size for case–control studies, including M'Lan, Joseph, and Wolfson (2006), Hanley, Csizmadi, and Collet (2005), De Santis, Pacifico, and Sambucini (2004), Gauderman (2002), Qiu, Moeschberger, Cooke, and Goldschmidt-Clemont (2000), Garcia-Closas and Lubin (1999), Foppa and Spiegelman (1997), Nam (1992), Hwang, Beaty, Liang, Coresh, and Khoury (1994), and Lubin, Gail, and Ershow (1987).

Sample Size Determination and Power, First Edition. Thomas P. Ryan.
© 2013 John Wiley & Sons, Inc. Published 2013 by John Wiley & Sons, Inc.

11.2   EPIDEMIOLOGY

Cheng, Branscum, and Stamey (2010b) examined the effect of measurement error and misclassification of a response variable and advised researchers to account for these (potential) problems in sample size determination and power calculations of epidemiologic data. See also Smith (1997), who considered sample size determination and power for epidemiologic surveillance. Luan, Wong, Day, and Wareham (2001) considered sample size determination for investigating potential gene–gene and gene–environment interactions. See also Kasiulevičius, Šapoka, and Filipaviciute (2006), which is a somewhat general paper.

11.3   LONGITUDINAL STUDIES

Longitudinal studies are studies of a group of subjects over time, with the group typically being small because of the cost of such studies, which can last for years and sometimes decades. Therefore, it is obviously important that sample sizes should only be as large as necessary for the stated objectives of the study.

Much of the work on sample size determination for longitudinal studies has been performed by Basagaña and Spiegelman (2010a,b, 2011a,b), with a User's Manual for an R program that is available at `http://hsph.harvard.edu/spiegelman/optitxs/optitxs_user_manual.pdf`. Shieh (2003) considered power and sample size calculations for repeated measures and longitudinal studies within the framework of a multivariate general linear model. See also sample size for longitudinal studies as discussed by Barrera-Gomez, Spiegelman, and Basagaña (2012), Donohue, Edland, and Gamst (2010), Lu, Mehrotra, and Liu (2009), Roy, Bhaumik, Aryal, and Gibbons (2007), Tu, Kowalski, Zhang, Lynch, and Crits-Christoph (2004), and Hedeker, Gibbons, and Waternaux (1999). Dawson (1998) illustrated sample size determination using summary statistics and how sample size is affected by summary statistic choice and other factors using an example with longitudinal data.

A case–cohort study is a form of a longitudinal study. Cai and Zeng (2004) considered sample size and power calculations for such studies. See also Kubota (2011). Falagas, Kouranos, Michalopoulos, Rodopoulou, Athanasoulia, and Karageorgopoulos (2010) reported that many comparative cohort studies have not had adequate power. Musonda, Farrington, and Whitaker (2006) derived several sample size formulas for the self-controlled case series method, which is a modified cohort method.

The LBPOWER module in Stata can be used to calculate either sample size or approximate power for longitudinal studies with a binary response and two treatment groups of equal size, provided that the log odds can be assumed to be linear and there is a constant correlation between repeated measurements.

11.4 MICROARRAY STUDIES

One strategy in determining sample size in microarray experiments is to look at each gene separately and determine the desired sample size for that gene, then combine the results to determine the overall sample size relative to the desired overall power. Mukherjee, Tamayo, Rogers, Rifkin, Engle, Campbell, Golub, and Mesirov (2004) considered estimating dataset size requirements for classifying microarray data using learning curves.

As far as multiple comparison tests are concerned, microarray experiments do present special problems because of the sheer volume of data that is involved. Müller, Parmigiani, Robert, and Rousseau (2004) considered the determination of optimal sample size for experiments that involve, in their words, "massive" multiple comparisons. Shao and Tseng (2007) also considered sample size determination for multiple comparisons, as did Jung, Bang, and Young (2005). Orr and Liu (2009) described a package in R, `ssize.fdr`, that can be used for determining sample size.

For additional information on sample sizes for microarray studies, see Liu and Hwang (2007), Tibshirani (2006), Dobbin and Simon (2005), Wei, Li, and Bumgartner (2004), Hwang, Schmitt, Ge. Stephanopoulos, and Gr. Stephanopoulos (2002), Lee and Whitmore (2002), and Chapter 12 of Chow, Shao, and Wang (2008b).

11.5 RECEIVER OPERATING CHARACTERISTIC ROC CURVES

Obuchowski and McClish (1997) considered sample size determination when ROC curves are used in diagnostic accuracy studies. See also Obuchowski (1998).

11.6 META-ANALYSES

Computation of power in a meta-analysis involves similar steps as in power computations for which a single sample is to be obtained (Hedges and Pigott, 2001, 2004). For example, we need the number of studies in the review (the "sample size"), the anticipated overall mean effect size, and the criterion for statistical significance. Meta-analysis in clinical trials is covered in Section 7.6 and power analysis for meta-analysis is covered in detail in Chapter 29 of Borenstein, Hedges, Higgins, and Rothstein (2009). See also Cohn and Becker (2003), who showed that fixed-effects meta-analysis does increase power.

11.7 SEQUENTIAL SAMPLE SIZES

In many statistical applications a single sample size is not determined. This was discussed in Chapter 6 for the use of a sequence of at least two experimental designs. Sequential samples are also popular in clinical trial work, as group sequential trials were covered briefly in Section 7.1.12.

11.8 SAMPLE SURVEYS

Surveys are conducted every day, ranging from surveys to gauge consumer preferences to approval ratings for the President of the United States. Because survey results can be highly influential, it is important that they be well designed. Of course, sample size determination is very important in sample surveys, just as it is in sampling in general.

The following quote from Lohr (1999, p. 8) is important.

> But large unrepresentative samples can perform as badly as small unrepresentative samples. A large unrepresentative sample may do more harm than a small one because many people think that large samples are better than small ones. The design of the survey is far more important than the absolute size of the sample.

As discussed by Lohr (1999, p. 241), "design effects are extremely useful for estimating the sample size needed for a survey. The term "design effect" is due to Kish (1965) and is defined as the variance of the estimator (for whatever is being estimated, such as the population mean) under the sampling plan divided by what the variance of that estimator would have been if simple random sampling had been used with the same sample size. Thus, it is a measure of the efficiency of the sampling plan. Lohr (1999, p. 241) stated that if the design effect for a previous, similar survey is known, the sample size if a simple random sample were to be taken could be estimated and the design effect value then multiplied times that number to obtain the sample size necessary for the complex survey design to be used for the survey that is to be conducted.

Tian, Tang, Liu, Tan, and Tang (2011) considered sample size determination for surveys that contain sensitive questions and Bankier (1988) addressed the problem of determining sample sizes for subnational areas in surveys. Johnson, Su, Gardner, and Christensen (2004) developed a Bayesian approach to sample size computations for surveys that are designed to show evidence of freedom from a disease or infectious agent.

Sample size formulas for various types of sampling (ratio estimation, cluster sampling, etc.) are given by Scheaffer, Mendenhall, and Ott (1979). We discuss sample size determination for cluster sampling in Section 11.9. See also the discussion of sample size determination in survey research in Bartlett, Kotrik, and Higgins (2001).

11.8.1 Vegetation Surveys

Sparks, Mountford, Manchester, Rothery, and Treweek (1997) considered sample size determination for estimating species lists in vegetation surveys.

11.9 CLUSTER SAMPLING

When subjects/objects in a population have some common characteristics, data obtained using these subjects will likely be correlated. One consequence of this is that a sample of correlated observations provides less information than a sample obtained from a population of subjects that are relatively heterogeneous. Accordingly, it is desirable to form clusters of heterogeneous objects and to have clusters that are similar. Sampling would be performed by selecting a sample of clusters from the population of clusters that has been formed and then use every element in each sampled cluster.

■ EXAMPLE 11.1

Kerry and Bland (1998) gave an example with the objective to lower cholesterol readings in patients. A new approach was to be studied relative to the standard approach, with the new approach consisting of intensive dietary intervention by practice nurses using a behavioral approach and the standard approach being the usual practice care. The outcome measure was the average cholesterol reading among patients attending each practice after one year. The study participants will have different medical providers and the number of such providers to sample must be determined, as well as the number of patients per medical practice.

Kerry and Bland (1998) started with the sample size formula when two means are to be compared, which they gave as $n = 21s^2/d^2$, where s^2 denotes the variance of the outcome measure, d is the difference between the means that is to be detected, power $= .90$, and $\alpha = .05$. [*Note:* Although this formula has not been given in previous chapters, it results, as was explained in Section 3.6, from Eq. (3.6) if we set $\sigma_1^2 = \sigma_2^2 = s^2$ and use the Z-values for power $= .90$ and $\alpha = .05$; namely, 1.28155 and 1.95996, respectively. Doing so produces $n = 21.0148$, which of course is virtually equal to 21.]

When clusters are involved, there will be a variance between clusters and a variance within each cluster. Kerry and Bland (1998) let s_w^2 denote the within-cluster variance and s_c^2 the variance of a cluster mean from cluster to cluster. With m subjects in each cluster, the variance of a cluster mean is thus s_w^2/m. The total variance is thus $s_w^2/m + s_c^2$, which is the "within" variance plus the "between" variance, using analysis of variance terminology. They obtained estimates of s_w^2 and s_c^2 from a previous study so that $s^2 = s_w^2/m + s_c^2 = 0.0046 + 1.28/50 = 0.0302$. With this estimate, the required sample size is thus $n = 21(0.0302)/(0.1)^2 = 63$. Thus, 63 groups would be sampled with 50 practices in each group for a total of 3150 patients in each group. ■

See also Tokola, Larocque, Nevalainen, and Oja (2011), who addressed sample size determination, power, and sampling costs when there is clustered data and Kumar and Indrayan (2002), who considered determination of the number of clusters for single-stage cluster-sample surveys.

11.10 FACTOR ANALYSIS

Factor analysis is a statistical method for uncovering the latent structure in a set of variables and is essentially a dimension-reduction technique. There are two types of factor analysis: exploratory and confirmatory. Many different views have been expressed about a minimum sample size for factor analysis and these are summarized here: `http://www.encorewiki.org/display/~nzhao/ The+Minimum+Sample+Size+in+Factor+Analysis`. Kline (2005) stated that sample size should depend on the number of parameters that are to be estimated. That recommendation was investigated by Jackson (2007). See also Marsh, Balla, and McDonald (1988), Marsh, Hau, Balla, and Grayson (1998), and Jackson (2001). Muthén and Muthén (2002) discussed how to use a Monte Carlo study to determine sample size, using confirmatory factor analysis and a growth model for illustration.

11.11 MULTIVARIATE ANALYSIS OF VARIANCE AND OTHER MULTIVARIATE METHODS

Multivariate methods are applied when there is more than one response variable. Hardly any sample size determination software can be used for determining sample size for multivariate methods, however, and D'Amico, Neilands, and Zambarano (2001) lamented this, while explaining how SPSS can be used to compute power. PASS goes further and can be used to determine both sample size and power for various multivariate methods. Specifically, PASS has capability for Hotelling's T^2 (either one sample or two samples, each with p variables) and MANOVA (Multivariate Analysis of Variance). Thus, there are several multivariate methods that are not included (e.g., cluster analysis and factor analysis) and "multivariate" is not a menu item and the multivariate methods are thus not easy to find, but at least some well-known methods are included. G*Power also has the capability for Hotelling's T^2 and MANOVA. Efird and Alimineti (2004) derived a generalized method for computing the exact power of Hotelling's T^2 test and provided SAS code for accomplishing it. Estimating the covariance matrix with good precision is of paramount important and Gupta and Gupta (1987) gave closed-form sample size formulas for the case of a diagonal matrix and gave an integral equation for use in the general case.

The one-sample T^2 test is the extension of the univariate t-test to more than two means, and in fact the PASS Hotelling's T^2 procedure for one sample could, if desired, be used to determine sample size for a univariate one-sample t-test since one response variable with one group is one of the options. This will be illustrated later.

The MANOVA procedure allows the user to choose one of the following test statistics: the Wilk's Lambda, the Pillai–Bartlett Trace, or the Hotelling–Lawley Trace.

The output of PASS for Hotelling's T^2 procedure includes the "effect size," which is defined, in their notation, as

$$\Delta = \sqrt{\left(\mu_A - \mu_0\right)' \sum^{-1} \left(\mu_A - \mu_0\right)}$$

with $\mu = \mu_0$ being the multivariate mean under the null hypothesis, μ_A denoting the multivariate mean that ones wishes to detect with a specified power, and $\sum$ being the assumed variance–covariance matrix, which the user can enter in the spreadsheet.

Power is computed using the noncentrality parameter, which is defined as $\lambda = N\Delta^2$, with power computed using the noncentral F-distribution.

To illustrate, consider the following example.

■ **EXAMPLE 11.2**

Assume that we wish to test the equality of three means—μ_1, μ_2 and μ_3—with the random variables Y_1, Y_2, and Y_3 assumed to be jointly distributed as a multivariate normal distribution with the following variance–covariance matrix:

$$\begin{bmatrix} \sigma_1^2 & \sigma_{12} & \sigma_{13} \\ & \sigma_2^2 & \sigma_{23} \\ \text{sym.} & & \sigma_3^2 \end{bmatrix} = \begin{bmatrix} 10 & 5 & 6 \\ 5 & 15 & 10 \\ 6 & 10 & 18 \end{bmatrix}$$

with "sym" denoting that the matrix is symmetric.

In PASS, Hotelling's T^2 would be accessed by selecting "Means," the "Multivariate Means," then "Hotelling's T-Squared." Use "1" for the number of groups, $\alpha = .05$, 3 for the number of response variables, then click the "Covariance" tab, then click "Spreadsheet," then enter the variance–covariance matrix given above, using the first 3 columns and first 3 rows of the spreadsheet. For "Mean Differences," enter " 2 2 2," signifying that the three means differ from the hypothesized means by two units each. For "Power," enter .80. The result is a sample size of 27 and a power of .8088.   ■

Hotelling's T^2 is the multivariate generalization of the univariate one-sample t-test, and the former can be used in PASS to solve for the sample size of the univariate test. Of course, we wouldn't do that in practice, but it is instructive to see the relationship. For example, for Hotelling's T^2 procedure, specify "1" for both the number of groups and the number of response variables, and enter 2 for the mean differences. Use the same values for power and α as before and enter the number "10" in the first row and first column of the spreadsheet. The output shows $n = 22$ and power $= .8075$. Now select "Means" followed by "One Mean" from the menu and then select "Inequality Tests" and "Specify Using Differences." Enter $3.162(= \sqrt{10})$ for the standard deviation, .80 for power, $\alpha = .05$, 0 for the hypothesized mean, 2 for the alternative mean, and indicate a two-sided test. The sample size is $n = 22$ and the power $= .80752$—in agreement with Hotelling's T^2 results.

Other work on sample size determination in a multivariate setting includes Liu and Liang (1997), who gave a multivariate extension of the work of Self and Mauritsen (1988) for generalized linear models that was cited in Chapter 5, and Wolynski (2005), who considered sample size determination for a Bayes classification procedure. Efird and Alimineti (2005) derived a method for computing power, based on Hotelling's T^2 statistic, for a multivariate repeated measurements design. See also Muller and Peterson (1984), who examined methods of computing power for testing the multivariate general linear hypothesis and Maccallum, Browne, and Sugawara (1996), who considered sample size determination for covariance structure modeling. Muller, LaVange, Ramey, and Ramey (1992) considered power calculations for general linear multivariate models. O'Brien and Shieh (1999) provided an algorithm for computing power probabilities for commonly used F-tests of the multivariate general linear hypothesis. The user-written Stata command `mvsampsi` can be used to compute power or sample size for multivariate F-tests that are derived from Wilks' lambda.

11.12   STRUCTURAL EQUATION MODELING

Structural equation modeling is essentially a combination of factor analysis and path analysis (see, e.g., Olobatuyi, 2006, for the latter). As discussed by Westland (2010), sample size determination for structural equation modeling has been quite a challenge, so it is not surprising that this paper discusses lower bounds on sample size rather than the determination of specific sample sizes. Enders and Peugh (2004) considered the choice of an adjusted sample size for estimating structural equation models with missing data through the use of an EM covariance matrix. Hancock and Freeman (2001) considered sample size for use with an approximation test of not close fit in structural equation modeling. Jackson (2003) investigated the suggestion of some authors that an adequate sample size is related to the number of parameters to be estimated and found only weak support for this contention.

Although structural equation modeling is relatively popular, it is nonetheless a specialized topic and thus it is not surprising that there is almost no available software for determining sample size for such models. Daniel Soper (www.danielsoper.com) has developed many statistical applets, including many for sample size determination. This includes one for structural equation modeling, which can be accessed from www.danielsoper.com/statcalc3/calc.aspx?id=89. The input includes the anticipated effect size, target power, significance level, number of latent variables, and number of observed variables. For example, if these are input as 0.9, 0.8, .05, 2, and 8, respectively, the applet gives 2 as the minimum sample size to detect the effect, and 100 as both the minimum sample size for the model structure and the recommended minimum sample size.

11.13   MULTILEVEL MODELING

The term "multilevel," as in multilevel modeling, is used in different ways, including designating different levels of analysis, such as individuals that are nested within spatial units. Sample size and power issues in multilevel modeling are discussed here, `http://www.esourceresearch.org/eSourceBook/Mult ilevelModeling/17PowerandSampleSize/tabid/353/Default.aspx,` and in Maas and Hox (2005). See also Moerbeek and Wong (2008), Cohen (2005), Snijders (2005), and Snijders and Bosker (1993). MLPowSim is freeware that can be used for sample size and power calculations in multilevel modeling (see `http://www.bristol.ac.uk/cmm/software/mlpowsim`). A recommended book source for information on multilevel modeling is Goldstein (2011).

11.14   PREDICTION INTERVALS

Prediction intervals are frequently used since a predicted value is of limited use without knowing the uncertainty associated with the predicted value, and that uncertainty is built into a prediction interval, just as it is built into a confidence interval. As is true with a confidence interval, a wide prediction interval is of limited value.

Wallis (1980) quoted W. Edwards Deming (1900–1993) as stating: "The only useful function of a statistician is to make predictions, and thus to provide a basis for action." Many users of statistics know prediction intervals only as an interval about a predicted value in regression analysis but there are other types of prediction intervals.

Assume that observations have approximately a normal distribution and there is interest in obtaining a prediction interval for a single future observation. If σ is assumed unknown and to be estimated from a sample, the prediction interval has lower bound given by $\bar{x} - t_{\alpha,n-1}s\sqrt{(1 + 1/n)}$ and an upper bound obtained from $\bar{x} + t_{\alpha,n-1}s\sqrt{(1 + 1/n)}$. (This result is derived in the chapter Appendix.) The width of the interval is thus the upper bound minus the lower bound, with that expression being $2t_{\alpha/2,n-1}s\sqrt{(1 + 1/n)}$. Of course, the general idea is to select the sample size so that the result for whatever is being computed will be acceptable. Here we have the same type of problem that is encountered in trying to determine the sample size for hypothesis tests: the width depends on s, which would be computed *from* a sample, not *before* the sample is taken. This problem might be addressed by estimating σ from the range of possible observations, as was discussed in Section 2.1. If that is done, $t_{\alpha/2,n-1}$ would be replaced by $z_{\alpha/2}$. The sample size expression would then be

$$n = \frac{4\,z_{\alpha/2}^2\,\widehat{\sigma}^2}{w^2 - 4\,z_{\alpha/2}^2\,\widehat{\sigma}^2}$$

with w denoting the width of the prediction interval.

11.15   MEASURES OF AGREEMENT

Sample size for testing a Pearson correlation coefficient was given in Section 5.7, with tests on the equality of two Pearson correlations given in Section 5.7.2 and for intraclass correlation in Section 5.7.1. The Spearman rank correlation coefficient and Kendall's tau were covered in Section 10.8. Correlation coefficients are in the category of *measures of agreement* and there are many such measures. Another such measure is the *kappa coefficient* for testing agreement between two raters. Donner and Rotondi (2010) considered sample size determination when the kappa statistic is used with multiple raters. Flack, Afifi, Lachenbruch, and Schouten (1988) gave a method for determining a sample size that will give a specified bound on the width of a confidence interval for kappa and also presented a table of sample sizes for a power of .80. Sample size determination for testing agreement is available in PASS, SiZ, and nQuery Advisor.

11.16   SPATIAL STATISTICS

Spatial statistics is a relatively new area of statistics. Before the issue of sample size determination can be addressed, the determination must first be made of the effective sample size in the presence of spatial correlations. There appears to be ongoing research on that problem (http://www.am2v.cl/index.php?option=com_jresearch&view=researcharea&id=7&task=show&Itemid=154).

11.17   AGRICULTURAL APPLICATIONS

Agricultural infestations in California, for example, can be a serious problem. Schwertman and Smith (1998) addressed the question of determining an optimal sample size for early detection of the problem. Yamamura and Ishimoto (2009) considered the determination of sample size for estimating the proportion of pecky rice grains when there is composite sampling with subsampling.

11.18 ESTIMATING THE NUMBER OF UNSEEN SPECIES

There has long been a need for estimating the total number of unseen species of various types, such as the number of deer in a forest. Zhang and Stern (2009) addressed the issue of sample size determination for finding unseen species and used a Bayesian approach.

11.19 TEST RELIABILITY

Test reliability refers generally to the ability of a test instrument to measure what it purports to measure. The coefficient alpha (α) is a commonly used index of test reliability. Sample size determination for estimating alpha has been considered by Bonett (2002), with Bonett (2003) and Feldt and Ankenmann (1999) considering sample size determination for comparing two alpha coefficients. See also sample size determination for test reliability as discussed by Shoukri, Asyali, and Donner (2004) and Walter, Eliasziw, and Donner (1998).

11.20 AGREEMENT STUDIES

Agreement studies are similar to test reliability in the sense that measurement methods, say, can be compared with agreement of course being the objective. Liao (2010) proposed a method of determining sample size for such studies.

11.21 GENOME-WIDE ASSOCIATION STUDIES

The objective of a genome-wide association study is to find genetic variations associated with a particular disease. Sample size determination for genome-wide association studies has been considered by Xie, Cai, and Li (2011) and other authors. Pirinen, Donnelly, and Spencer (2012) show that the inclusion of known covariates in a model such as a logistic regression model can, in the case of rare diseases, reduce the power to detect new genetic associations, whereas the power can be increased when a disease is common. Wang and Zhao (2003) discussed sample size requirements for detecting gene–gene interactions. See also Edwards, Haynes, Levenstien, Finch, and Gordon (2005) and Kozlitina, Xing, Pertsemlidis, and Schucany (2010).

11.22   NATIONAL SECURITY

Biometrics have been used during the past several years in national security work. Wu and Wilson (2005) considered sample size determination when biometrics are used with fingerprint data.

11.23   MISCELLANEOUS

Pennington and Volstad (1991) showed that a smaller sampling unit can be more efficient than a larger unit in marine abundance surveys and determined the sample size that produces the most precise density estimate given a fixed amount of survey resources or the sample size that minimizes the cost for a given level of precision. Bochmann, Johnson, and Azuara-Blanco (2007) reported that sample size calculations were not being reported in the ophthalmology literature for diagnostic performance studies. Branscum, Johnson, and Gardner (2007) developed a Bayesian approach to determining sample size for evaluating diagnostic test accuracy and Buderer (1996) considered sample size determination for estimating the sensitivity and specificity of a diagnostic test. Carley, Dosman, Jones, and Harrison (2005) stated that sample size calculations are performed infrequently in diagnostic studies and provided some simple nomograms as aids in sample size determination. Kosinski, Chen, and Lyles (2010) provided a method for determining sample size for evaluating a diagnostic test when the gold standard for the test is missing at random. Liu, Schisterman, Mazumbar, and Hu (2005) considered power and sample size calculation of diagnostic studies with multiple correlated test results.

Cheng, Branscum, and Stamey (2010a) developed a Bayesian procedure for determining sample size and power for cross-sectional studies designed to evaluate and compare continuous medical tests. Although the worth of internal pilot studies in designed experimentation is well accepted, Gurka, Coffey, and Gurka (2010) demonstrated how they can also have value in observational studies.

Analysis of molecular variance (AMOVA) is widely used in genetic data analysis for quantifying the contribution of various levels of population structure to patterns of genetic variation. Fitzpatrick (2009) considered power and sample size determination for nested AMOVA. Gadbury, Page, Edwards, Kayo, Prolla, Weindruch, Permana, Mountz, and Allison (2004) considered sample size and power estimation in high dimensional biology. Ein-Dor, Zuk, and Domany (2006) discussed the need for thousands of samples to generate a robust gene list for predicting cancer outcomes in clinical research.

Cai, Lin, and Lee (2010) considered sample size determination for high-dimensional data analyses and Edwards, Mohai, Halverson, and DeWalle (1989) considered sample size determination for throughfall chemistry. Meadows-Shropshire, Gennings, and Carter (2005) considered the determination of sample size for detecting interactions of drugs or chemicals. Specifically, they determined the number of observations to use at specific mixture points of interest. Hayasaka, Peiffer, Hugenschmidt, and Laurienti (2007) considered power and sample size in neuroimaging studies and Li and Fine (2004) considered sample size for sensitivity and specificity in prospective accuracy studies. Liu, Schisterman, and Teoh (2004) developed procedures for power and sample size and power calculations for planning a study comparing the accuracy of biomarkers in diagnosing diseases. Noble, Bailer, Kunkel, and Straker (2006) considered sample size determination for estimating parameters in small populations.

Voting irregularities and miscounts unfortunately often occur, necessitating some type of audit. McCarthy, Stanislevic, Lindeman, Addona, and Batcher (2008) addressed the question of whether percentage-based audits should be used, or if it is preferable to take a power-based approach to determining sample size. They defined the power of an audit as being equal to the probability of sampling at least one miscounted precinct whenever there are enough precincts with miscounts to have altered the outcome. They pointed out that percentage audits (such as a 10% audit) have limited power and urged the use of power-based audits.

The QT interval is a type of heart measurement. Zhang, Dmitrienko, and Luta (2008) and Chow, Cheng, and Cosmatos (2008a) considered sample size determination for QT studies.

Although a distribution must be specified when sample size determination software is used, Mahnken (2009) presented a method for determining sample size and power for moderate-to-large studies that use quasi-likelihood methods, with the only requirement being that the variance as a functional proportion of the mean be known.

Moon, Lee, Ahn, and Nikolova (2002) gave a Web-based simulator for determining sample size and power in animal carcinogenicity studies. Figueroa, Zeng-Treitler, Kandula, and Ngo (2012) considered sample size determination for predicting a classifier's performance and Guo, Graber, McBurney, and Balasubramanian (2010) considered sample size and power for comparing classification algorithms. Greselin and Maffenini (2007) considered minimum sample sizes for constructing confidence intervals for Gini's mean difference.

Bartolucci, Bae, and Singh (2006) considered sample size determination for stratified random sampling of pond water using a Bayesian approach.

11.24 SUMMARY

Sample size determination in conjunction with many statistical methods and tests has been presented in this chapter and previous chapters. Some familiarity with sample size determination and power is desirable for people in a wide variety of professions and tutorials have been given in the literature to provide the basics (see, e.g., Rempher and Miller, 2008).

REFERENCES

Bankier, M. D. (1988). Power allocation: Determining sample sizes for subnational areas. *The American Statistician*, **42**(3), 174–177.

Barrera-Gomez, J., D. Spiegelman, and X. Basagaña (2012). Optimal combination of number of participants and number of repeated measurements in longitudinal studies with time-varying exposure. Submitted to *Statistics in Medicine*.

Bartlett, J. E. II, J. W. Kotrik, and C. C. Higgins (2001). Organizing research: Determining appropriate sample size in survey research. *Information Technology, Learning, and Performance Journal*, **19**(1), 43–50.

Bartolucci, A. A., S. J. Bae, and K. P. Singh (2006). A Bayesian method of computing sample size and cost requirements for stratified random sampling of pond water. *Environmental Modelling & Software*, **21**(9), 1319–1323.

Basagaña, X. and D. Spiegelman (2010a). Power and sample size calculations for longitudinal studies estimating a main effect of a time-varying exposure. *Statistical Methods in Medical Research*, **19**(3), 1–17.

Basagaña, X. and D. Spiegelman (2010b). Power and sample size calculations for longitudinal studies comparing rates of change with a time-varying exposure. *Statistics in Medicine*, **29**(2), 181–192.

Basagaña, X, and D. Spiegelman (2011a). The design of observational longitudinal studies with a time-invariant exposure. Submitted for publication, *International Statistical Review*, July 2011.

Basagaña, X. and D. Spiegelman (2011b). The design of observational longitudinal studies. Manuscript. Part of doctoral thesis of first author, Harvard School of Public Health. (Available at `http://www.hsph.harvard.edu/donna-spiegelman/files/opt ixs_the_design_of_observational_longitudinal_studies.pdf`).

Basagaña, X., X. Liao, and D. Spiegelman (2011). Power and sample size calculations for longitudinal studies estimating a main effect of a time-varying response. *Statistical Methods in Medical Research*, **20**, 471–487.

Bochmann, F., Z. Johnson, and A. Azuara-Blanco (2007). Sample size in studies on diagnostic accuracy in ophthalmology: A literature survey. *British Journal of Ophthalmology*, **91**, 898–900.

Bonett, D. G. (2002). Sample size requirements for testing and estimating coefficient alpha. *Journal of Educational and Behavioral Statistics*, **27**(4), 335–340.

Bonett, D. G. (2003). Sample size requirements for comparing two alpha coefficients. *Applied Psychological Measurement*, **27**, 72–74.

Borenstein, M., L. V. Hedges, J. P. T. Higgins, and H. R. Rothstein (2009). *Introduction to Meta-Analysis*, Chapter 29. Hoboken, NJ: Wiley.

Branscum, A. J., W. O. Johnson, and I. A. Gardner (2007). Sample size calculations for studies designed to evaluate diagnostic test accuracy. *Journal of Agricultural, Biological, and Environmental Statistics*, **12**(1), 112–127.

Buderer, N. M. (1996). Statistical methodology: 1. Incorporating the prevalence of disease into the sample size calculation for sensitivity and specificity. *Academic Emergency Medicine*, **3**(9), 895–900.

Cai, J. and D. Zeng (2004). Sample size/power calculation for case–cohort studies. *Biometrics*, **60**, 1015–1024.

Cai, G., X. Lin, and K. Lee (2010). Sample size determination with false discovery rate adjustment for experiments with high-dimensional data. *Statistics in Biopharmaceutical Research*, **2**(2), 165–174.

Carley, S., S. Dosman, S. R. Jones, and M. Harrison (2005). Simple nomograms to calculate sample size in diagnostic studies. *Emergency Medical Journal*, **22**, 180–181.

Cheng, D., A. J. Branscum, and J. D. Stamey (2010a). A Bayesian approach to sample size determination for studies designed to evaluate continuous medical tests. *Computational Statistics and Data Analysis*, **54**, 298–307.

Cheng, D., A. J. Branscum, and J. D. Stamey (2010b). Accounting for response misclassification and covariate measurement error improves power and reduces bias in epidemiologic studies. *Annals of Epidemiology*, **20**(7), 562–567.

Chow, S.-C., B. Cheng, and D. Cosmatos (2008a). On power and sample size calculation for QT studies with recording replicates at given time point. *Journal of Biopharmaceutical Statistics*, **18**(3), 483–493.

Chow, S.-C., J. Shao, and H. Wang (2008b). *Sample Size Calculations in Clinical Research*, 2nd edition. Boca Raton, FL: Chapman & Hall/CRC.

Cohen, M. P. (2005). Sample size considerations for multilevel surveys. *International Statistical Review*, **73**(3), 279–287.

Cohn, L. D. and B. J. Becker (2003). How meta-analysis increases statistical power. *Psychological Methods*, **8**(3), 243–253.

D'Amico, E. J., T. B. Neilands, and R. Zambarano (2001). Power analysis for multivariate and repeated measures designs: A flexible approach using the SPSS MANOVA procedure. *Behavior Research Methods, Instruments, and Computers*, **33**(4), 479–484.

Dawson, J. D. (1998). Sample size calculations based on slopes and other summary statistics. *Biometrics*, **54**, 323–330.

De Santis, F., M. P. Pacifico, and V. Sambucini (2004). Optimal predictive sample size for case–control studies. *Journal of the Royal Statistical Society, Series C*, **53**, 427–441.

Dobbin, K. and R. Simon (2005). Sample size determination in microarray experiments for class comparison and prognostic classification. *Biostatistics*, **6**(1), 27–38.

Donohue, M. C., S. D. Edland, and A. C. Gamst (2010). Power for linear models of longitudinal data with applications to Alzheimer's disease Phase II study design. Manuscript.

Donner, A. and M. A. Rotondi (2010). Sample size requirements for interval estimation of the kappa statistic for interobserver agreement studies with a binary outcome and multiple raters. *The International Journal of Biostatistics*, **6**(1), Article 31.

Dupont, W. (1988). Power calculations for matched case–control studies. *Biometrics*, **44**, 1157–1168.

Edwards, B. J., C. Haynes, M. A. Levenstien, S. J. Finch, and D. Gordon (2005). Power and sample size calculations in the presence of phenotype errors for case/control genetic association studies. *BMC Genetics*, **6**(18). (Available at http://www.biomedcentral.com/1471-2156/6/18.)

Edwards, P. J., P. Mohai, H. G. Halverson, and D. R. DeWalle (1989). Considerations for throughfall chemistry sample-size determination. *Forest Science*, **35**(1), 173–182.

Efird, J. T. and K. Alimineti (2004). Computing exact power and sample size for Hotelling's T^2-test and related multivariate procedures. WUSS 2004 Proceedings, SAS Institute, Pasadena, CA.

Efird, J. T. and K. Alimineti (2005). Computing exact power for multivariate repeated measurements design. WUSS Proceedings, SAS Institute, San Jose, CA.

Ein-Dor, L., O. Zuk, and E. Domany (2006). Thousands of samples are needed to generate a robust gene list for predicting outcome in cancer. *Proceedings of the National Academy of Sciences*, **103**(15), 5923–5928.

Enders, C. K. and J. L. Peugh (2004). Using an EM covariance matrix to estimate structural equation models with missing data: Choosing an adjusted sample size to improve the accuracy of inferences. *Structural Equation Modeling*, **11**, 1–19.

Falagas, M. E., V. D. Kouranos, A. Michalopoulos, S. P. Rodopoulou, A. P. Athanasoulia, and D. E. Karageorgopoulos (2010). Inadequate statistical power of published comparative cohort studies on ventilator-associated pneumonia to detect mortality differences. *Clinical Infectious Diseases*, **50**(4), 468–472.

Feldt, L. S. and R. D. Ankenmann (1999). Determining sample size for a test of the equality of alpha coefficients when the number of part tests is small. *Psychological Methods*, **4**(4), 366–377.

Ferreira, J. A. and A. H. Zwinderman (2006). Approximate sample size calculations with microarray data: An illustration. *Statistical Applications in Genetics and Molecular Biology*, **5**(1), article 25.

Figueroa, R. L., Q. Zeng-Treitler, S. Kandula, and L. H. Ngo (2012). Predicting sample size required for classification performance. *BMC Medical Informatics and Decision Making*, **12**(8), electronic journal.

Fitzpatrick, B. M. (2009). Power and sample size for nested analysis of molecular variance. *Molecular Ecology*, **18**, 3961–3966.

Flack, V. F., A. A. Afifi, P. A. Lachenbruch, and H. J. A. Schouten (1988). Sample size determinations for the two rater Kappa statistic. *Psychometrika*, **53**(3), 321–325.

Foppa, I. and D. Spiegelman (1997). Power and sample size calculations for case–control studies of gene–environment interactions with a polytomous exposure variable. *American Journal of Epidemiology*, **146**(7), 596–604.

Gadbury, G. L., G. P. Page, J. Edwards, T. Kayo, T. A. Prolla, R. Weindruch, P. A. Permana, J. D. Mountz, and D. B. Allison (2004). Power and sample size estimation in high dimensional biology. *Statistical Methods in Medical Research*, **13**(4), 325–338.

Garcia-Closas, M. and J. H. Lubin (1999). Power and sample size calculations in case–control studies of gene–environment interactions: Comments on different approaches. *American Journal of Epidemiology*, **149**, 689–692.

Gauderman, W. J. (2002). Sample size requirements for matched case–control studies of gene–environment interaction. *Statistics in Medicine*, **21**, 35–50.

Goldstein, H. (2011). *Multilevel Statistical Models*, 4th edition. Hoboken, NJ: Wiley

Greselin, F. and W. Maffenini (2007). Minimum sample sizes for confidence intervals for Gini's mean difference: A new approach for their determination. *Statistica and Applicazioni*, **5**, 103–122.

Guo, Y., A. Graber, R. N. McBurney, and R. Balasubramanian (2010). Sample size and statistical power considerations in high-dimensionality data settings: A comparative study of classification algorithms. *BMC Bioinformatics*, **11**, Article 447.

Gupta, P. L. and R. D. Gupta (1987). Sample size determination in estimating a covariance matrix. *Computational Statistics & Data Analysis*, **5**, 185–192.

Gurka, M. J., C. S. Coffey, and K. K. Gurka (2010). Internal plots for observational studies. *Biometrical Journal*, **52**(5), 590–603.

Hancock, G. R. and M. J. Freeman (2001). Power and sample size for the root mean square error of approximation test of not close fit in structural equation modeling. *Educational and Psychological Measurement*, **61**(5), 741–758.

Hanley, J. A., I. Csizmadi, and J.-P. Collet (2005). Two-stage case–control studies: Precision of parameter estimates and consideration in selecting sample size. *American Journal of Epidemiology*, **162**, 1225–1234.

Hayasaka, S., A. M. Peiffer, C. E. Hugenschmidt, and P. J. Laurienti (2007). Power and sample size calculation for neuroimaging studies by noncentral random field theory. *NeuroImage*, **37**(3), 721–730.

Hedeker, D., R. D. Gibbons, and C. Waternaux (1999). Sample size estimation for longitudinal designs with attrition: Time-related concepts between two groups. *Journal of Educational and Behavioral Statistics*, **24**(1), 70–93.

Hedges, L. V. and T. D. Pigott (2001). The power of statistical tests in meta-analysis. *Psychological Methods*, **6**(3), 203–217.

Hedges, L. V. and T. D. Pigott (2004). The power of statistical tests for moderators in meta-analysis. *Psychological Methods*, **9**(4), 424–445.

Hwang, D., W. A. Schmitt, Ge. Stephanopoulous, and Gr. Stephanopolous (2002). Determination of minimum sample size and discriminatory expression patterns in microarray data. *Bioinformatics*, **18**, 1184–1193.

Hwang, S.-J., T. H. Beaty, K.-Y. Liang, J. Coresh, and M. J. Khoury (1994). Minimum sample size estimation to detect gene–environment interaction in case–control designs. *American Journal of Epidemiology*, **140**, 1029–1037.

Jackson, D. L. (2001). Sample size and number of parameter estimates in maximum likelihood confirmatory factor analysis: A Monte Carlo investigation. *Structural Equation Modeling*, **8**(2), 205–223.

Jackson, D. L. (2003). Revisiting sample size and number of parameter estimates: Some support for the N-q hypothesis. *Structural Equation Modeling*, **10**, 128–141.

Jackson, D. L. (2007). The effect of the number of observations per parameter in misspecified confirmatory factor analytic models. *Structural Equation Modeling*, **14**(1), 48–76.

Johnson, W. O., C.-L. Su, I. A. Gardner, and R. Christensen (2004). Sample size calculations for surveys to substantiate freedom of populations from infectious agents. *Biometrics*, **60**, 165–171.

Jung, S. H., H. Bang, and S. S. Young (2005). Sample size calculation for multiple testing in microarray data analysis. *Biostatistics*, **6**, 157–159.

Kasiulevičius, V., V. Šapoka, and R. Filipaviciute (2006). Sample size calculation in epidemiological studies. *Gerontologija*, **7**(4), 225–231.

Kerry, S. M. and J. M. Bland (1998). Statistics notes: Sample size in cluster randomization. *British Medical Journal*, **316**, 549.

Kish, L. (1965). *Survey Sampling*. New York: Wiley.

Kline, R. B. (2005). *Principles and Practice of Structural Equation Modeling*. New York: Guilford.

Kosinski, A. S., Y. Chen, and R. H. Lyles (2010). Sample size calculations for evaluating a diagnostic test when the gold standard is missing at random. *Statistics in Medicine*, **29**, 1572–1579.

Kozlitina, J., C. Xing, A. Pertsemlidis, and W. S. Schucany (2010). Power of genetic association studies with fixed and random genotype frequencies. *Annals of Human Genetics*, **74**(5), 429–438.

Kubota, K. (2011). Sample-size formula for case–cohort studies. *Epidemiology*, **22**(2), 279.

Kumar, R. and A. Indrayan (2002). A nomogram for single-stage cluster-sample surveys in a community for estimation of a prevalence rate. *International Journal of Epidemiology*, **31**(2), 463–467.

Lee, M. L. and G. A. Whitmore (2002). Power and sample size for DNA microarray studies. *Statistics in Medicine*, **21**(23), 3543–3570.

Li, J. and J. Fine (2004). On sample size for sensitivity and specificity in prospective diagnostic accuracy studies. *Statistics in Medicine*, **23**, 2537–2550.

Liao, J. J. Z. (2010). Sample size calculation for an agreement study. *Pharmaceutical Statistics*, **9**, 125–132.

Liu, A., E. F. Schisterman, and E. Teoh (2004). Sample size and power calculation in comparing diagnostic accuracy of biomarkers with pooled assessments. *Journal of Applied Statistics*, **31**(1), 49–59.

Liu, A., E. F. Schisterman, M. Mazumbar, and J. Hu (2005). Power and sample size calculation of comparative diagnostic accuracy studies with multiple correlated test results. *Biometrical Journal*, **47**(2), 140–150.

Liu, G. and K. Liang (1997). Sample size calculations for studies with correlated observations. *Biometrics*, **53**, 937–947.

Liu, J.-P., H. Hsueh, and J. J. Chen (2002). Sample size requirements for evaluation of bridging evidence. *Biometrical Journal*, **44**, 969–981.

Liu, P. and J. T. G. Hwang (2007). Quick calculation for sample size while controlling false discovery rate with application to microarray analysis. *Bioinformatics*, **23**(6), 739–746.

Lohr, S. L. (1999). *Sampling: Design and Analysis*. North Scituate, MA: Duxbury.

Lu, K., D. V. Mehrotra, and G. Liu (2009). Sample size determination for constrained longitudinal data analysis. *Statistics in Medicine*, **28**, 679–699.

Luan, J. A., M. Y. Wong, N. E. Day, and N. J. Wareham (2001). Sample size determination for studies of gene–environment interaction. *International Journal of Epidemiology*, **30**(5), 1035–1040.

Lubin, J. H., M. H. Gail, and A. G. Ershow (1987). Sample size and power for case–control studies when exposures are continuous. *Statistics in Medicine*, **7**(3), 363–376.

M'Lan, C. E., L. Joseph, and D. B. Wolfson (2006). Bayesian sample size determination for case–control studies. *Journal of the American Statistical Association*, **101**(474), 760–772.

Maas, C. J. and J. J. Hox (2005). Sufficient sample sizes for multilevel modeling. *Methodology*, **1**(3), 86–92.

Maccallum, R. C., M. W. Browne, and H. M. Sugawara (1996). Power analysis and determination of sample size for covariance structure modeling. *Psychological Methods*, **1**(2), 130–149.

Mahnken, J. D. (2009). Power and sample size calculations for models from unknown distributions. *Statistics in Biopharmaceutical Research*, **1**, 328–336.

Marsh, H. W., J. R. Balla, and R. P. McDonald (1988). Goodness of fit indices in confirmatory factor analysis: The effect of sample size. *Psychological Bulletin*, **103**, 391–410.

Marsh, H. W., K.-T. Hau, J. R. Balla, and D. Grayson (1998). Is more ever too much? The number of indicators per factor in exploratory factor analysis. *Multivariate Behavioral Research*, **33**, 181–220.

McCarthy, J., H. Stanislevic, H. M. Lindeman, V. Addona, and M. Batcher (2008). Percentage-based versus statistical-power-based vote tabulation audits. *The American Statistician*, **62**(1), 11–16.

Meadows-Shropshire, S. L., C. Gennings, and W. H. Carter, Jr. (2005). Sample size and power determination for detecting interactions in mixtures of chemicals. *Journal of Agricultural, Biological, and Environmental Statistics*, **10**(1), 104–117.

Moerbeek, N. and W. K. Wong (2008). Sample size formula for trials comparing group and individual treatments in a multilevel model. *Statistics in Medicine*, **27**, 2850–2864.

Moon, H., J. J. Lee, H. Ahn, and R. G. Nikolova (2002). A web-based simulator for sample size and power estimation in animal carcinogenicity studies. *Journal of Statistical Software*, **7**, 1–36.

Mukherjee, S., P. Tamayo, S. Rogers, R. Rifkin, A. Engle, C. Campbell, T. R. Golub, and J. P. Mesirov (2004). Estimating dataset size requirements for classifying DNA microarray data. *Journal of Computational Biology*, **10**(2), 119–142.

Muller, K. E. and B. L. Peterson (1984). Practical methods for computing power in testing the multivariate general linear hypothesis. *Computational Statistics and Data Analysis*, **2**, 143–158.

Muller, K. E., L. LaVange, S. L. Ramey, and C. T. Ramey (1992). Power calculations for general linear multivariate models including repeated measures applications. *Journal of the American Statistical Association*, **87**, 1209–1226.

Müller, P., G. Parmigiani, C. Robert, and J. Rousseau (2004). Optimal sample size for multiple testing: The case of gene expression microarrays. *Journal of the American Statistical Association*, **99**(468), 990–1001.

Müller, P., C. Robert, and J. Rousseau (2006). Sample size choice for microarray experiments. In *Bayesian Inference for Gene Expression and Proteomics* (K.-A. Do, P. Müller, and M. Vannucci, eds.) Cambridge, UK: Cambridge University Press.

Musonda, P., C. P. Farrington, and H. J. Whitaker (2006). Sample sizes for self-controlled case series studies. *Statistics in Medicine*, **25**, 2618–2631.

Muthen, L. K. and B. Muthen (2002). How to use a Monte Carlo study to decide on sample size and power. *Structural Equation Modeling*, **4**, 599–620.

Nam, J.-M. (1992). Sample size determination for case–control studies and the comparison of stratified and unstratified analyses. *Biometrics*, **48**, 389–395.

Noble, R. B., J. A. Bailer, S. R. Kunkel, and J. K. Straker (2006). Sample size requirements for studying small populations in gerontology research. *Health Services & Outcomes Research Methodology*, **6**, 59–67.

O'Brien, R. G. and G. Shieh (1999). Pragmatic, unifying algorithm gives power probabilities for common F tests of the multivariate general linear hypothesis. Unpublished manuscript. (Available at www.bio.ri.ccf.org/UnifyPow.all/ PowerMVGLH990908.pdf.)

Obuchowski, N. A. (1998). Sample size calculations in studies of test accuracy. *Statistical Methods in Medical Research*, **7**, 371–392.

Obuchowski, N. A. and D. K. McClish (1997). Sample size determination for diagnostic studies involving binormal ROC curve indices. *Statistics in Medicine*, **16**(13), 1529–1542.

Olobatuyi, M. E. (2006). *A User's Guide to Path Analysis*. Lanham, MD: University Press of America.

Orr, M. and P. Liu (2009). Sample size estimation while controlling false discovery rate for microarray experiments using ssize.fdr package. *The R Journal*, **1**(1), 47–53.

Pennington, M. and J. H. Volstad (1991). Optimum size of sampling unit for estimating the density of marine populations. *Biometrics*, **47**, 717–723.

Pirinen, M., P. Donnelly, and C. C. A. Spencer (2012). Including known covariates can reduce power to detect genetic effects in case–control studies. *Nature Genetics*, **44**, 848–851.

Qiu, P., M. L. Moeschberger, G. E. Cooke, and P. J. Goldschmidt-Clemont (2000). Sample size to test for interaction between a specific exposure and a second risk factor in a pair-matched case–control study. *Statistics in Medicine*, **19**(7), 923–935.

Rempher, K. J. and S. Miller (2008). Making sense of statistical power. *American Nurse Today*, June.

Roy, A., D. K. Bhaumik, S. Aryal, and R. D. Gibbons (2007). Sample size determination for hierarchical longitudinal designs with differential attrition rates. *Biometrics*, **63**(3), 699–707.

Satten, G. A. and L. L. Kupper (1990). Sample size requirements for interval estimation of the odds ratio. *American Journal of Epidemiology*, **99**, 381–384.

Scheaffer, R. L., W. Mendenhall, and L. Ott (1979). *Elementary Survey Sampling*, 2nd edition. North Scituate, MA: Duxbury. (The current edition is the 6th edition, 2005.)

Schwertman, N. C. and D. K. Smith (1998). Optimal sample size for detection of an infestation. *Journal of Agricultural, Biological, and Environmental Statistics*, **3**(4), 359–369.

Self, S. and R. Mauritsen (1988). Power/sample size calculations for generalized linear models. *Biometrics*, **44**, 79–86.

Shao, Y. and C. Tseng (2007). Sample size calculation with dependence adjustment for FDR-control in microarray studies. *Statistics in Medicine*, **26**, 4219–4237.

Shieh, G. (2003). A comparative study of power and sample size calculations for multivariate general linear models. *Multivariate Behavioral Research*, **38**(3), 285–307.

Shoukri, M. M., M. H. Asyali, and A. Donner (2004). Sample size requirements for the design of reliability study: Review and new results. *Statistical Methods in Medical Research*, **13**(4), 251–271.

Smith, P. J. (1997). Power and sample size considerations for detecting deviations from secular trends in surveillance surveys. *The Statistician*, **46**(3), 423–432.

Snijders, T. A. B. (2005). Power and sample size in multilevel modeling. In *Encyclopedia of Statistics in Behavioral Science*, **3**, 1570–1573.

Snijders, T. A. B. and R. J. Bosker (1993). Standard errors and sample sizes for two-level research. *Journal of Educational Statistics*, **18**(3), 237–259.

Sparks, T. H., J. O. Mountford, S. J. Manchester, P. Rothery, and J. R. Treweek (1997). Sample size for estimating species lists in vegetation surveys. *The Statistician*, **46**(2), 253–260.

Taylor, J. M. G. (1986). Choosing the number of controls in a matched case–control study, some sample size, power and efficiency considerations. *Statistics in Medicine*, **5**(1), 29–36.

Tian, G.-L., M.-L. Tang, Z. Liu, M. Tan, and N.-S. Tang (2011). Sample size determination for the non-randomised triangular model for sensitive questions in a survey. *Statistical Methods in Medical Research*, **20**, 159–173.

Tibshirani, R (2006). A simple method for assessing sample sizes in microarray experiments. *BMC Bioinformatics*, **7**, 106.

Tokola, K., D. Larocque, J. Nevalainen, and H. Oja (2011). Power, sample size and sampling costs for clustered data. *Statistics and Probability Letters*, **81**, 852–860.

Tu, X. M., J. Kowalski, J. Zhang, K. G. Lynch, and P. Crits-Christoph (2004). Power analyses for longitudinal trials and other clustered designs. *Statistics in Medicine*, **23**(18), 2799–2815.

Ury, H. K. (1975). Efficiency of case–control studies with multiple controls per case: Continuous or dichotomous data. *Biometrics*, **31**, 643–649.

Wallis, W. A. (1980). The Statistical Research Group, 1942–45. *Journal of the American Statistical Association*, **75**(370), 321.

Walter, S. D., M. Eliasziw, and A. Donner (1998). Sample size and optimal designs for reliability studies. *Statistics in Medicine*, **17**(1), 101–110.

Wang, S. and H. Zhao (2003). Sample size needed to detect gene–gene interactions using association designs. *American Journal of Epidemiology*, **158**, 899–914.

Wei, C., J. Li, and R. E. Bumgartner (2004). Sample size for detecting differentially expressed genes in microarray experiments. *BMC Genomics*, **5**(1), 87.

Westland, J. C. (2010). Lower bounds on sample size in structural equation modeling. *Electronic Commerce Research and Applications*, **9**(6), 476–487.

Wolynski, W. (2005). Minimal sample size in the group classification problem. *Journal of Classification*, **22**, 49–58.

Wu, J. C. and C. L. Wilson (2005). Using Chebyshev's inequality to determine sample size in biometric evaluation of fingerprint data. NISTIR 7273, National Institute of Technology, Gaithersburg, MD.

Xie, J., T. T. Cai, and H. Li (2011). Sample size and power analysis for sparse signal recovery in genome-wide association studies. *Biometrika*, **98**(2), 273–290.

Yamamura, K. and M. Ishimoto (2009). Optimal sample size for composite sampling with subsampling, when estimating the proportion of pecky rice grains in a field. *Journal of Agricultural, Biological, and Environmental Statistics*, **14**(2), 135–153.

Zhang, H. and H. Stern (2009). Sample size calculation for finding unseen species. *Bayesian Analysis*, **4**, 763–792.

Zhang, L., A. Dmitrienko, and G. Luta (2008). Sample size calculations in thorough QT studies. *Journal of Biopharmaceutical Statistics*, **18**, 468–482.

Answers to Selected Exercises

CHAPTER 1

1.1. A p-value is the probability that the value of the test statistic is more extreme than the value that was computed if the null hypothesis were true.

1.2. A very small difference in two population means is generally not going to be of any practical interest.

1.6. The statement is misleading because the significance level is the probability of rejecting the null hypothesis if the null hypothesis were true.

CHAPTER 2

2.5. Using Eq. (2.5), we obtain Power $= 1 - \Phi\left[(Z_\alpha - \sqrt{n}(|\mu - \mu_0|)/\sigma)\right] = 1 - \Phi\left[(1.645 - \sqrt{100}(5)/10)\right]$ since σ would be estimated as $(70 - 10)/6 = 10$. Thus, Power $= 1 - \Phi\left[(1.645 - \sqrt{100}(5)/10)\right] = 1 - \Phi\left[-3.355\right] = 1 - .00039 = .9996$. The experimenter should not have arbitrarily selected the number of observations because the power is far higher than necessary or desirable. Next time the experimenter should use software to determine the sample size to use or, if preferred, perform the computation by hand.

2.8. No, because sigma might have been overestimated by at least enough to make up the difference.

Sample Size Determination and Power, First Edition. Thomas P. Ryan.
© 2013 John Wiley & Sons, Inc. Published 2013 by John Wiley & Sons, Inc.

CHAPTER 3

3.1. Using the PASS software, the required minimum sample size is 56. If $n = 100$ is used, the power is .95434. Since such a power value would generally be considered excessive, this illustrates why sample size should not be arbitrarily chosen.

3.2. It is never logical or practical to use hand computation when iteration is required, as is the case if Eq. (3.4) were used to solve for a sample size. So the use of software is imperative.

3.8. The power will probably be less because it is more difficult to detect a small difference than a large difference. A definite answer cannot be given, however, because the standard deviations are almost certainly unknown and will not be estimated precisely, so it depends on the magnitudes and direction of the misestimation.

CHAPTER 4

4.1. Using

$$ n = \left[\frac{z_\alpha \sqrt{(p_1 + p_2)(1 - p_1 + 1 - p_2)/2} + z_\beta \sqrt{p_1(1 - p_1) + p_2(1 - p_2)}}{p_1 - p_2} \right]^2 $$

we have

$$ n = \left[\frac{1.645\sqrt{(.55 + .65)(1 - .55 + 1 - .65)/2} + 0.84\sqrt{.55(1 - .55) + .65(1 - .65)}}{.55 - .65} \right]^2 $$

so that $n = 295.365$ and $n = 296$ would thus be used. It is desirable to see how sample sizes are obtained, but once that understanding is achieved, it is preferable to use software to determine sample size when the necessary hand calculation would be somewhat mathematically laborious.

4.5. Using the PASS software, we obtain $n = 35$. Of course, the use of software is almost imperative, because there is no equation for the sample size, as stated in Section 4.5.

CHAPTER 5

5.2. Using the Demidenko applet, a sample size of $n = 275$ is obtained.

5.3. Since the minimum acceptable R^2 value was stated, let's start with that and the relationship between R^2 and the calculated t-statistic for testing the null hypothesis that $\beta_1 = 0$, with that relationship being $R^2 = t^2/(n - 2 + t^2)$. We know that we need to do more than just barely reject the null hypothesis in order to have a good model, so let's combine this expression with the Wetz criterion. If the latter is just barely met, then $R^2 = 4t^2_{\alpha/2,n-2}/(n - 2 + 4t^2_{\alpha/2,n-2})$. Substituting .75 for R^2 and solving for n gives $n = \frac{4}{3} t^2_{\alpha/2,n-2} + 2$. Unfortunately, this doesn't give us a simple solution since n is on both sides of the equation. We can, however, write a small program to produce the value of each side of the equation for a range of n values and see where approximate equality occurs. This will give us, at the very least, a starting point for determining n. Doing so and using $\alpha = .05$ produces the following results.

n	$\frac{4}{3} t^2_{.025,n-2} + 2$
5	15.5040
6	12.2782
7	10.8105
8	9.9832
9	9.4553
10	9.0902
11	8.8231
12	8.6195

This leads us to zero in on $n = 9$ or 10 because if a fractional value for n were possible, equality between the left side and the right side would occur between 9 and 10. If we used $n = 10$ and the Wetz criterion is just barely met, then $R^2 = .73$. Similarly, $n = 9$ gives $R^2 = .76$. Thus, $n = 9$ or 10 is a reasonable choice for this problem, in general accordance with the Draper and Smith rule-of-thumb and in recognition of the cost of sampling. Of course, this says nothing about whether the Wetz criterion will actually be met, as that will depend on the relationship between X and Y.

5.4. The use of a sample size of 10 may be acceptable, depending on the expected variability of the data, but the use of retrospective power is not acceptable.

CHAPTER 6

6.4. This would make it impossible to determine the sample size. If MINITAB is used, for example, the user must enter the "values of the maximum difference between means." If Power and Precision were used, the user would enter the "effect size f." The user of nQuery Advisor must enter either the effect size or both the variance of the means and the common standard deviation. And so on.

6.12. (a) The required sample sizes are 97, 81, and 50 for $a = 19$, 20, and 22, respectively.

(b) The required sample sizes are 693, 709, and 740 for $a = -19$, -20, and -22, respectively.

CHAPTER 7

7.1. Using PASS 11, the required sample size for the clinical trial is 55. The null hypothesis will be rejected if the number of responses is at least 10.

7.2. There should be concern because some survey articles have shown that a very high percentage of clinical trials have been underpowered. This should be alarming since human subjects are involved in the experimentation.

CHAPTER 8

8.1. These values are obtained by first computing

$$Z = \left(\mu + 3\sigma/\sqrt{n} - (\mu + a\sigma)\right) / \left(\sigma/\sqrt{n}\right)$$
$$= 3 - a\sqrt{n}$$

with $a = 1$. Thus, for $n = 4$, $Z = 1$ and $P(Z > 1) = .15866$, as can be obtained using statistical software. The other values in Table 8.1 would be obtained by substituting each of the other values of n in the expression for Z.

CHAPTER 9

9.1. PASS gives the sample size for each group as 328 and the power as .8001. The number of events is given as 214 for the first group and 213 for the second group. This is important information as these numbers of events must occur in order for the desired power to be attained.

CHAPTER 10

10.2. In PASS, for example, the routine for a test of one mean with a Wilcoxon test is the same routine as is used when normality is assumed. The difference is that for the Wilcoxon test the user specifies a "nonparametric adjustment" and selects either the uniform, double exponential, or logistic distribution. This is necessary for determining the power of the test. If the true distribution were known, however, then there would not be a need to use a nonparametric test, as a user could work directly with that distribution, as indicated in Section 10.1. Thus, determining sample size for nonparametric tests can very easily be a less-than-satisfying exercise.

Index

Sample Size Determination and Power, First Edition. Thomas P. Ryan.
© 2013 John Wiley & Sons, Inc. Published 2013 by John Wiley & Sons, Inc.

WILEY SERIES IN PROBABILITY AND STATISTICS
ESTABLISHED BY WALTER A. SHEWHART AND SAMUEL S. WILKS

Editors: *David J. Balding, Noel A. C. Cressie, Garrett M. Fitzmaurice,*
Harvey Goldstein, Iain M. Johnstone, Geert Molenberghs, David W. Scott,
Adrian F. M. Smith, Ruey S. Tsay, Sanford Weisberg
Editors Emeriti: *Vic Barnett, J. Stuart Hunter, Joseph B. Kadane, Jozef L. Teugels*

The **Wiley Series in Probability and Statistics** is well established and authoritative. It covers many topics of current research interest in both pure and applied statistics and probability theory. Written by leading statisticians and institutions, the titles span both state-of-the-art developments in the field and classical methods.

Reflecting the wide range of current research in statistics, the series encompasses applied, methodological and theoretical statistics, ranging from applications and new techniques made possible by advances in computerized practice to rigorous treatment of theoretical approaches.

This series provides essential and invaluable reading for all statisticians, whether in academia, industry, government, or research.

† ABRAHAM and LEDOLTER · Statistical Methods for Forecasting
AGRESTI · Analysis of Ordinal Categorical Data, *Second Edition*
AGRESTI · An Introduction to Categorical Data Analysis, *Second Edition*
AGRESTI · Categorical Data Analysis, *Second Edition*
ALTMAN, GILL, and McDONALD · Numerical Issues in Statistical Computing for the
Social Scientist
AMARATUNGA and CABRERA · Exploration and Analysis of DNA Microarray and
Protein Array Data
ANDĚL · Mathematics of Chance
ANDERSON · An Introduction to Multivariate Statistical Analysis, *Third Edition*
* ANDERSON · The Statistical Analysis of Time Series
ANDERSON, AUQUIER, HAUCK, OAKES, VANDAELE, and WEISBERG ·
Statistical Methods for Comparative Studies
ANDERSON and LOYNES · The Teaching of Practical Statistics
ARMITAGE and DAVID (editors) · Advances in Biometry
ARNOLD, BALAKRISHNAN, and NAGARAJA · Records
* ARTHANARI and DODGE · Mathematical Programming in Statistics
* BAILEY · The Elements of Stochastic Processes with Applications to the Natural
Sciences
BAJORSKI · Statistics for Imaging, Optics, and Photonics
BALAKRISHNAN and KOUTRAS · Runs and Scans with Applications
BALAKRISHNAN and NG · Precedence-Type Tests and Applications
BARNETT · Comparative Statistical Inference, *Third Edition*
BARNETT · Environmental Statistics
BARNETT and LEWIS · Outliers in Statistical Data, *Third Edition*
BARTHOLOMEW, KNOTT, and MOUSTAKI · Latent Variable Models and Factor
Analysis: A Unified Approach, *Third Edition*
BARTOSZYNSKI and NIEWIADOMSKA-BUGAJ · Probability and Statistical
Inference, *Second Edition*
BASILEVSKY · Statistical Factor Analysis and Related Methods: Theory and
Applications
BATES and WATTS · Nonlinear Regression Analysis and Its Applications
BECHHOFER, SANTNER, and GOLDSMAN · Design and Analysis of Experiments for
Statistical Selection, Screening, and Multiple Comparisons

*Now available in a lower priced paperback edition in the Wiley Classics Library.
†Now available in a lower priced paperback edition in the Wiley–Interscience Paperback Series.

BEIRLANT, GOEGEBEUR, SEGERS, TEUGELS, and DE WAAL · Statistics of
   Extremes: Theory and Applications

BELSLEY · Conditioning Diagnostics: Collinearity and Weak Data in Regression

† BELSLEY, KUH, and WELSCH · Regression Diagnostics: Identifying Influential Data
   and Sources of Collinearity

BENDAT and PIERSOL · Random Data: Analysis and Measurement Procedures, *Fourth
   Edition*

BERNARDO and SMITH · Bayesian Theory

BHAT and MILLER · Elements of Applied Stochastic Processes, *Third Edition*

BHATTACHARYA and WAYMIRE · Stochastic Processes with Applications

BIEMER, GROVES, LYBERG, MATHIOWETZ, and SUDMAN · Measurement Errors
   in Surveys

BILLINGSLEY · Convergence of Probability Measures, *Second Edition*

BILLINGSLEY · Probability and Measure, *Anniversary Edition*

BIRKES and DODGE · Alternative Methods of Regression

BISGAARD and KULAHCI · Time Series Analysis and Forecasting by Example

BISWAS, DATTA, FINE, and SEGAL · Statistical Advances in the Biomedical Sciences:
   Clinical Trials, Epidemiology, Survival Analysis, and Bioinformatics

BLISCHKE and MURTHY (editors) · Case Studies in Reliability and Maintenance

BLISCHKE and MURTHY · Reliability: Modeling, Prediction, and Optimization

BLOOMFIELD · Fourier Analysis of Time Series: An Introduction, *Second Edition*

BOLLEN · Structural Equations with Latent Variables

BOLLEN and CURRAN · Latent Curve Models: A Structural Equation Perspective

BOROVKOV · Ergodicity and Stability of Stochastic Processes

BOSQ and BLANKE · Inference and Prediction in Large Dimensions

BOULEAU · Numerical Methods for Stochastic Processes

* BOX and TIAO · Bayesian Inference in Statistical Analysis

BOX · Improving Almost Anything, *Revised Edition*

* BOX and DRAPER · Evolutionary Operation: A Statistical Method for Process
   Improvement

BOX and DRAPER · Response Surfaces, Mixtures, and Ridge Analyses, *Second Edition*

BOX, HUNTER, and HUNTER · Statistics for Experimenters: Design, Innovation, and
   Discovery, *Second Editon*

BOX, JENKINS, and REINSEL · Time Series Analysis: Forcasting and Control, *Fourth
   Edition*

BOX, LUCEÑO, and PANIAGUA-QUIÑONES · Statistical Control by Monitoring and
   Adjustment, *Second Edition*

* BROWN and HOLLANDER · Statistics: A Biomedical Introduction

CAIROLI and DALANG · Sequential Stochastic Optimization

CASTILLO, HADI, BALAKRISHNAN, and SARABIA · Extreme Value and Related
   Models with Applications in Engineering and Science

CHAN · Time Series: Applications to Finance with R and S-Plus®, *Second Edition*

CHARALAMBIDES · Combinatorial Methods in Discrete Distributions

CHATTERJEE and HADI · Regression Analysis by Example, *Fourth Edition*

CHATTERJEE and HADI · Sensitivity Analysis in Linear Regression

CHERNICK · Bootstrap Methods: A Guide for Practitioners and Researchers, *Second
   Edition*

CHERNICK and FRIIS · Introductory Biostatistics for the Health Sciences

CHILÈS and DELFINER · Geostatistics: Modeling Spatial Uncertainty, *Second Edition*

CHOW and LIU · Design and Analysis of Clinical Trials: Concepts and Methodologies,
   Second Edition

CLARKE · Linear Models: The Theory and Application of Analysis of Variance

CLARKE and DISNEY · Probability and Random Processes: A First Course with
   Applications, *Second Edition*

*Now available in a lower priced paperback edition in the Wiley Classics Library.

†Now available in a lower priced paperback edition in the Wiley–Interscience Paperback Series.

---

*Now available in a lower priced paperback edition in the Wiley Classics Library.

†Now available in a lower priced paperback edition in the Wiley–Interscience Paperback Series.

FELLER · An Introduction to Probability Theory and Its Applications, Volume I, *Third Edition,* Revised; Volume II, *Second Edition*

FITZMAURICE, LAIRD, and WARE · Applied Longitudinal Analysis, *Second Edition*

* FLEISS · The Design and Analysis of Clinical Experiments

FLEISS · Statistical Methods for Rates and Proportions, *Third Edition*

† FLEMING and HARRINGTON · Counting Processes and Survival Analysis

FUJIKOSHI, ULYANOV, and SHIMIZU · Multivariate Statistics: High-Dimensional and Large-Sample Approximations

FULLER · Introduction to Statistical Time Series, *Second Edition*

† FULLER · Measurement Error Models

GALLANT · Nonlinear Statistical Models

GEISSER · Modes of Parametric Statistical Inference

GELMAN and MENG · Applied Bayesian Modeling and Causal Inference from ncomplete-Data Perspectives

GEWEKE · Contemporary Bayesian Econometrics and Statistics

GHOSH, MUKHOPADHYAY, and SEN · Sequential Estimation

GIESBRECHT and GUMPERTZ · Planning, Construction, and Statistical Analysis of Comparative Experiments

GIFI · Nonlinear Multivariate Analysis

GIVENS and HOETING · Computational Statistics

GLASSERMAN and YAO · Monotone Structure in Discrete-Event Systems

GNANADESIKAN · Methods for Statistical Data Analysis of Multivariate Observations, *Second Edition*

GOLDSTEIN · Multilevel Statistical Models, *Fourth Edition*

GOLDSTEIN and LEWIS · Assessment: Problems, Development, and Statistical Issues

GOLDSTEIN and WOOFF · Bayes Linear Statistics

GREENWOOD and NIKULIN · A Guide to Chi-Squared Testing

GROSS, SHORTLE, THOMPSON, and HARRIS · Fundamentals of Queueing Theory, *Fourth Edition*

GROSS, SHORTLE, THOMPSON, and HARRIS · Solutions Manual to Accompany Fundamentals of Queueing Theory, *Fourth Edition*

* HAHN and SHAPIRO · Statistical Models in Engineering

HAHN and MEEKER · Statistical Intervals: A Guide for Practitioners

HALD · A History of Probability and Statistics and their Applications Before 1750

† HAMPEL · Robust Statistics: The Approach Based on Influence Functions

HARTUNG, KNAPP, and SINHA · Statistical Meta-Analysis with Applications

HEIBERGER · Computation for the Analysis of Designed Experiments

HEDAYAT and SINHA · Design and Inference in Finite Population Sampling

HEDEKER and GIBBONS · Longitudinal Data Analysis

HELLER · MACSYMA for Statisticians

HERITIER, CANTONI, COPT, and VICTORIA-FESER · Robust Methods in Biostatistics

HINKELMANN and KEMPTHORNE · Design and Analysis of Experiments, Volume 1: Introduction to Experimental Design, *Second Edition*

HINKELMANN and KEMPTHORNE · Design and Analysis of Experiments, Volume 2: Advanced Experimental Design

HINKELMANN (editor) · Design and Analysis of Experiments, Volume 3: Special Designs and Applications

HOAGLIN, MOSTELLER, and TUKEY · Fundamentals of Exploratory Analysis of Variance

* HOAGLIN, MOSTELLER, and TUKEY · Exploring Data Tables, Trends and Shapes

* HOAGLIN, MOSTELLER, and TUKEY · Understanding Robust and Exploratory Data Analysis

---

*Now available in a lower priced paperback edition in the Wiley Classics Library.

†Now available in a lower priced paperback edition in the Wiley–Interscience Paperback Series.

HOCHBERG and TAMHANE · Multiple Comparison Procedures

HOCKING · Methods and Applications of Linear Models: Regression and the Analysis of Variance, *Third Edition*

HOEL · Introduction to Mathematical Statistics, *Fifth Edition*

HOGG and KLUGMAN · Loss Distributions

HOLLANDER, WOLFE, and CHICKEN · Nonparametric Statistical Methods, *Third Edition*

HOSMER and LEMESHOW · Applied Logistic Regression, *Second Edition*

HOSMER, LEMESHOW, and MAY · Applied Survival Analysis: Regression Modeling of Time-to-Event Data, *Second Edition*

HUBER · Data Analysis: What Can Be Learned From the Past 50 Years

HUBER · Robust Statistics

† HUBER and RONCHETTI · Robust Statistics, *Second Edition*

HUBERTY · Applied Discriminant Analysis, *Second Edition*

HUBERTY and OLEJNIK · Applied MANOVA and Discriminant Analysis, *Second Edition*

HUITEMA · The Analysis of Covariance and Alternatives: Statistical Methods for Experiments, Quasi-Experiments, and Single-Case Studies, *Second Edition*

HUNT and KENNEDY · Financial Derivatives in Theory and Practice, *Revised Edition*

HURD and MIAMEE · Periodically Correlated Random Sequences: Spectral Theory and Practice

HUSKOVA, BERAN, and DUPAC · Collected Works of Jaroslav Hajek— with Commentary

HUZURBAZAR · Flowgraph Models for Multistate Time-to-Event Data

JACKMAN · Bayesian Analysis for the Social Sciences

† JACKSON · A User's Guide to Principle Components

JOHN · Statistical Methods in Engineering and Quality Assurance

JOHNSON · Multivariate Statistical Simulation

JOHNSON and BALAKRISHNAN · Advances in the Theory and Practice of Statistics: A Volume in Honor of Samuel Kotz

JOHNSON, KEMP, and KOTZ · Univariate Discrete Distributions, *Third Edition*

JOHNSON and KOTZ (editors) · Leading Personalities in Statistical Sciences: From the Seventeenth Century to the Present

JOHNSON, KOTZ, and BALAKRISHNAN · Continuous Univariate Distributions, Volume 1, *Second Edition*

JOHNSON, KOTZ, and BALAKRISHNAN · Continuous Univariate Distributions, Volume 2, *Second Edition*

JOHNSON, KOTZ, and BALAKRISHNAN · Discrete Multivariate Distributions

JUDGE, GRIFFITHS, HILL, LÜTKEPOHL, and LEE · The Theory and Practice of Econometrics, *Second Edition*

JUREK and MASON · Operator-Limit Distributions in Probability Theory

KADANE · Bayesian Methods and Ethics in a Clinical Trial Design

KADANE AND SCHUM · A Probabilistic Analysis of the Sacco and Vanzetti Evidence

KALBFLEISCH and PRENTICE · The Statistical Analysis of Failure Time Data, *Second Edition*

KARIYA and KURATA · Generalized Least Squares

KASS and VOS · Geometrical Foundations of Asymptotic Inference

† KAUFMAN and ROUSSEEUW · Finding Groups in Data: An Introduction to Cluster Analysis

KEDEM and FOKIANOS · Regression Models for Time Series Analysis

KENDALL, BARDEN, CARNE, and LE · Shape and Shape Theory

KHURI · Advanced Calculus with Applications in Statistics, *Second Edition*

KHURI, MATHEW, and SINHA · Statistical Tests for Mixed Linear Models

* KISH · Statistical Design for Research

*Now available in a lower priced paperback edition in the Wiley Classics Library.

†Now available in a lower priced paperback edition in the Wiley–Interscience Paperback Series.

---

*Now available in a lower priced paperback edition in the Wiley Classics Library.

†Now available in a lower priced paperback edition in the Wiley–Interscience Paperback Series.

*Now available in a lower priced paperback edition in the Wiley Classics Library.
†Now available in a lower priced paperback edition in the Wiley–Interscience Paperback Series.

† SEBER · Multivariate Observations

SEBER and LEE · Linear Regression Analysis, *Second Edition*

† SEBER and WILD · Nonlinear Regression

SENNOTT · Stochastic Dynamic Programming and the Control of Queueing Systems

* SERFLING · Approximation Theorems of Mathematical Statistics

SHAFER and VOVK · Probability and Finance: It's Only a Game!

SHERMAN · Spatial Statistics and Spatio-Temporal Data: Covariance Functions and Directional Properties

SILVAPULLE and SEN · Constrained Statistical Inference: Inequality, Order, and Shape Restrictions

SINGPURWALLA · Reliability and Risk: A Bayesian Perspective

SMALL and McLEISH · Hilbert Space Methods in Probability and Statistical Inference

SRIVASTAVA · Methods of Multivariate Statistics

STAPLETON · Linear Statistical Models, *Second Edition*

STAPLETON · Models for Probability and Statistical Inference: Theory and Applications

STAUDTE and SHEATHER · Robust Estimation and Testing

STOYAN · Counterexamples in Probability, *Second Edition*

STOYAN, KENDALL, and MECKE · Stochastic Geometry and Its Applications, *Second Edition*

STOYAN and STOYAN · Fractals, Random Shapes and Point Fields: Methods of Geometrical Statistics

STREET and BURGESS · The Construction of Optimal Stated Choice Experiments: Theory and Methods

STYAN · The Collected Papers of T. W. Anderson: 1943–1985

SUTTON, ABRAMS, JONES, SHELDON, and SONG · Methods for Meta-Analysis in Medical Research

TAKEZAWA · Introduction to Nonparametric Regression

TAMHANE · Statistical Analysis of Designed Experiments: Theory and Applications

TANAKA · Time Series Analysis: Nonstationary and Noninvertible Distribution Theory

THOMPSON · Empirical Model Building: Data, Models, and Reality, *Second Edition*

THOMPSON · Sampling, *Third Edition*

THOMPSON · Simulation: A Modeler's Approach

THOMPSON and SEBER · Adaptive Sampling

THOMPSON, WILLIAMS, and FINDLAY · Models for Investors in Real World Markets

TIERNEY · LISP-STAT: An Object-Oriented Environment for Statistical Computing and Dynamic Graphics

TSAY · Analysis of Financial Time Series, *Third Edition*

TSAY · An Introduction to Analysis of Financial Data with R

UPTON and FINGLETON · Spatial Data Analysis by Example, Volume II: Categorical and Directional Data

† VAN BELLE · Statistical Rules of Thumb, *Second Edition*

VAN BELLE, FISHER, HEAGERTY, and LUMLEY · Biostatistics: A Methodology for the Health Sciences, *Second Edition*

VESTRUP · The Theory of Measures and Integration

VIDAKOVIC · Statistical Modeling by Wavelets

VIERTL · Statistical Methods for Fuzzy Data

VINOD and REAGLE · Preparing for the Worst: Incorporating Downside Risk in Stock Market Investments

WALLER and GOTWAY · Applied Spatial Statistics for Public Health Data

WEISBERG · Applied Linear Regression, *Third Edition*

WEISBERG · Bias and Causation: Models and Judgment for Valid Comparisons

WELSH · Aspects of Statistical Inference

*Now available in a lower priced paperback edition in the Wiley Classics Library.

†Now available in a lower priced paperback edition in the Wiley–Interscience Paperback Series.

WESTFALL and YOUNG · Resampling-Based Multiple Testing: Examples and Methods for *p*-Value Adjustment

* WHITTAKER · Graphical Models in Applied Multivariate Statistics

WINKER · Optimization Heuristics in Economics: Applications of Threshold Accepting

WOODWORTH · Biostatistics: A Bayesian Introduction

WOOLSON and CLARKE · Statistical Methods for the Analysis of Biomedical Data, *Second Edition*

WU and HAMADA · Experiments: Planning, Analysis, and Parameter Design Optimization, *Second Edition*

WU and ZHANG · Nonparametric Regression Methods for Longitudinal Data Analysis

YIN · Clinical Trial Design: Bayesian and Frequentist Adaptive Methods

YOUNG, VALERO-MORA, and FRIENDLY · Visual Statistics: Seeing Data with Dynamic Interactive Graphics

ZACKS · Stage-Wise Adaptive Designs

* ZELLNER · An Introduction to Bayesian Inference in Econometrics

ZELTERMAN · Discrete Distributions—Applications in the Health Sciences

ZHOU, OBUCHOWSKI, and McCLISH · Statistical Methods in Diagnostic Medicine, *Second Edition*

*Now available in a lower priced paperback edition in the Wiley Classics Library.
†Now available in a lower priced paperback edition in the Wiley–Interscience Paperback Series.

Printed in Poland
by Amazon Fulfillment
Poland Sp. z o.o., Wrocław
04 December 2020

ae11382d-5052-40c9-af47-76fdd218a9deR02